The Self and Society in Aging Processes

Carol D. Ryff, Ph.D., is Director of the Institute on Aging and Professor of Psychology at the University of Wisconsin-Madison. She is a member of the MacArthur Research Network for Successful Midlife Development, a Fellow of the American Psychological Association (Division 20-Adult Development and Aging) and the Gerontological Society of America, a Consulting Editor for two major APA journals (*Journal of Personality and Social Psychology, Psychology and Aging*). Her work has been supported by the National Institute on Aging, the National Institute of Mental Health, and the MacArthur Foundation.

Dr. Ryff's research centers on the study of psychological well-being, an area in which she has generated a theory-driven, empirically based approach to assessment of multiple dimensions of positive psychological functioning. These assessment procedures have been translated into over 15 different languages and are used in diverse studies in fields of psychology, sociology, demography, epidemiology, and health. Her own studies have documented sociodemographic correlates of well-being (i.e., how positive mental health varies by age, gender, social class, and ethnic/minority status) and have examined how individuals' life experiences and their interpretations of them account for variations in well-being.

Victor W. Marshall, Ph.D., is Director of the Institute on Aging of the University of North Carolina at Chapel Hill, where he is also Professor of Sociology. Prior to 1999, he was Professor of Public Health Sciences and Director of the Institute for Human Development, Life Course and Aging at the University of Toronto. Active in the study of aging for over thirty years, he has published widely on social theories of aging, family and intergenerational relations, health and health care issues for the aged. His current research focuses on older workers and the transition into retirement and on aging policy issues. His interests in social policy and aging have been expressed as a member of the Canada Pension Plan Advisory Board, and currently as Chair of the Gerontology Advisory Council of Veterans Affairs Canada.

The Self and Society in Aging Processes

Carol D. Ryff, *PhD*
Victor W. Marshall, *PhD*
Editors

 Springer Publishing Company

Copyright © 1999 by Springer Publishing Company, Inc.

Springer Publishing Company, Inc.
536 Broadway
New York, NY 10012–3955

Cover design by James Scotto-Lavino
Acquisitions Editor: Helvi Gold
Production Editor: Jeanne Libby

99 00 01 02 03 / 5 4 3 2 1

Library of Congress Cataloging-in-Publication Data

The self and society in aging processess / Carol D. Ryff and Victor W. Marshall, editors.
    p.   m.
    Includes bibliographical references and index.
    ISBN 0-8261-1267-6 (hardcover)
    1. Aging—Society aspects. 2. Aging—Psychological aspects. 3. Aged—Social conditions. 4. Aged—psychology. 5. Gerontology. I. Ryff, Carol D. II. Marshall, Victor W.
    HQ1061.S438 1999
    305.26—dc21   99-25933
                                           CIP

Contents

Contributors   ix

Part 1   Theoretical Perspectives on Self and Society Linkages

1. **Linking the Self and Society in Social Gerontology:
   Crossing New Territory via Old Questions**   3
   *Carol D. Ryff, Victor W. Marshall,
   & Philippa J. Clarke*

2. **Social Perspectives on the Self in Later Life**   42
   Linda K. George

3. **Neoteny, Naturalization, and Other Constituents
   of Human Development**   67
   Dale Dannefer

4. **Continuity Theory, Self, and Social Structure**   94
   Robert C. Atchley

5. **Identity and Adaptation to the Aging Process**   122
   Susan Krauss Whitbourne

6. **Self-Development in Adulthood and Aging:
   The Role of Critical Life Events**   150
   Manfred Diehl

Part 2 Socioeconomic Structures and the Self

7. **Practical Consciousness, Social Class,
   and Self-Concept: A View From Sociology**   187
   Jon Hendricks

8. **Educational Attainment and
   Self-Making in Later Life**   223
   *Melissa M. Franks, A. Regula Herzog,
   Diane Holmberg, & Hazel R. Markus*

9. **Forging Macro-Micro Linkages
   in the Study of Psychological Well-Being**   247
   *Carol D. Ryff, William J. Magee,
   Kristen C. Kling, & Edgar H. Wing*

10. **Income and Subjective Well-Being
    Over the Life Cycle**   279
    Richard A. Easterlin & Christine M. Schaeffer

Part 3 Contexts of Self and Society: Work and Family

11. **Structure and Agency in the Retirement Process:
    A Case Study of Montreal Garment Workers**   305
    Julie A. McMullin & Victor W. Marshall

12. **Gender and Distress in Later Life: The Importance
    of Lifelong Employment and Familial Experiences**   339
    Lorraine Davies

13. **The Caregiving Context: The Intersection of
    Social and Individual Influences in the
    Experience of Family Caregiving**   362
    Marsha Mailick Seltzer & Jan S. Greenberg

14. **Linking Social Structure and Self-Concept:
    Variations in Sense of Mastery**   398
    Marilyn McKean Skaff

15. **Intersections of Society, Family, and Self Among
    Hispanics in Middle and Later Life**   423
    Sonia Miner & Julian Montoro-Rodriguez

16. **The Social Psychology of Values: Effects of Individual Development, Social Change, and Family Transmission Over the Life Span**   453
Robert E. L. Roberts & Vern L. Bengtson

Index   483

Contributors

Robert C. Atchley
The Naropa Institute
Department of Gerontology
2130 Arapahoe Ave.
Boulder, CO 80302-6697

Vern L. Bengtson
University of Southern California
Andrus Gerontology Center
University Park MC-0191
Los Angeles CA 90089-0191

Philippa J. Clarke
University of Toronto
Institute on Human Development,
    Life Course and Aging
222 College Street, Suite 106
Toronto, Ontario, Canada M5T 3J1

Dale Dannefer
University of Rochester
Warner Graduate School of Education
    and Human Development
Lattimore Hall
Rochester, NY 14627

Lorraine Davies
The University of Western Ontario
Department of Sociology
Social Science Center
London, Ontario N6A 5C2, Canada

Manfred Diehl
University of Colorado-Colorado Springs
Psychology Department
1420 Austin Bluffs Parkway
P.O. Box 7150
Colorado Springs, CO 80933-7150

Richard A. Easterlin
University of Southern California
Department of Economics
University Park,
Los Angeles, CA 90007

Melissa Franks
Wayne State University
Institute on Gerontology
87 East Ferry
226 Knapp Building
Detroit, MI 48202

Linda K. George
Duke University Medical Center
Center for the Study of Aging and
    Human Development
P.O. Box 3003
Durham, NC 27710

Jan S. Greenberg
University of Wisconsin-Madison
School of Social Work
1350 University Ave.
Madison, WI 53706

Jon Hendricks
Oregon State University
University Honors College
229 Strand Hall
Corvallis, OR 97331-2221

A. Regula Herzog
University of Michigan
Institute of Social Research
P.O. Box 1248
Ann Arbor MI 48106-1248

Diane Holmberg
Acadia University
Department of Psychology
Wolfville, N.S.
Canada BOP 1XO

Kristen C. Kling
University of Minnesota
Psychology Department
Elliott Hall
75 E. River Rd.
Minneapolis, MN 55455

William J. Magee
University of Toronto
Department of Sociology
203 College St.
Toronto, Ontario M5T 1P9 Canada

Hazel R. Markus
Stanford University
Department of Psychology
420 Jordan Hall, Room 256
Stanford, CA 94305

Victor W. Marshall
108 Bolinwood Drive
Chapel Hill, NC 27514

Julie A. McMullin
The University of Western Ontario
Department of Sociology
Social Science Center
London, Ontario N6A 5C2, Canada

Sonia Miner
University of Utah
Department of Family and Consumer
    Studies
228 Alfred E. Emery Bldg.
Salt Lake City, UT 84112

Julian Montoro-Rodriguez
Case Western Reserve University
Department of Sociology
11477 Mayfield Road, Suite 806
Cleveland OH 44106

Robert E. L. Roberts
California State University
Sociology Program
San Marcos, CA 92096-0001

Carol D. Ryff
University of Wisconsin-Madison
Department of Psychology
1300 University Ave. #2245 MSC
Madison, WI 53706

Christine M. Schaeffer
21701 Prairie St.
Chatsworth, CA 91311

Marsha Mailick Seltzer
University of Wisconsin-Madison
School of Social Work
S102 Waisman Center
1500 Highland Ave.
Madison, WI 53706

Marilyn McKean Skaff
University of California- San Francisco
School of Medicine
Department of Family & Community
  Medicine
500 Parnassus Ave., Box 0900
San Francisco, CA 94143-0990

Susan Krauss Whitbourne
University of Massachusetts
Department of Psychology
Tobin Hall
Amherst, MA 01003

Edgar H. Wing
University of Wisconsin-Madison
Department of Psychology
1202 W. Johnson St.
Madison, WI 53706

PART 1

Theoretical Perspectives on Self and Society Linkages

Linking the Self and Society in Social Gerontology: Crossing New Territory via Old Questions

Carol D. Ryff, Victor W. Marshall, & Philippa J. Clarke

S ocial gerontology is a broad field in which a number of disciplines come together to advance understanding of aging individuals and societies. These disciplines range from psychology, with its traditional emphasis on the individual, to sociology and anthropology, which focus much of their attention on large-scale social structures and on cultures. Because social gerontology attempts to bring together this wide array into a common enterprise, it faces important theoretical and methodological challenges in linking the micro and the macro, or self and society.

Our primary objectives in this chapter are twofold. The first is to provide a historical overview of prior efforts to link individual and social structural factors in social gerontology. The nexus between micro- and macro-levels of analysis has been a leading intellectual theme, not only in prior gerontological theorizing and research, but in the social sciences more generally. The disciplines in social gerontology, and in broader theoretical work, have approached this challenge with differing theoretical assumptions and emphases on the micro level, the macro level, or the link-age between the two. The premise of this volume is that we are entering a new era in scientific discourse about such micro-macro linkages in social gerontology.

Over the last three decades, much of the best theory construction in social gerontology has occurred in efforts to map the intersection of indi-vidual and social structural factors that shape the aging process. We review these prior attempts and also examine efforts outside social gerontology, specifically work in the personality and social structure tradition that embraced similar broad scientific territory. Our aim is to bring to mind the notable contributions of these traditions as well as their limitations. This section concludes with an overview of new developments in social geron-tology and beyond (e.g., recent scholarship on the self), designed to move the self-society linkage forward. Our intent is to take the best from past and current work to chart new courses through the expansive territory ahead.

The second objective of the introductory chapter is to provide an in-depth overview of the chapters that follow. Written by social gerontolo-gists trained in different disciplinary contexts (psychology, sociology, social work, economics, human development), some are oriented toward individual-level processes, while others incline toward social-structural questions. All, however, share a commitment to bridge the two levels of analysis. Collectively, their questions represent exciting diversity in the content of current questions about micro-macro linkages.

SOCIAL GERONTOLOGY'S FASCINATION: THE LINKAGE OF INDIVIDUALS AND SOCIAL STRUCTURE

Dominant gerontological theories of the 1960s and 1970s were explicitly about efforts to link the aging of the individual to societal influences (Bengtson, Burgess, & Parrott, 1997; Marshall 1996a, 1996b). Disengage-ment and activity theories offered contrasting perspectives on the optimal adjustment of the individual to the social order. Subsequent formulations, such as role perspectives on aging (Rosow, 1974, 1976), or the social breakdown syndrome (Kuypers & Bengtson, 1973), continued to elaborate social-structural influences and their consequences for individual func-tioning. Modernization theory (Burgess, 1960; Cowgill, 1974), in contrast, pursued the "fit" between the aging individual and the society from a macro-level perspective.

Concern with the link between individual and society can be traced to early social scientific interest in aging—specifically, adaptation of the aging individual to society. In a 1940 memo to the Social Sciences Research Council Committee on Social Adjustment, Ernest Burgess argued that there was a poor fit between older individuals and modern society. He argued that the problem could be rectified by adjusting the society to the needs of the older individual, or conversely, by helping the older individual adjust to modern society (Calhoun, 1978). This committee, which Burgess chaired, played a key role in the development of social gerontology, through stimulating research at major U.S. universities (Shanas, 1971).

How well did these early efforts fare in bridging the gap between individual and social structural levels? Generally, hindsight judgment has been fairly negative. Marshall and Tindale (1978–9) castigated social gerontology for its individualism and neglect of social structure, particularly the political economy of aging and socioeconomic forces. Modernization theory, in contrast, was been faulted for ignoring the individual as well as failing to recognize the complexities of societal modernization processes and how societies are located within a world socioeconomic system (Quadagno, 1982; Stearns, 1977; Thomas, 1976).

Disengagement theory (Cumming & Henry, 1961), which postulated that with age there is a mutual severing of the ties between the individual and society, is illustrative of the former problem. That is, the theory and its refinements (Williams & Wirths, 1965) had strongly micro-level conceptualizations of social structure (i.e., measuring it by counts of social role occupancy, number of interactions, and subjective ratings of time spent in normatively governed interaction with others). Marshall (1994) summarized the general program of research as follows:

> The major independent variables entered over this period into models to predict variability in life satisfaction were either themselves dispositional or personality factors, or largely restricted to three domains: health, income security, and social integration. These, in turn, were largely unexamined variables. Few scholars theorized about the causes of variability in health, wealth, or social integration. To do so would have shifted attention away from the social psychological levels toward a social structural level of analysis (p. 771)

Ironically, disengagement theory, despite its micro-level focus, did not adequately characterize the self, viewing the individual largely as a collection of social roles. In reaction to the individualism of disengagement theory, later approaches, such as the age stratification perspective (Riley, 1971; Riley, Foner, & Waring, 1988; Riley, Johnson, & Foner, 1972), shifted the focus to social structure; but did so without reference to intentionality at the individual level (Hendricks, 1992; Hendricks & Leedham, 1992). Through processes of socialization and role allocation, age stratification postulated explicit links between the individual and society. Social structure in this formulation did not address macro levels of social power and domination in allocation of resources, and the individual was conceived largely as passive or reactive (i.e., being socialized). Complex, multilayered selves were missing; the focus was on individuals comprised as role constellations and need dispositions. The "individual-structure dialectic" (Hendricks, 1992; Hendricks & Leedham, 1992), seeking to bridge the gap between social structure and individual life worlds, was never brought explicitly to the fore, and remains a major challenge in contemporary social gerontology (Bengtson et al., 1997).

Social structure has thus been undertheorized in social gerontology (as in the broader field of sociology) and all too rarely dealt with macro-level social relations of power, domination, and allocation of opportunities and resources, while simultaneously avoiding the reification fallacy (i.e., treating social structure as if it exists independently of the actions of human beings). Anthony Giddens (1993) views social structure in terms of complex rules and resources, which are as much constrained by, as constitutive of, individual action. He argues, "Structures . . . have to be treated for purposes of analysis as specifically 'impersonal'; but . . . it is essential to recognize that structures only exist as the reproduced conduct of situated actors with definite intentions and interests" (1993, p. 134). Social structure is therefore not a stable, external object (although it can be usefully theorized as such), nor, of course, is the self or identity.

Running in parallel over the past two decades have been efforts by developmental psychologists and sociologists to link the individual and society in theories of life course development (Baltes, 1987; Dannefer & Perlmutter, 1990; Elder, 1991, 1997; Lerner, 1984; Riegel, 1975). These scholars saw human development as extending beyond adolescence and generated conceptual frameworks to study it. Their perspectives gave attention to the dynamic interrelationships between the developing individual and the *changing sociocultural context*. That is, selves and societies were brought together with an explicit goal of tracking processes of change at both the micro and macro levels of analysis. Much focus was given to research designs and analytic methods that could disentangle age, cohort, and period effects (Schaie & Baltes, 1975). The challenges of dealing with temporally complex data that links individuals to surrounding societal contexts persist into the present (see Roberts and Bengtson, Chapter 16).

At the conceptual level, theories of human development were criticized for their failure to specify "the ways in which social structures and human beings mutually influence one another" (Dowd, 1990, p. 138). Extant models of human development were also faulted for failing to give sufficient attention to the differential distribution of the "opportunities" for human development, which occur via the "allocation of economic and cultural resources that are the enabling requisite of development" (p. 150). Human subjectivity—"the tendency for workers to truncate their aspirations in the face of obdurate social reality" (p. 150) was deemed a critical route of influence on developmental trajectories. Dowd thus reconceptualized human development as a process of self-realization, which requires both opportunities and desire.

Taken together, work in social gerontology and life course development addressed both the individual and social structural factors, although invariably, one side was more richly elaborated than the other, and none theorized the link itself adequately. Outside these realms were other efforts to build micro-macro linkages; specifically, research in the personality and social structure tradition.

THE PERSONALITY AND SOCIAL STRUCTURE RESEARCH

Work in this tradition had disciplinary origins in anthropology, psychology, and sociology. Emphasis was placed jointly on personality, defined as enduring characteristics of the individual (e.g., values, attitudes, beliefs, needs) and social structure, defined as normative characteristics of social systems (e.g., roles, norms, organizational features, socialization processes). The goal was to bring these levels of analysis together.

Historical reviews (e.g., House, 1981) point to Marx and Weber as foremost theorists in this tradition. Marx's conceptions of alienation and class consciousness inherently concerned the relation (both actual and ideal) of societal institutions (industry, government, economy) to individual beliefs,

motivations, and behaviors. Similarly, Weber was concerned with the relation between position in the social structure and individual values,
motives, and beliefs. His thesis that secular ideology caused the rise of
capitalism in Western Europe viewed values, motives, and beliefs playing
an autonomous role in society and leading to dramatic changes in social
structure. Personality and social structure were also evident in Durkheim's
studies of suicide, where personality was introduced as an intervening
variable between integration of the social structure and suicide rates
(Inkeles, 1959).

Within psychology, Freud (1930/1961) was interested in how civilization demanded the suppression of sexual and aggressive instincts in
exchange for a measure of security. Through the work of Kardiner (1939),
psychoanalysis became central to the study of culture and personality,
which emphasized that members of society share a basic personality structure, which is the product of societal institutions, especially childrearing
practices. These ideas were elaborated in anthropological work on culture
and personality (e.g., Levine, 1973; Whiting & Child, 1953).

Major global events (i.e., world wars) also spurred studies of "national
character", whose goal was to identify the basic motives, beliefs, and psychological attributes shared by members of a given society (e.g., enemy
nations such as Japan, Germany, Russia). The widely disseminated
description of the "authoritarian personality" (Adorno, Frenkel-Brunswik,
Levinson, & Sanford, 1950) was a product of such inquiry. After the war,
psychologists maintained interest in personality and social structure.
Allport (1968) addressed how individuals are both created by their cultural
surroundings and create new cultural forms for the guidance of new generations. White (1966) probed how values and ideals of the American culture affected the course of individual development. McClelland (1961)
studied achievement motivation as an expression of the relationship
between the individual and society.

On the whole, this early literature was faulted for not being strongly
empirical, for failing to explicate the hows and whys of relationships
between individuals and society, and for the fragmented nature of its
inquiries (House, 1981; Ryff, 1987). From the perspective of experimental psychology, the work was also faulted for its inaccessible and heavily
philosophic style, which did not lend itself to overt behavioral observations
(Pepitone, 1981). Thus, questions of social structural influence were
notably absent in American social psychology. Markus and Kitayama's
(1991) major treatise on "culture and the self", documenting the decidedly
Western flavor of much psychological inquiry about personality, cognition,

motivation, and emotion, sharply challenged the pervasive neglect of broad cultural influence. Such queries are essential to elaborate the societal structures that impinge on individual actions, attitudes, and behaviors, including those observed in the laboratory (Ryff, 1987).

Although social norms and cultural forces are seen as influences on individual behaviors, attitudes, and values, the actual macro-level influences and how their effects occur have rarely been explicated. For example, position in the socioeconomic hierarchy has been descriptively related to numerous behaviors and beliefs (e.g., political party preference, sexual behavior, church membership, child-rearing practices) (Kohn, 1969), but how these associations come about is rarely addressed. One attempt to provide a process account of how macro and micro level variables are associated is Rosenberg and Pearlin's (1978) efforts to explain the developmental linkage of social class and self-esteem. In childhood, these two variables are not correlated, but they show modest association in adolescence, and even stronger ties in adulthood.

Four possible theoretical mechanisms were proffered to explain the pattern. The first emerges from the observation that the socioeconomic environments of children are more homogenous than those of adults. Because adults are exposed to greater social inequities, they are more likely to evaluate themselves via social comparison with others on SES-related dimensions. Such comparisons, largely irrelevant to children's self-evaluations, are thus hypothesized to influence the self-esteem of adults. The second mechanism argues that people come to see themselves as they believe others see them. Because the child's role set is primarily from his or her own level of socioeconomic status, these reflected appraisals from significant others are unlikely to incorporate class-linked feedback. The diversity of the adults' social environment, however, makes it more likely that they see themselves as viewed by significant others in social status terms, with related consequences for self-esteem.

Behavioral self-perceptions, the third mechanism, clarified that for the adult, SES status is a product of one's efforts, actions, and behaviors; while for the child, such status is conferred. Thus, SES is more salient for adults because they engage in more behaviors relevant to it. The final theoretical explanation was based on the idea of psychological centrality, which argues that self-concept is complex, with some components at the center of attention, and others at the periphery. For children, social class is seen as more peripheral and thus unimportant to self-esteem, but adults are hypothesized to be more aware of and concerned about socioeconomic status. Later research provided further empirical support, particularly with regard to the three latter theories (Demo & Savin-Williams, 1983), but work was largely restricted to adolescents.

Overall, the personality and social structure research tradition reveals similar strengths and limitations to those evident in social gerontology. While both research fields are to be applauded for their joint emphasis on individual and social structural factors, the individual and social structure are narrowly or inadequately theorized, and there has been all too little elaboration as to the how of these micro-macro linkages. To overcome deficiencies of earlier studies, it is thus imperative to theorize the meaning of individual and social structure and to explain the linkages between individuals and surrounding social forces.

> Thus, personality and social structure research needs to be revived at a more sophisticated level of analysis that is more theoretically informed, more empirically substantiated, and more concerned with explanatory processes. (Ryff, 1987, p. 1201)

This is fundamentally a call for interdisciplinary dialogue (Stryker, 1983) and for recognition of the complementarity between micro- and macro-level research approaches. Nearly 40 years ago, Wrong (1961) faulted contemporary sociology for its "oversocialized" conception of mankind, arguing that the person is both more and less than an acceptance seeker, a follower of social norms and expectations. Contemporary psychology has likewise suffered from an "overpsychologized" conception of human nature (Ryff, 1987) that sees individuals as cognitive processors operating independently of their ties to the social world, including family, neighborhood, community, and culture. Social structure, which is not just a set of pervasive social norms and expectations, has also been inadequately conceptualized. As we argue below, it has features of durability, control over resources, coercion and constraint that go well beyond shared norms. How to respond to these prior concerns and imbalances is the challenge at hand.

NEW DIRECTIONS IN LINKING INDIVIDUALS AND SOCIETIES IN LIFE COURSE STUDIES

The preceding sections illustrate literatures, in the field of aging and beyond, that tried to weave individuals and societies together. We build on these traditions, hoping to address their shortcomings. In this section, we distill key directives to advancing knowledge of micro-macro linkages in aging processes. Two broad issues guide our formulation of new directions: (1) the importance of attending simultaneously to both levels of analysis, individual and social structural; and (2) the need to elaborate mechanisms of linkage, recognizing that both selves and societies are dynamic processes.

Simultaneous Consideration of Individual and Social Structural Factors

All of the preceding literature takes as a given that both individual and social structural factors are essential to gain comprehensive understanding of human adaptation, both in old age and throughout the life course. Nonetheless, surprisingly few strong examples illustrate a joint focus, conceptually or empirically. One attempt was N. J. Smelser and W. T. Smelser's *Personality and Social Systems* (1970), which emphasized the usefulness of defining personality and social structure as jointly independent and dependent variables. When considering personality as outcome, they presented studies dealing with the influences of family, the school environment, the peer group, adult roles, social class, and social change on individuals. Conversely, other sections looked at how individuals influence group processes, family environments, community and social roles, and social change. Unfortunately, much of the literature in these works is dated: personality, for example, is conceptualized almost exclusively from a Freudian perspective.

N. J. Smelser and W. T. Smelser's (1970) collection remains an important contribution for clarifying the likely reciprocal relations between personality and social structure. Subsequent formulations of the individual-society linkages elaborated that social reality acts on the individual not simply through socialization processes, but also through a variety of "reality maintenance" devices, which are often conversational, maintained by ritual, and relying on traces embodied in written and other institutional formats (N. J. Smelser, 1988). More recent work distinguishes between micro-, meso-, macro-, and global levels of analysis (N. J. Smelser, 1997). Reflecting roots in structural-functionalism, emphasis has largely been on social roles in a normative context, thereby providing a somewhat static conceptualization of social structure that is removed from concerns with power, coercion, and constraints on people's opportunity structures.

Viewed in the context of social gerontology, most prior theorizing did not formulate the individual and society as reciprocally related (i.e., both acting and being acted upon). Moreover, rarely did guiding conceptual frameworks keep both sides of the dialectic in focus. Much of the work in the Kansas City studies essentially *reduced the macro-level to the micro-level* (Marshall, 1995). Social structure was redefined as attributes of the individual, thereby losing sight of influence and change occurring at the institutional and structural level. Keeping both levels of analysis simultaneously in focus requires conceptual frameworks *and* related operational definitions that represent micro and macro factors. This can occur via "parallel form" approaches (Marshall, 1995), which postulate similar constructs operative on both sides (e.g., individual needs, societal needs). Such an approach was exemplified by the Kansas City studies, with the joint focus on needs of the individual and the society for disengagement. Despite the dual emphasis on individuals and social structure, the formulation of disengagement theory was problematic because it assumed a harmonious and self-regulating equilibrium system that can occur only via abstractions largely disconnected from actual lives and institutional dynamics. Tensions, contradictions, and inconsistencies between micro and macro levels must be considered.

As illustrated by many chapters in this volume, parallel-form analyses are the likely exception, rather than the rule, in integrating analyses of selves and societies. A more typical approach examines structures at the macro-level (e.g., economic changes) for their impact on individual factors (e.g., subjective well-being) (e.g., Chapter Ten). The critical task therein is to not lose sight of the social processes that link these levels.

The Need to Postulate Mechanisms of Linkage

We elaborate below four avenues for explicating mechanisms of linkage, namely, how the nexus between individuals and the social order come about. Some of these are closer, both theoretically and empirically, to the social structural side of the equation, while others are more aligned with the "self" side of the query. *All* delineate processes that bridge macro-micro-levels, thereby responding to the call for theory-driven research in social gerontology (Bengtson et al., 1997).

Mediating Meso-Structures

Marshall (1995) clarified that modernization theory and the age stratification perspective relied on meso-level social structures, such as the family or the work group, to link the individual to the social structure. In modernization theory, as articulated by Cowgill (1974), structures such as the labor market or the family intervene between broad patterns of socioeconomic development (e.g., urbanization, technological change) and social status. In the age stratification perspective, age-graded social statuses are found within the economic system, the legal system, or the family system, and these social institutions channel the impact of the age stratification system on the individual.

Life in institutions such as families or work settings, however, cannot be reduced to bundles or clusters of roles, and the social patterns in these meso-level institutions cannot be adequately explained by assuming that role incumbents will internalize widely shared values and behavioral expectations through some putatively efficient socialization mechanisms. To the extent that a Parsonian perspective is adopted,

> The potential for conflict and change might be overlooked. Structural-functionalism tends to view society as built up from institutions which are, in turn, built up from roles. There is a presumed isomorphism between individual and society, as mediated through social institutions at the meso level (Marshall, 1995, p. 362).

Thus, there is a need to pay greater attention to these intermediary social structures (e.g., family, work, community) as well as the great variability and complexity of the players in these settings, including their proactive capacities. George (Chapter 2) sharpens appreciation of these points by drawing attention to the ways in which individuals select themselves into particular social environments of the meso level, and the extent to which meso-environments themselves facilitate or diminish self-direction. Greater attention must be paid to discerning the social organizational features of these meso-levels (i.e., what are the critical dimensions of work and family structures to examine?) and how they come about (i.e., what macro-level variables shape these influences?). How such structures affect, and are affected by, individual behavior and belief in such settings is the critical remaining piece in connecting the self and society via the intermediary meso level.

Role Allocation and Socialization

These are the processes hypothesized to link individuals and the social order in structural-functionalist perspectives, such as the age stratification approach (see also Chapter 2, this volume, George, 1983; Marshall, 1995). Role allocation refers to "a set of mechanisms for the continual assignment and reassignment of individuals of given ages to the appropriate roles" (Riley et al., 1972, p. 11). Socialization is a process that "serves to teach individuals at each stage of the life course how to perform new roles, how to adjust to changing roles, and how to relinquish old ones" (Riley et al., 1972, p. 11).

We distinguish these processes from the above meso-structures to differentiate the settings from the activities that occur in them. Both are requisite to a comprehensive understanding of social-structural influences, but emphasis on one typically overshadows the other. Moreover, while socialization and role allocation can occur via the meso level, they are not restricted to such levels. Beyond proximal work, family, and community settings are broader societal influences (e.g., normative expectations, public policies) impinging on older persons.

As noted earlier, the age stratification perspective emphasized socialization and role allocation processes. However, of structural functionalist assumptions that social systems tend toward equilibrium, the age stratification approach was faulted for weakly developed formulations of change (in societies and in individuals) as well as for construing individuals as uniformly passive and reactive (i.e., ideal candidates for smooth socialization).

More recently, emphasis on the structural lag hypothesis (Riley, Kahn, & Foner, 1994) has underscored the general absence of relevant social institutional structures that surround the added years of life many elders now experience. If social structures do lag behind such added years of life, socialization and role allocation processes are unlikely to be significant operative influences on aging, apart from how their absence undermines optimal later life adjustment.

A key limitation of prior efforts to elaborate socialization and role allocation mechanisms of linkage has been the failure to provide empirical evidence for the hypothesized processes. While structural-functionalist perspectives formulate socialization as a mechanism connecting individuals and social structures, few operational definitions have been provided of how such processes at work in the middle and later years. One example of how social structures (especially via social roles and normative guidance, or lack of both) impinge on aging individuals was Kuypers and Bengtson's (1973) "social breakdown syndrome." The social system changes postulated to occur in old age that lead to negative self-attitudes and a reduced sense of competence in the elderly were: loss of normative guidelines (absence of clear, positive behavioral expectations in old age, presence of negative expectations); shrinkage of roles (many former roles terminate in old age, few alternative roles are developed); and lack of appropriate reference groups (lack of shared, positive values and attitudes about the aged). The counter-scenario emphasized the maintenance of later life competence and well-being via positive social integration and accompanying roles, socialization, and normative guidance. An operational translation of part of this formulation (Heidrich & Ryff, 1993a) showed that positive social integration mediated the effects of declining physical health on psychological well-being. Additional empirical tests of key socialization and role allocation processes, at both meso- and macro-structural levels, are critical to advancement of the self and society agenda.

Self-Processes

The last two decades have witnessed dramatic proliferation of scientific research on the self and self-related processes (e.g., self-evaluation, self-enhancement, self-discrepancy). This work builds on scholarly traditions in psychology and sociology (see Markus & Cross, 1990) that underscore the fundamentally social, interpersonal nature of how selves come to be and how they function. However, rather than deal exclusively with the content or structure of selves (prominent in prior inquiries), the new era of research elaborates the role of the self in basic activities of how individuals process information (Markus & Sentis, 1982) (e.g., documenting that processing speed is more efficient when the information central to the self).

Implications of these conceptual and empirical refinements in self scholarship have been translated to the field of aging. Earlier, Breytspraak (1984) argued that the self had not had a prominent position in social gerontology, and when considered, it was seldom viewed dynamically. Rather, the focus was on the content of the self, the "me". More agentic features of the self are, however, strongly evident in Markus and Herzog's (1992) examination of "The Role of the Self-Concept in Aging." Key proactive functions of the self are described, such as organizing experience, regulating affect, and motivating behavior. Self-content and functions are also seen as having consequences for adjustment, such as levels of well-being and life satisfaction, or choice of activities. Importantly, Markus and Herzog emphasize the temporal dynamics of the self via the formulation of "possible selves" which include one's conception of self in the past as well as anticipated in the future. Past selves are seen to play key roles in self-evaluative processes, while future selves reflect desired or feared changes, which can also prompt action in the present. Empirical studies have translated these temporal evaluations of self to the study of health (Hooker, 1992) and well-being (Ryff, 1991).

Additional self-processes pertain to social comparisons, reflected appraisals, and psychological centrality (see preceding discussion of Rosenberg & Pearlin, 1978, as well as Markus & Cross, 1990). These mechanisms address how individuals evaluate themselves via comparison with key others, perceptions of feedback from others, and designations of what is and is not central to one's self-conception. Ryff and Essex (1992) examined the role of these self-evaluative processes in how older persons negotiate their way through various life transitions (e.g., community relocation), or how they deal with the physical challenges (e.g., emerging chronic conditions) of aging (Heidrich & Ryff, 1993b, 1996). Suls and Mullen (1982) also examined how social comparisons influence self-evaluation across the life-span. These perspectives draw on advances occurring in mainstream social psychology, which clarify that the goal of social comparison is not always accurate self-evaluation (as Festinger (1954) originally suggested), but may be self-enhancement (Wood, 1989; Wood & Taylor, 1991). Such motives underscore the proactive, agentic role of the self in maintaining positive adjustment.

Because much of the above theorizing and research has taken place in psychology, the linkage between these self-processes and social structure has rarely been a question of interest. However, the need for such inquiry has been noted. Markus and Herzog (1992) emphasize that social structural factors, such as culture, gender, race, and socioeconomic status, have "a significant direct impact on the self and further influence how the self may be modified across the life span" (p. 127). For example, they argue that those with higher levels of education will have different expectations and theories about later life health. "Incorporated into possible selves, this information can facilitate health behaviors, and these, in turn, influence both the onset and the course of various diseases" (p. 128). How position in the educational or income hierarchies of society impacts these self-evaluative processes is a central question for multiple contributors to this volume (see Chapters 7, 8, and 10).

Forging linkages between meaning-making activities of the self and surrounding social structural influences is a key future challenge that fundamentally requires reaching across disciplinary boundaries (i.e., connecting the proactive features of self-construction and self-evaluation with position in the social order and larger societal forces). While early social gerontology was nearly exclusively focussed on personal adjustment as the individual-level variable of interest, the new era of self scholarship points to a host of agentic features of self-processing that may be critical mediators and moderators of the link between social structure and individual health and well-being.

Life Events as Nexus

Another fruitful mechanism for linking selves and societies focuses analytical attention on the actual events occurring in the lives of individuals as they age. This event focus, implicit or explicit, has longstanding presence in the social sciences, such as literatures on critical life events or life transitions (Elder, Pavalko, & Hastings, 1991; George, 1993; Holmes & Rahe, 1967). Life event studies have addressed the impact of such experiences on health and well-being, or the timing and sequencing of major transitions. What this volume brings into high relief is the role of life events as a nexus between social structural influences and individual functioning. Diehl (Chapter 6) makes the argument explicit by advocating that researchers should make greater efforts to examine how critical life events are linked to the micro- and macro-structures of individuals' life contexts. In this regard, Diehl draws extensively on the work of a key theorist who attempted to link individual or psychological and sociocultural levels of analysis: Klaus Riegel. In Riegel's formulation, critical life events are the key dynamic forces that prompt the changes required for continued adult development.

It is important to recognize, however, that the occurrence of life events can be examined from both the social-structural (e.g., are life stresses more prevalent among the poor?) and individual angles (e.g., how do critical events affect adjustment? Do individuals differ in their coping responses?). As such, the experiential substance of people's lives becomes a profitable context for joint focus on how life opportunities and life difficulties are distributed across the social order, and what their consequences are for individual functioning. Mindful of prior tendencies to construe individuals as exclusively passive, reactive players in the social-structural arena, the new work draws distinctions between self-selected versus imposed life events. The former address the proactive, self-negotiated occurrence of key transitions and experiences, while the latter refer to events beyond the individual's control and personal preferences.

Numerous chapters in this volume elaborate the life event theme that serves as a vital linkage between individual and social-structural levels of analysis. Before previewing these chapters, we conclude this section with two observations. First, we want to emphasize dynamics of the self-society linkage in our proposed mechanisms. It goes without saying that change processes are fundamental to understanding how these work. Selves are evolving, changing, and developing over the course of life, as are social structures and institutions changing over historical time. Efforts to forge macro-micro linkages must incorporate such dynamics. Elder (1991) proposes the concept of "control cycle" to describe how social change sets in motion efforts to regain control and adapt, with such efforts serving to construct and reconstruct the life course. Concepts such as "situational imperatives" or the "accentuation principle" emphasize how large-scale social changes can constrain human action. Thus, individuals are simultaneously actors in, and reactors to, social change, with both agency, and constraints on it, operative. Elder (1997; Elder & O'Rand, 1995) summarizes these connections as a form of "loose coupling" which "reflects the agency of people even in constrained situations as well as their accomplishments in rewriting their journeys in the course of aging" (Elder, 1997, p. 965).

Elder's intellectual ancestry brings into life-course theorizing a strong strain of symbolic interactionism, recognizing that both agency and process are important. Speaking of individuals in a Meadian framework emphasizes the processual and fundamentally social nature of the self, formed by the individual reflecting on the reaction of others. Both the self and social structure are seen as processes not states. We also invoke Berger and Luckmann's exemplary work *The Social Construction of Reality* (1966), which starts with action and interaction and moves up to the macro-level, not setting the latter apart from the social interaction which constitutes it. The individual and society are thus in a dialectical relationship in which social reality assumes an objectivated status beyond the constitutive actions which constructed it. As N. J. Smelser (1988) notes, this objectivated reality acts back on the individual not simply through the socialization important in structural-functionalist perspectives, but also through a variety of "reality maintenance" devices, which are themselves processual, often conversational, often maintained by ritual, and often relying on traces embodied in written and other institutional forms.

Our second observation is the need to consider the intersections and interactions between our proposed mechanisms of linkage. Self-evaluative processes, for example, will be more richly understood vis-à-vis the mediating meso-structures of individual lives (e.g., work and family contexts). Socialization and role allocation processes, in turn, are both set in motion by, as well as prescribe, the life events that individuals experience. While few of our contributors work simultaneously across these levels, we underscore the need for future inquiries that probe the intersections among them, as each captures various aspects of the self-society dialectic.

PREVIEW OF CHAPTERS

Contributors to this volume reveal diverse questions, content areas, and strategies for capturing the dynamics in evolving selves and changing societies. We organize the chapters into three primary groups. Those in the first section address largely conceptual issues in the linkage of self and society. These chapters reveal the diversity in disciplinary backgrounds of our contributors and the wide range of approaches brought to core questions of how to bring together individual and social structural levels of analysis. The second group of chapters explores, from differing vantage points, the nexus of socioeconomic structures and the self, defining the latter broadly in terms of self-described content, including levels of well-being, and for some, attending to the self as process. The third cluster of chapters anchors the self-and-society dialectic in specific life contexts, thereby invoking the emphasis on mediating meso-structures described above. To varying degrees, these chapters investigate the dynamic processes which constitute these meso-structures and their relations to the individual and to more macro aspects of social structure. Family and work comprise the primary contextual settings for these final six chapters. Below, we preview individual chapters in each of these three organizing categories.

SECTION 1: THEORETICAL PERSPECTIVES ON THE SELF AND SOCIETY LINKAGES

In Chapter 2, "Social Perspectives on the Self in Later Life", Linda George reminds us of the abiding sociological premise, namely that the self is established, modified, and sustained in social context. As such, there should be "strong and predictable links between characteristics of social environments in which individuals are embedded and their self-attributions and evaluations of themselves." She contrasts two major sociological paradigms on the self: structural or determinist views, and interactionist or proactive perspectives. Research on the former tends to focus on social location (especially SES position) and further posits socialization as a major mechanism whereby structural factors affect the self. George underscores the causal ambiguities in established links between individuals' social roles and their identities—rarely is there clarity as to whether the dominant influence runs from social roles to identity, or whether individuals, with particular identities, self-select into specific roles.

Interactionist perspectives, underscoring the latter possibility, view people as architects of their own lives, and thereby, place greater emphasis on human agency, including how individuals interpret and give meaning to their social lives. In sociology, interactionist research tends to rely on observational and/or qualitative studies. George argues that a more complete understanding would come from integrating the structural/determinist perspective, in which the self is seen to be shaped by various social structures, with the interactionist view, wherein the self is viewed as more proactive in shaping or modifying the effects of social structure on the lived experience: "It seems to me that by failing to better integrate the two paradigms, we miss the opportunity to observe the fundamental dynamics of self and society—the dialectic rhythm in which the self cannot be divorced from the social context and the social structure cannot be severed from its inhabitants." Such integration underscores a key objective described above, namely, keeping both social structure and the self simultaneously in focus.

Adding specificity to the task of integration, George discusses two targeted areas for future inquiry. The first examines processes of self-selection into social environments, a topic ideally studied in longitudinal designs. She asks, for example, whether the maintenance of life satisfaction in later life might be due, in part, to self-selection into preferred environments? The second area calls for a focus on social environments themselves and the extent to which they reveal evidence of self-direction. Here George elaborates how social structural and interactional paradigms have dealt with questions of self-direction and offers suggestions for refinements in both. She concludes with a call for structuralists to take a broader view of the self and interactionists to take social structure more seriously.

Chapter 3, by Dale Dannefer, entitled "Neoteny, Naturalization, and Other Constituents of Human Development," brings an evolutionary and developmental perspective to the task of linking individuals to their surrounding worlds. He distinguishes two dramatically different ways of conceiving the relations between the individual organism and the environment. The first parallel process model conceives of individuals born into structured, fixed environments where the essential task is to survive to reproduction. The second interactive, dialectical model, focuses on how organisms and environments continuously shape and influence each other through time. The "fixed requirements" of the former are inappropriate for studying human development, argues Dannefer. Speaking from an evolutionary, species-wide perspective, he calls for emphasis on the interactive paradigm prominent in the formulation provided by George.

Using the examples of exterogestation (organismic developments taking place in infants after separation from the womb) and neoteny (retention of juvenile characteristics into adulthood through deceleration of physical development), Dannefer argues that "what distinguishes the human being is an openness and responsiveness to the environment that is necessary for human development to occur." The resulting indeterminancy and contingency in human development requires attention to, not just internal programming of the organism, but environmental influences. Illustrating such ideas, Dannefer describes occupational and educational differentials in risk of Alzheimer's disease and, in so doing, suggests possible links between social organization (e.g., cognitively stimulating jobs) and later life biological changes.

Underscoring the recurrent theme of human agency, Dannefer describes the purposeful, intentional aspects of human behavior, but is mindful that social systems contour such intentionality. "Thus, while engaging in purposeful activity, human beings co-construct the social systems they live within at the same time that each person's own being, self, personhood is being constituted in social interaction. The essence of self-society relations is that an irreducible reciprocity through which both human development and social systems are constitute in the course of social interaction." Dannefer then elaborates two basic social system processes involved in this co-constitution of social relations and human development.

Social relation production (the externalization of human intentionality) is the first process, which typically occurs at the micro level in face-to-face interaction. Social allocation (fitting people into roles), the second process, occurs at the micro level and in the larger system. With compelling examples, Dannefer illuminates how developmental theory (rooted as it is in evolutionary concepts) has ignored the dynamics and reciprocities between these macro-micro forces. "Because of the flexibility of the human organism, manifested in neoteny and world-openness, micro-interaction is inevitably constitutive of development. At the same time, and especially in modern and postmodern societies, key parameters of micro-interaction are unavoidably and, indeed, increasingly shaped by much broader political

and cultural forces, including centralized and imposed state practices."
Micro-macro linkages are thus central to Dannefer's developmental/evo-
lutionary perspective.

In Chapter 4, "Continuity Theory, Self and Social Structure", Robert
Atchley addresses adult development and adaptation by asking how continuity theory helps advance understanding of the relations between aging,
self, and social structure. This theory emerged from the observation that
despite "widespread changes in health, functioning, and social circumstances, a large proportion of older adults showed considerable consistency over time in their patterns of thinking, activity profiles, and social
relationships." Continuity theory postulates that the self is constantly
developing through feedback processes, but also maintains a high degree
of consistency over time. Continuity is thus not (as in structural functionalist theory) a state of equilibrium, but a long-term, evolving set of probabilistic relationships between past, present, and anticipated patterns of
thought, behavior, and social arrangements. The assumption about human
nature is that persons actively engage the world, motivated by a desire to
provide continuity to the self in adapting to new life circumstances.

One emergent life circumstance that affects many persons in later life
is the loss of functional ability. Atchley views functional disability as a
property of social structure, akin to social class, gender, and education.
With longitudinal data he asks to what extent social structural factors
influence the sense of agency, and to what extent disability, in particular,
influences three components of the self: personal agency, emotional
resilience, and personal goals. Over the period 1981–1991, he found substantial continuity in personal agency, but that neither age, education, nor
gender influenced this continuity. This suggests that the successful use of
continuity strategies is not contingent on lifelong antecedent social structural factors.

Atchley compared respondents who did and did not become disabled
during a longer, 16-year period, and again found strong continuity,
although disability did influence some self-referent dimensions, leading to
a diminished sense of personal agency in a minority of respondents, but in
others, showing either continuity or improvement in their sense of personal
agency. Emotional resiliency was not generally lessened as a result of disability; and regardless of disability, the great majority maintained their personal goals over time. Atchley concludes that most aging people are able
to "neutralize the effects of these disadvantages for the self" this because,
over the course of their lives, they have developed "robust frameworks of
ideas, adaptive skills, relationships, and activities that create internal and

external environments—life worlds—that insulate them" from difficult changes of aging and ageism in our culture.

In Chapter 5, "Identity and Adaptation to the Aging Process," Susan Krauss Whitbourne explores the continuity of the self vis-à-vis the physiological, psychological, and contextual challenges of aging. The extent to which age-related change is slowed down, prevented, or compensated for depends, in part, on proactive efforts to use personal capacities. These, in turn, depend on past histories: "Whether individuals take advantage of positive steps to regulate their own aging may be seen as a function of past adaptational strategies to their health and functioning," thereby underscoring the need for tracking the use of such strategies longitudinally. Resilience in the face of the stresses associated with aging is again emphasized: "Not only are older adults seen as able to navigate the often stormy waters of later life, but they are increasingly seen as creating new challenges, goals, and opportunities for themselves."

Identity is presented as a major organizing principle within personality and as the link between individual and society. Multiple domains (physical, cognitive, personality) are described as comprising the content of identity. The key processes of identity are assimilation (interpretation of life events in terms of cognitive and affective schema that are already incorporated in identity) and accommodation (changes in one's identity in response to identity- relevant experience). The most desirable state is that of dynamic balance so that alternation takes place between assimilation and accommodation. "In this state, the individual's identity is flexible enough to change when warranted but not so unstructured so that every new experience causes the person to question fundamental assumptions about the self's integrity and unity." Those with limited access to resources may have to make greater use of accommodation because "they have not typically been able to effect change in the desired direction."

For older adults, physical identity becomes strongly linked with health status. Whitbourne presents the multiple threshold model as a way of relating age change in the body to psychological adaptation. Threshold refers to the individual's point at which age-related change is recognized. Once recognized, "heightened vigilance leads to behavior that offsets the aging process, thus reducing the dreaded outcome of loss, but also leads the individual to become acutely sensitive to signs that loss has occurred." Whitbourne concludes the chapter with an examination of how identity processes of assimilation and accommodation (prompted by the recognition of age-related change) interact with control orientations and coping strategies to comprise favorable psychological responses to physical aging.

In Chapter 6, "Self-Development in Adulthood and Aging: The Role of Critical Life Events", Manfred Diehl brings a life-span developmental perspective to the volume and reiterates themes raised by Dannefer regarding the dynamic interrelatedness of the developing individual and the changing sociocultural context. Diehl examines the role of critical life events in linking adults' development to micro- and macro-structures of the surrounding sociocultural context. He draws extensively on Riegel's dialectical view of adult development, which called for an explicit "focus on states of disequilibrium and discontinuity as constructive confrontations that may serve as impetus for further development." Riegel argued that developmental progressions are initiated by asynchronies among major dimensions (inner biological, individual psychological, cultural sociological, outer physical). When two or more of these dimensions are out of step, there is a constructive confrontation, an existential challenge. Individuals use these "disequilibria in a constructive manner and become producers of their own development."

Diehl offers a valuable extension and critique of this dialectical formulation by noting that the emphasis on "constructive confrontations" is perhaps overly optimistic in its assumptions that opportunities for positive growth are equally distributed. This observation, also elaborated in Dowd's (1990) sociological critique of theories of human development, underscores the "dramatic differences in individual's choice options and coping repertoires depending on position in the social order." Disequilibrium may, for some, prompt new developmental strides, but for others, it may constitute a threat that catalyzes little more than stress and disruption.

Emphasizing that individuals are both proactive producers and reactive responders in developmental processes, Diehl contrasts life-span developmental perspectives, which have elevated producer themes, and stressful life event research, which frequently adopts reactive models. Both orientations have typically failed to delineate the specific characteristics of the individual (e.g., self-appraisals, perceived competencies, efficacy beliefs, coping styles, personality), the sociocultural environment (e.g., economic and political forces, class standing, family, and educational and occupational structures), and interrelationships between the two. He calls for a comparable level of complexity on the individual and the social-structural side. Diehl's chapter illustrates these dialectical themes with a focused examination of two kinds of critical life events: those in which the occurrence is self-determined, and uncontrollable events. Empirical evidence linking both types of events to adult self-development is summarized.

SECTION 2: SOCIOECONOMIC STRUCTURES AND THE SELF

The chapters in Section 2 focus largely on the import of social class standing, educational levels, and income differentials for individual well-being. These chapters invoke, implicitly or explicitly, various aspects of the role identity or self-processes proposed earlier as key mechanisms for linking social structural and individual levels of analysis. Jon Hendricks begins this section with "Practical Consciousness, Social Class, and Self-Concept" (Chapter 7). Calling for a blend of the macro-level tradition in sociology with the individual-level focus of psychologists, he emphasizes that self-concept is both an expression of personal agency and an outgrowth of social participation. Personal agency in sociology is among those "stalled revolutions", Hendricks argues. He revisits the philosophical origins of intentionality and illustrates the "distillation of meaning" via personal interpretations of caregiving burdens. Referring to the counterintuitive relationship between race and caregiving burden, which shows that Black Americans experience lower perceived burden and less depression, Hendricks underscores the importance of understanding the actor's reading of his/her own situation.

Calling for an ecological perspective on self and social class, he reminds us that "the norms implicit in class membership are woven into the fabric of life. Far from being simply a mosaic of occupational, educational, and financial resources, social class wields considerable sway over all aspects of an actor's situation, including what they discern as meaningful or how they age." Social class permeates numerous noneconomic areas including psychological processes, linguistic and moral practices, lifestyles, worldviews, and normative expectations, "all of which are leavened into self-concept." With this formulation, Hendricks examines heterogeneity among the aged, including distinctions between usual and successful aging.

What most people regard as successful aging, he suggests, may be essentially the benefits accruing from advantaged social circumstances. Critically needed is research on "social experience shaped by access to opportunity, normative roles, transitions, and timetables" to see if "it is causally implicated in tracking people down disparate pathways." These ideas are illustrated with the sequencing of adult benchmarks, such as going to work early in the life course versus staying in school. What are the unfolding sequelae, Hendricks asks, such as longer work life, earlier

marriage, earlier parenthood, differential retirement, and earlier grandparenthood? In this framework, self-concept reflects a "complex coterie of
roles, awareness of age norms, age-appropriate behavior, social and anticipated timetables, interaction patterns, and personal priorities." These elements, fundamental to understanding the life course dynamics of the self
and society dialectic, are center stage in explicating later life variability.

Chapter 8, by Melissa Franks, Regula Herzog, Diane Holmberg, and
Hazel Markus, entitled "Educational Attainment and Self-Making in Later
Life" further probes the class and self-concept questions raised by
Hendricks. Viewing the self as a multidimensional, dynamic entity, they
construe the "self-system" as an ongoing interpretive process influenced
not only by the individual's own thoughts, feelings, and desires, but also
by cultural imperatives and social expectations. Their focus is on how
social structure sets the stage for important life experiences which "facilitate or impede the construction of the self into later life." They address
one key aspect of social structure that may alter life trajectories: "we focus
on educational attainment and its relevance to the richness of the self-
system in older adulthood."

Franks et al. clarify that their formulation of the self and successful
aging rests on the premise that multiple role identities enhance mental
health. They allow for greater opportunities for positive self-evaluation as
well as a forum within which to offset failures. "A more diverse self offers
advantages through the protection of high valued domains of self and the
selection of positive self-aspects for social comparison." They ask what is
the role of educational attainment in supporting a rich, multifaceted self-
system throughout the life course? Education, they suggest, communicates
that the self is worthy of study and provides tools for construing and com-
municating about diverse (possibly abstract) features of the self. In older
age, education also promotes better cognitive functioning, higher sense of
control, and better health.

Franks et al. summarize data from their self-portraits survey of nearly 1500
adults. Their respondents, aged 65 and older, reported (via self-generated
descriptors) multidimensional selves. Supporting their hypotheses, the
authors found that having higher educational standing was related to a
broader, more differentiated conception of self, not only in the present, but
also with regard to descriptions of past, recalled selves, and anticipated, future
selves. Some evidence suggested that income mediated the relationship
between education and the current self. They conclude with a call for future
work on the import of these differences in self-construal for later life health
and well-being (i.e., do more complex selves promote successful aging?)

In "Forging Macro-Micro Linkages in the Study of Psychological Well-Being" (Chapter 9), Carol Ryff, William Magee, Kristen Kling, and Edgar Wing ask how a micro-level variable, psychological well-being, is shaped by macro-level influences. Their objective is to steer clear of the "over-psychologized" nature of the person that pervades much contemporary psychology and the "over-socialized" view that prevails in sociology. They argue that the "central question is not whether to bridge the self and social structure realms, but *how* to do it." Ryff et al. propose social comparison processes as one route through which structural and individual factors are connected. "As a linking mechanism, such comparisons follow, in part, from one's location in the social structure *and* they have impact on self-evaluated well-being." Location in structural hierarchies creates unavoidable contrasts with those in lower or higher positions. And, such contrasts are consequential for how individuals assess their own worth, competence, and success.

Ryff et al. summarize the prior research on psychological well-being, showing how it varies by age, and how it is influenced by various life experiences or life transitions (e.g., parenthood, community relocation). They acknowledge that most prior inquiries in this line of research, including their own, have kept social structure in the background, frequently obviating its influence via statistical controls for sociodemographic variables (e.g., gender, education, income, and marital status). Recent studies investigating social inequalities in health have, however, revealed a strong socioeconomic gradient in psychological well-being (using multiple measures of SES and well-being). The authors conclude that these results for positive mental health "are particularly informative because they show, for the first time, that lower socioeconomic position not only increases the likelihood of ill health, it also decreases chances for well-being. Possessing these features of positive functioning constitutes an important window on quality of life, but in addition, their presence may provide important protective mechanisms in the face of life stresses, and their absence creates vulnerability."

The central question, however, is how do these effects come about? While prior investigations have examined health behaviors, work conditions, family life, and neighborhood environments as intervening mechanisms, these authors focus on more phenomenological, interpretive mechanisms. "Beyond life conditions and behavioral actions are the ways in which individuals perceive themselves in their social contexts." They offer empirical findings via two studies. The first documents linkages between educational attainment and psychological well-being in midlife, and further shows that social comparison with significant others (i.e., parent, sibling) mediate the influence of educational standing on well-being. The second reports selective findings from the recent national survey conducted by the MacArthur Research Network on Successful Midlife Development. Education is again demonstrated to be a prominent predictor of psychological well-being, but in addition, perceived inequalities (the extent to which individuals have an awareness of an unequal distribution of life resources) were found to mediate the education/well-being linkage. Their studies document that position in the educational hierarchy is linked with differential levels of well-being and underscore the role of interpretive activities (social comparisons, perceived inequalities) in bridging these macro and micro levels of analysis.

Richard Easterlin and Christine Schaeffer continue the socioeconomic emphasis with their investigation of "Income and Subjective Well-Being Over the Life Course" (Chapter 10). Prior cross-sectional linkages of income with subjective well-being "suggest that the increase in material goods per person brought about by higher income leads, on average, to feelings of enhanced well-being." They ask whether life-cycle income, which typically increases up to retirement, is accompanied by a growth in subjective well-being. The empirical findings show, however, that happiness over the life cycle does not grow as income increases (even though the point-in-time relationship between income and happiness is positive). They suggest that "a macro-micro link neglected in traditional economic theory is the key to the paradox; this link is the effect of the growth of society's income on the *material norms* of the individual."

Easterlin and Schaeffer challenge the emphasis on revealed preference (e.g., what people buy) in much economic theory, clarifying that in such an approach the "judgment on a person's well-being is made, not by the person himself, but by an outsider who is observing the person's consumption choices." For those who believe that the most authoritative observations on a person's well-being come from the person him or herself, standard utility theory is superior to revealed preference theory. Both, however, postulate that an increase in income of society as a whole would lead, other things being constant, to greater well-being.

Breaching the wall of "behavioral positivism in economics," Easterlin and Schaeffer report data from the General Social Survey, conducted yearly between 1972 and 1993, to illuminate relationships between income and reported happiness. The main conclusion is that happiness tends to be remarkably stable over the entire course of the life cycle. At the individual level, there may be trends up or down, but for the cohort as a whole, happiness remains constant, despite the fact that economic well-being increases to around ages 55 to 60 and then levels off. Neither improvement in material living up to retirement, nor the leveling off of income following retirement appear to be accompanied by changes in average happiness. The authors invoke comparative processes and norms to explain this effect: "This is because judgments of personal well-being are made by comparing one's objective status with a subjective living level norm, which is significantly influenced by the average level of living of others in society." Happiness is thus influenced, not by absolute levels of income, but by judgments made by actors through comparison processes, just as Ryff and colleagues articulate in the preceding chapter.

SECTION 3: CONTEXTS OF SELF AND SOCIETY: WORK AND FAMILY

The concluding section of the book includes six chapters describing self and society in the two specific, meso-level contexts of work and the family. Within these contexts, the contributors focus on particular life event transitions (e.g., retirement), past work and family histories, ongoing life experiences (caregiving), and the intersection of culture and familial beliefs and expectations. Many examine individual well-being or adjustment as an outcome or consequence of these work and family influences. One addresses, via the study of human values, the analytic task of putting together multiple levels of analysis (macro, meso, and micro).

Chapter 11, by Julie McMullin and Victor Marshall, entitled "Structure and Agency in the Retirement Process: A Case Study of Montreal Garment Workers", explores the dialectic between retirement as a life transition controlled by governments, employers, and unions and a life change allowing for elements of individual choice. Although it is known that individual and social structural factors play a role in determining retirement outcomes, little is known "about how workers make retirement timing decisions or what their subjective views of these decisions are. We know little of how human agency—the way in which individuals interpret and act within their worlds—interacts with the social structure in framing the retirement process." Setting the conceptual context, McMullin and Marshall first examine what is meant by social structure among age stratification and political economy researchers and further consider how human agency has been handled in aging research.

The view of agency and social structure McMullin and Marshall set forth is grounded in the theorizing of Berger and Luckmann (1966) and Giddens (1991, 1993). Berger and Luckmann see the relationship of self and social structure as dialectical: individuals produce the world through their actions (externalization), this world takes on a reality that is partly independent of the actions which constitute it (objectivation, which is similar to reification), and social reality in turn is incorporated in human consciousness through socialization and internalization. For Giddens, social structure is both the medium and the outcome of social activity. Action and structure presuppose one another and co-constitute one another in a "duality of structure". Thus, McMullin and Marshall do not start with the assumption that structure ultimately or fully determines individual action—"Individuals are not passive objects who conform to structural forces in their day to day lives. Nor do we start with the assumption that individuals act freely in a world that is left untouched by structural pressures. Indeed, the options that are available to individuals vary and are constrained by a host of structural factors."

Their conceptual framework is applied to older women in the garment industry in Montreal. At the macro level, this industry in Canada is experiencing severe global economic pressures as well as considerable technological change. Owners and managers of the mostly small manufacturing establishments that make up the industry face external constraints, and the women who work as sewers have limited opportunities to work outside the industry because they have little educational attainment and are often illiterate. The skills attained through their work are also not transferable to other types of work, and they face gender discrimination, with more highly paid jobs (e.g., cutter) being reserved for men. Yet these women do make choices and act strategically, with even constrained choices reflecting human agency: "Their choices ... are nevertheless active, involving knowledge of the range of options before them, calculation of which of these options is feasible and desirable, and, at times, the development of innovative strategies ... to facilitate an economically viable retirement." Their union representatives, reflecting collective agency, also negotiate retirement policies that serve the interests of the workers. The individual and collective choices they make in turn contribute to the maintenance of the very social structure that constrains (but does not wholly eliminate) these choices. Thus, when the majority of garment workers choose to retire at age 65, even though they could continue working to age 70, they reproduce the institutionalized, "normal" age of retirement.

Chapter 12, "Gender and Distress in Later Life: The Importance of Lifelong Employment and Familial Experiences," by Lorraine Davies examines how paid work and family arrangements over the life course illuminate later life gender differences in psychological distress. She argues, "the nature of the paid and unpaid work performed by women shapes the degree to which they have control over their daily lives, both inside and outside the family domain, which in turn has an impact on their mental health." Drawing on the life course perspective, she argues that the different distress profiles of women and men in later life are partially conditioned by the accumulation of life experiences which are, themselves, gendered. Davies challenges the view that the reduction of work and childcare responsibilities in later life reduce the salience of gender, and thereby, female disadvantage among older married women.

Davies utilizes data from the National Survey of Families and Households (USA) to operationalize questions of how gendered employment and familial experiences over a lifetime shape the mental health of older wives and husbands. She first shows that women report significantly higher levels of distress in later life than men. Whereas an approach that neglected the life course would be content to examine these differences in relation to current family status, she links them to the differentially unfolding labor force histories and differences in child-rearing responsibilities, both seen as grounded in changing sociohistorical and ideological factors shaping normative roles for men and women. Illustrative of this fact, older wives were less likely than older husbands to have been employed and more likely to have been unemployed.

Among employed women, the greater the percentage of life spent employed, the higher the distress reported. Women who worked both full- and part-time also reported more distress than those who worked only full-time. Number of children was negatively linked to distress. For men, only the number of work periods was significantly related to distress. Davies summarizes these findings by stating that different lifelong work patterns matter to the mental health of men and women. The most distressed men were those with more work interruptions, while for women, it was those with both full- and part-time histories who had higher distress, perhaps reflecting their experience with jobs having fewer promotion opportunities, fewer intrinsic rewards, and less control. The data revealed no support for the view that juggling work and family responsibilities would translate to more positive mental health for women.

Chapter 13, entitled "The Caregiving Context: The Intersection of Social and Individual Influences in the Experience of Family Caregiving," is written by Marsha Mailick Seltzer and Jan Greenberg. They argue that in most caregiving research, social-structural factors are in the background (controlled for) and primary emphasis is given to how caregiving affects the well-being of the caregiver. However, "the larger social context in which the stress occurs affects the success of one's coping efforts and the usefulness of social support in mitigating the effects of stress." Their work defines the caregiving context by variations in type of disability of the care recipient (mental retardation, mental illness, problems of aging) and the kinship relationship of care provider to care recipient (mother, daughter, wife). These are selected "because of their connection to larger social factors that shape the individual's experience of caregiving."

For example, community-based services are more extensive for those with mental retardation than for those with mental illness. Such differences reflect underlying cultural beliefs and attitudes about the etiology of these disabilities (i.e., retardation and Alzheimer's are not viewed as the fault of the family, although more blame is associated with mental illness). Wives and daughters may also experience service systems differently, and the systems may different expectations of them. Daughters may have more roles, and thereby, expect more from supportive services. "Wives, in contrast, may be more reluctant to interact with the service system, both because of the perception that caregiving is a natural extension of the wife role and because of cohort-specific attitudes regarding the appropriateness of formal services."

Seltzer and Greenberg utilize data from three longitudinal studies to contrast these differences in type of disability and type of kinship relationship. The first contrast between aging mothers of adults with mental retardation and aging mothers of adults with mental illness shows higher risk of depressive symptoms, more caregiving burden, and more feelings of pessimism about the child's future among mothers of adults with mental illness. They then explore differences in coping strategies, finding that problem-focused coping strategies did not buffer the effects of stress for these mothers, due in part to the unpredictable nature of the behavior problems of their adult son or daughter with mental illness. "These effects are exacerbated by social and institutional structures that stigmatize families of persons with mental illness and that have in the past tended to blame rather than support them in their caregiving efforts."

A further contrast between wives and daughters caring for an aging husband or parent focused on how two dimensions of social support, namely, social participation and emotional support, affect the well-being of the caregiver. They hypothesized that social participation would have more positive effects on the well-being of daughters but not wives, but that emotional support would buffer caregiving stress for both groups. These predictions were largely supported. Seltzer and Greenberg conclude their chapter with a call for more research on how social services influence individuals coping efforts and on the impact of social stigma for certain types of caregiving. Both avenues represent inroads to explicit linkage of the personal experience of caregiving with the institutional and normative structures that surround it.

Marilyn McKean Skaff, in "Linking Social Structure and the Self-Concept: Variations in Sense of Mastery" (Chapter 14), also examines family caregiving, but with a specific focus on providing care for a relative with Alzheimer's disease. She asks what effects such caregiving has on the caregiver's sense of mastery and how such linkages are influenced by one's location in the social structure (i.e., income). Skaff formulates the inquiry as linking three conceptual levels: the macro/social structural level (income), the meso level (the caregiving role), and the micro level (individual sense of mastery). Relevant prior findings showing linkages between socioeconomic indicators and stress or sense of control are reviewed. Social roles are posited as the linking mechanisms between the social structural factors and the individual outcomes. Importantly, it is not just role occupancy, but experience in the role that is relevant.

Skaff elaborates the experience of caregiving (seen as the mediating context between SES and mastery) via measurement of caregiving conditions (objective stressors), subjective assessments of hardship, emotional and instrumental resources, and coping. The objective is to look at "how income affects psychosocial resources (social support and cognitive coping), as well as the perception of stress in the context of the caregiving role, and how those factors help explain the relationship between income and sense of mastery." She notes that while caregiving might be assumed to be easier for those with greater economic resources, the inexorable progression of decline accompanying Alzheimer's could be even more challenging for those who are used having control and tractable life problems.

Using the first wave of a longitudinal study of spouses and children caring for a family member with Alzheimer's disease, she finds that mastery was significantly related to income and education. Instrumental and emotional support were positively correlated with income and mastery, while subjective sense of burden (overload) was negatively related to both income and mastery. Path analysis suggests that the effects of income on mastery appear to operate through subjective sense of burden and emotional support (with emphasis on the combined effects of the latter). She concludes that "income cannot prevent or control cognitive decline of the person with Alzheimer's disease; however, it does provide choices, alternative security." Those with more money are less likely to be involved in the daily care of the relative and may have more time to cultivate supportive relationships.

Chapter 15 by Sonia Miner and Julian Montoro-Rodriguez is entitled "Intersections of Society, Family, and Self Among Hispanics in Middle and Later Life." These authors bring issues of culture to the self/society linkage and ask how perceived well-being among aging Hispanics in the U.S. is influenced by acculturation and familistic beliefs. "For Hispanics, issues of acculturation, discriminatory barriers, family support patterns and norms of familism often compound the more commonly experienced society factors to shape the sense of self in later life." Distinctions between individualistic, collectivistic, independent, and interdependent constructions of self in society are reviewed, with evidence that Hispanic immigrants have more collectivistic attitudes with regard to family support norms and self-definitions than U.S. natives.

Their conceptual framework posits that "micro-level psychological adjustment is affected by macro societal variables (acculturation level, cultural familistic beliefs, ethnicity) and meso factors (family structure and contact)." Inconsistencies in prior work on acculturation and the self (i.e., does it enhance or hinder well-being?) are noted, and familism, a cultural belief system that refers to feelings of loyalty, reciprocity, and solidarity toward members of the family, is described as a core value shared in Hispanic culture. Miner and Montoro-Rodriguez utilize data from the National Survey of Families and Households to explore how several substantive aspects of the self (perceived happiness, depression, self-esteem) are linked with various indicators of acculturation (length of time in U.S., speaking Spanish in the interview) and familism (adherence to norms of intergenerational reciprocity in time of need). Acculturation was a significant predictor of familism and self-esteem: those in the U.S. longer had lower levels of familism, and those who spoke Spanish in the interview had higher self-esteem. The authors call for more research focusing on the family as a mediating link between social structure and the self.

Robert Roberts and Vern Bengtson conclude this section with "The Social Psychology of Values: Effects of Individual Development, Social Change, and Family Transmission over the Life Span" (Chapter 16). Values are conceptualized as standards of the desirable, which at both the micro-social level of individuals and macro level of social structures, can lead to important outcomes for individuals and collective behavior. Emphasizing the critical theme of dynamic change, they look at stability and change in two value orientations, individualism and materialism, over 23 years in three generations of family members. While psychological processes may promote or inhibit intrapsychic consistency over time, "value orientations cannot be reduced completely to individual psychology because conceptions of the desirable are learned socially and are shaped under the press of influences spanning one's interpersonal relationships, social statuses, historical period, and cultural milieu."

Roberts and Bengtson highlight structural complexity, viewed as "the interdependent and hierarchical linkages that connect the micro- and macro-social contexts within which individual development takes place." Micro structures are embedded or "nested" within progressively larger and more comprehensive structures. Change in any one level "reverberates across adjacent levels, promoting change throughout the system." This formulation requires analytic techniques capable of handling such structural and temporal complexity. Roberts and Bengtson suggest that innovations in hierarchical linear models have rendered such problems more tractable by allowing one to incorporate measures gathered at different levels of analysis (individual, contextual, sociohistorical) into single-level prediction equations.

Based on data from the USC Longitudinal Study of Generations, Roberts and Bengtson reveal significant intergenerational differences in values, with a shift from individualism to greater collectivism as one moves from the oldest to the youngest generation, and greater instability with respect to the dimension of humanism versus materialism. The hierarchical modelling techniques found secular trends towards both greater individualism and greater materialism; but that individuals tended to become more collectivist as they aged, even while society became more individualist. With respect to materialism, they found a large shift toward materialism during the 1970s and 1980s, and a smaller shift in the same direction moving to the 1990s. Most of the change towards greater materialism reflected sociohistorical changes and was not reducible to individual-level developmental change. The authors conclude, "by isolating influences across three levels of analysis—individual, familial, and socio-historical—we were able to document how stability and change in individual orientations was related to stability and change in others. More importantly, our findings illuminate bi-directional flows of influence linking individuals and their socio-historical contexts."

SUMMARY COMMENTS: THE ROAD AHEAD

The central aim of our collective enterprise is to forge linkages between the expansive literatures on meaning-making activities of the self and surrounding social structural influences. We have looked carefully at prior attempts to connect macro and micro levels of analysis so as to understand the limitations of past work, and what they point to regarding needed advances. Of particular significance, we argue, is the task of elaborating how these levels of social reality and individual experience are connected. We put forth an array of linking mechanisms (mediating meso-structures, role allocation and socialization, self processes, life events) to elaborate the middle ground connecting the individual to social structure. Our authors illustrate the utility of these directions across a diverse array of content areas, and in so doing, offer important new strides in building bridges between selves and society.

We are mindful that our enterprise is but an approximation of the larger objective of integrating the multiple levels of analysis required to understand the complex experience of human aging. For example, in delineating mechanisms of linkage, we add precision, focus, and empirical substance to the macro-micro research agenda, but because the linking tools are derived largely from the social-structural, sociological side, or individual, psychological accounts, there is danger in perpetuating more intra- rather than interdisciplinary inquiries. Approaches which postulate mediating meso-structures are useful, but too often fail to articulate the complex social dynamics at the institutional level, or the ways in which that level interacts with either the individual or the broader social structure. Role allocation and socialization strategies, in and of themselves, are not wholly satisfactory because their structural functional foundations fail to credit individuals with much agency. The advancement of self-processes (e.g., social comparisons, reflected appraisals, self-directive activities) elaborates agency, but tends to overlooks larger structural constraints on proactive initiatives. Life events can more easily be differentiated between those that are selected for versus those imposed via external forces, but rarely have these experiential investigations kept larger social-structural factors (e.g., social class) and individual outcomes (e.g., well-being, distress) simultaneously in focus.

Thus, we conclude our introductory chapter with the observation that future inquiry in the self-and-society agenda be oriented toward incorporating multiple linking mechanisms (e.g., investigate aspects of self-processes, such as social comparisons or reflected appraisals, *in* mediating meso-level contexts of work or family; e.g., examine socialization influences on agentic self-processes in the context of life event transitions). As studies move toward greater explication of how these mechanisms intersect, it is equally critical to maintain connection (theoretically and empirically) with macro-level forces that comprise more distal levels of social structure (economic influences, social policy). Ultimately, this is a call for continuing refinement of the longstanding tradition in social gerontology for integrative, multidisciplinary science.

REFERENCES

Adorno, T., Frenkel-Brunswik, E., Levinson, D. J., & Sanford, R. N. (1950). *The authoritarian personality*. New York: Harper.

Allport, G. W. (1968). The historical background of modern social psychology. In G. Lindzey & E. Aronson (Eds.), *The handbook of social psychology* (Vol. 1, pp. 1–80). Reading, MA: Addison-Wesley.

Baltes, P. B. (1987). Theoretical propositions of life-span developmental psychology: On the dynamics of growth and decline. *Developmental Psychology, 23,* 611–626.

Bengtson, V. L., Burgess, E. O., & Parrott, T. M. (1997). Theory, explanation, and a third generation of theoretical development in social gerontology. *Journal of Gerontology: Social Sciences, 52B,* S72–S88.

Berger, P. L., & Luckmann, T. (1966). *The social construction of reality.* New York: Doubleday.

Breytspraak, L. M. (1984). *The development of self in later life.* Boston: Little, Brown.

Burgess, E. W. (1960). Aging in western culture. In E. W. Burgess (Ed.), *Aging in Western Societies* (pp. 3–28). Chicago: The University of Chicago Press.

Calhoun, R. B. (1978). *In search of the new old: Redefining old age in America, 1945–1970.* New York: Elsevier.

Cowgill, D. (1974). Aging and modernization: A revision of the theory. In J. Gubrium (Ed.), *Late life: Communities and environmental policy* (pp. 123–146). Springfield, IL: Charles C. Thomas.

Cumming, E., & Henry, W. E. (1961). *Growing old: The process of disengagement.* New York: Basic.

Dannefer, D., & Perlmutter, M. (1990). Development as a multidimensional process: Individual and social constituents. *Human Development, 33,* 108–137.

Demo, D. H., & Savin-Williams, R. C. (1983). Early adolescent self-esteem as a function of social class: Rosenberg and Pearlin revisited. *American Journal of Sociology, 88,* 763–774.

Dowd, J. J. (1990). Ever since Durkheim: The socialization of human development. *Human Development, 33*, 138–159.

Elder, G. H., Jr. (1991). Lives and social change. In W. R. Heinz (Ed.), *Theoretical advances in life course research: Status passage and the life course* (Vol. 1, pp. 558–586). Weinheim: Deutscher Studien Verlag.

Elder, G. H., Jr. (1997). The life course and human development. In R. M. Lerner (Ed.), *Handbook of child psychology: Vol. I. Theoretical models of human development* (pp. 939–991). New York: Wiley.

Elder, G. H., Jr., & O'Rand, A. M. (1995). Adult lives in a changing society. In K. S. Cook, G. A. Fine, & J. S. House (Eds.), *Sociological perspectives on social psychology* (pp. 452–475). Boston: Allyn and Bacon.

Elder, G. H., Jr., Pavalko, E. K., & Hastings, T. J. (1991). Talent, history, and the fulfillment of promise. *Psychiatry, 54*, 251–267.

Festinger, L. (1954). A theory of social comparison processes. *Human Relations, 7*, 117–140.

Freud, S. (1961). *Civilization and its discontents.* New York: Norton. (Original work published 1930).

Giddens, A. (1991). *Modernity and self-identity: Self and society in the late modern age.* Stanford: Stanford University Press.

Giddens, A. (1993). *New rules of sociological method* (2nd ed.). Stanford, CA: Stanford University Press.

George, L. K. (1983). Socialization, roles, and identity in later life. In A. C. Kerckoff (Ed.), *Research in the sociology of educational and socialization: Vol. 4. Personal change over the life course* (pp. 235–263). Greenwich, CT: JAI Press.

George, L. K. (1993). Sociological perspectives on life transitions. *Annual Review of Sociology, 19*, 353–373.

Heidrich, S. M., & Ryff, C. D. (1993a). Physical and mental health in later life: The self-system as mediator. *Psychology and Aging, 8*, 327–338.

Heidrich, S. M., & Ryff, C. D. (1993b). The role of social comparisons processes in the psychological adaptation of elderly adults. *Journal of Gerontology, 48*, P127–P136.

Heidrich, S. M., & Ryff, C. D. (1996). The self in later years of life: Changing perspectives on psychological well-being. In L. Sperry & H. Prosen (Eds.), *Aging in the twenty-first century: A developmental perspective* (pp. 73–102). New York: Garland.

Hendricks, J. (1992). Generations and the generation of theory in social gerontology. *International Journal of Aging and Human Development, 35*, 31–47.

Hendricks, J., & Leedham, C. (1992). Toward a moral and political economy of aging: An alternative perspective. *International Journal of Health Services, 22*, 125–137.

Holmes, T. H., & Rahe, R. H. (1967). The social readjustment rating scale. *Journal of Psychosomatic Research, 11*, 213–218.

Hooker, K. (1992). Possible selves and perceived health in older adults and college students. *Journal of Gerontology: Psychological Sciences, 47*, P85–P95.

House, J. S. (1981). Social structure and personality. In M. Rosenberg & R. H. Turner (Eds.), *Social psychology: Sociological perspectives* (pp. 525–561). New York: Basic.

Inkeles, A. (1959). Personality and social structure. In R. K. Merton, L. Broom, & L. S. Cottrell, Jr. (Eds.), *Sociology today: Problems and prospects* (pp. 249–276). New York: Basic.

Kardiner, A. (1939). *The individual and his society.* New York: Columbia University Press.

Kohn, M. L. (1969). *Class and conformity: A study in values.* Homewood, IL: Dorsey Press.

Kuypers, J. A., & Bengtson, V. L. (1973). Social breakdown and competence: A model of normal aging. *Human Development, 26*, 181–201.

Lerner, R. M. (1984). *On the nature of human plasticity.* New York: Cambridge University Press.

Levine, R. (1973). *Culture, behavior, and personality.* Chicago: Aldine.

Markus, H. R., & Cross, S. (1990). The interpersonal self. In L. Pervin (Ed.), *Handbook of personality theory and research* (pp. 576–608). New York: Guilford.

Markus, H. R., & Herzog, A. R. (1992). The role of the self-concept in aging. In K. W. Schaie & M. P. Lawton (Eds.), *Annual Review of Gerontology and Geriatrics* (Vol. 11, pp. 110–143). New York: Springer Publishing Company.

Markus, H. R., & Kitayama, S. (1991). Culture and the self: Implications for cognition, emotion, and motivation. *Psychological Review, 98*, 224–253.

Markus, H. R., & Sentis, K. (1982). The self in social information processing. In J. Suls (Ed.), *Psychological properties of the self* (Vol. 1, pp. 41–70). Hillsdale, NJ: Erlbaum.

Marshall, V. W. (1996a). The state of theory in aging and the social sciences. In R. H. Binstock & L. George (Eds.), *Handbook of aging and the social sciences* (4th ed., pp. 12–30). San Diego, CA: Academic Press.

Marshall, V. W. (1996b). Theories of aging: Social. In J. E. Birren (Ed.), *Encyclopedia of gerontology* (Vol. 2, pp. 569–572). San Diego, CA: Academic.

Marshall, V. W. (1994). Sociology, psychology, and the theoretical legacy of the Kansas City Studies. *The Gerontologist, 34*, 768–774.

Marshall, V. W. (1995). The micro-macro link in the sociology of aging. In C. Hummel & C. J. Lalive D'Epinay (Eds.), *Images of aging in Western societies* (pp. 337–371). Geneva: Centre for Interdisciplinary Gerontology, University of Geneva.

Marshall, V. W., & Tindale, J. A. (1978–9). Notes for a radical gerontology. *International Journal of Aging and Human Development, 9*, 163–175.

McClelland, D. C. (1961). *The achieving society.* Princeton, NJ: Van Nostrand.

Pepitone, A. (1981). Lessons from the history of social psychology. *American Psychologist, 36*, 972–985.

Quadagno, J. (1982). *Aging in early industrial society: Work, family, and social policy in nineteenth-century England.* New York: Academic Press.

Riegel, K. F. (1975). Toward a dialectical theory of development. *Human Development, 18*, 346–370.

Riley, M. W. (1971). Social gerontology and the age stratification of society. *The Gerontologist, 11*, 79–87.

Riley, M. W., Foner, A., & Waring, J. (1988). Sociology of age. In N. J. Smelser (Ed.), *Handbook of sociology* (pp. 243–290). Newbury Park, CA: Sage.

Riley, M. W., Johnson, M., & Foner, A. (Eds.) (1972). *Aging and society. Vol. 3: A sociology of age stratification.* New York: Russell Sage Foundation.

Riley, M. W., Kahn, R. L., & Foner, A. (1994). *Age and structural lag.* New York: Wiley.

Rosenberg, M., & Pearlin, L. I. (1978). Social class and self-esteem among children and adolescents. *American Journal of Sociology, 84*, 53–77.

Rosow, I. (1974). *Socialization to old age.* Berkeley, CA: University of California Press.

Rosow, I. (1976). Status and role change through the life-span. In R. H. Binstock & E. Shanas (Eds.), *Handbook of aging and the social sciences* (pp. 457–482). New York: Van Nostrand Reinhold.

Ryff, C. D. (1987). The place of personality and social structure research in social psychology. *Journal of Personality and Social Psychology, 53*, 1192–1202.

Ryff, C. D. (1991). Possible selves in adulthood and old age: A tale of shifting horizons. *Psychology and Aging, 6*, 286–295.

Ryff, C. D., & Essex, M. J. (1992). The interpretation of life experience and well-being: The sample case of relocation. *Psychology and Aging, 7*, 507–517.

Schaie, K. W., & Baltes, P. B. (1975). On sequential strategies in developmental research: Description or explanation? *Human Development, 18*, 384–390.

Schutz, A. (1964). The social world and the theory of action. In A. Broderson (Ed.), Alfred Schutz. Collected papers: II. Studies in social theory (pp. 3–19). The Hague: Martinus Nijhoff.

Shanas, E. (1971). The sociology of aging and the aged. *The Sociological Quarterly, 12*, 159–176.

Smelser, N. J. (1988). Social structure. In N. J. Smelser (Ed.), *Handbook of sociology* (pp. 103–129). Newbury Park, CA: Sage.

Smelser, N. J. (1997). *Problematics of sociology.* Berkeley, CA: University of California Press.

Smelser, N. J., & Smelser, W. T. (Eds.). (1970). *Personality and social systems* (2nd ed.). New York: Wiley.

Stearns, P. (1977). *Old age in European society.* London: Croom Helm.

Stryker, S. (1983). Social psychology from the standpoint of a structural symbolic interactionism: Toward an interdisciplinary social psychology. In L. Berkowitz (Ed.), *Advances in experimental social psychology* (Vol. 16, pp. 181–218). New York: Academic Press.

Suls, J., & Mullen, B. (1982). From the cradle to the grave: Comparison and self-evaluation across the life span. In J. Suls (Ed.), *Psychological perspectives on the self* (pp. 97–125). Hillsdale, NJ: Erlbaum.

Thomas, K. (1976). Age and authority in modern England. *Proceedings of the British Academy, 62*, 205–248.

White, R. W. (1966). The shaping of lives by social forces. In *Lives in progress: A study of the natural growth of personality* (2nd ed., pp. 107–142). New York: Holt, Rinehart & Winston.

Whiting, J. W. M., & Child, T. L. (1953). *Child training and personality: A cross-cultural study.* New Haven, CT: Yale University Press.

Williams, R. H., & Wirths, C. G. (1965). *Lives through the years: Styles of life and successful aging.* New York: Atherton Press.

Wood, J. V. (1989). Theory and research concerning social comparisons of personal attributes. *Psychological Bulletin, 106*, 231–248.

Wood, J. V., & Taylor, K. L. (1991). Serving self-relevant goals through social comparison. In J. Suls & T. A. Wills (Eds.), *Social comparison: Contemporary theory and research* (pp. 23–50). Hillsdale, NJ: Erlbaum.

Wrong, D. H. (1961). The oversocialized conception of man in modern sociology. *American Sociological Review, 26*, 183–193.

CHAPTER 2

Social Perspectives on the Self in Later Life

Linda K. George

W hat is variously called personhood, identity, or the self has been an important construct in multiple disciplines. The purpose of this chapter is to examine issues of self and identity in later life from a social perspective. Social scientists have contributed much to our understanding of the self and will, hopefully, make additional contributions in the future. Let me state for the record, however, that my intellectual allegiance is in with the basic premise of this volume: self and identity can be best understood when examined using the perspectives of multiple disciplines.

Social scientists are not known for their consensual approach to social phenomena. Conceptual and empirical competition tend to characterize sociology—and perhaps most other disciplines as well. Nonetheless, social perspectives on the self rest on several propositions that appear to be nearly universally accepted. The overarching sociological premise in this regard is that the self is established, modified, and sustained in social context (e.g., Cooley, 1902/1964; Gecas, 1982; Mead, 1934; Rosenberg, 1979; Stryker, 1980). The implication of this premise for empirical research is that there will be strong and predictable links between characteristics of the social environments in which individuals are embedded and their self-attributions and evaluations of themselves. Corollaries of this proposition include the view that early socialization, experienced largely in the family, is especially important in establishing core elements of the self (e.g., Mead, 1934; Rosenberg, 1965; Smith, 1968). But it also is recognized that the self is mutable and that both reinforcements and modifications of the self continue throughout life (e.g., Brim & Wheeler, 1966; Dion, 1985; Zurcher, 1977).

Beyond these consensual propositions, there has been divergence in sociological perspectives on the self, resulting in two major paradigms: (1) structural, deterministic views of the self and (2) interactionist, proactive perspectives on the self (e.g., Gecas & Burke, 1995; George, 1980, 1983; Rosenberg, 1981). It is worth noting, perhaps, that these two paradigms have been applied to many social phenomena in addition to the self and represent a major bifurcation among social scientists. Both paradigms have generated important knowledge about the self in social context; thus, I will review both briefly.

THE STRUCTURAL/DETERMINISTIC PARADIGM

In brief, the structural/deterministic perspective proposes that both the content of self-concept and the evaluative valence of self-esteem are determined by structural statuses and processes (e.g., Gecas & Burke, 1995; George, 1980; House, 1977; Stryker, 1980). From this perspective, social processes sort people into various social structures, which in turn shape the self. In practice, research in this tradition tends to focus on social location, especially socioeconomic position, and social roles as the proximate determinants of self and identity (e.g., Burke & Reitzes, 1991; Burke & Tully, 1977; Demo & Savin-Williams, 1983; Gecas & Seff, 1989; Kohn & Schooler, 1983; Rosenberg & Pearlin, 1978). Socialization is posited to be the major mechanism by which these structural factors exert their effects on the self. Advocates of this perspective note that successful socialization produces not only the skills and behaviors required to perform specific social roles or function more broadly as societal members, but also the attitudes and subjective commitments compatible with those behavioral outcomes (George, 1980; Rosow, 1965, 1985). Thus, successful socialization ultimately results in the individual having incorporated the socialization experience into personal identity.

An impressive body of research supports structural/deterministic perspectives on the self. Space limitations preclude even scratching the surface of this research base. Most of this research is based on two kinds of evidence. First, and most significant in terms of the sheer volume of research, there are strong links between individuals' social roles and their identities. For example, an especially fruitful part of this research focuses on the links between the demands of jobs and their predictable relationships with self and identity—including strong evidence that job-related identity "spills over" to other roles (e.g., Gecas & Seff, 1989; Kohn, 1977; Kohn & Schooler, 1983; Mortimer & Lorence, 1979; Spenner & Rosenfeld, 1990). Second, researchers have demonstrated quite convincingly that changes in social roles often trigger changes in identity (e.g., Ebaugh, 1988; George, 1985; Mutran & Reitzes, 1981). For example, some of the important aging research in this tradition has articulated the conditions under which widowhood leads to stronger versus weaker changes in identity (Goldberg, Comstock, & Sioban, 1988; Schuster & Butler, 1989; Wortman & Silver, 1990).

But nagging problems are associated with use of the structural/deterministic paradigm. First, and an issue addressed in more detail later, much of this research can be challenged on the issue of causal order. Phrased simply, it is not clear whether individuals with specific identity commitments self-select into specific roles or whether the dominant influence is from social roles to associated identity commitments. Obviously, research that examines the effects of role changes on self and identity is not as compromised in this regard. Unfortunately, however, most research of this kind has examined role changes that, by definition, cannot be the result of self-selection (e.g., widowhood).

Second, the assumption that socialization is the mechanism by which social structure influences self and identity has proven difficult to test in a straightforward manner. When investigators using this paradigm are asked to explain findings in which social location is unrelated to identity, they usually revert to attributions of socialization "failure." This explanation results in the inability to perform compelling tests of the effects of socialization because there is no way to disprove it. If expected links are found, it is evidence of successful socialization; if such links are not observed, it is evidence that socialization was incomplete or inadequate.

It appears that many scholars are aware of the problem of interpreting the effects of socialization on the basis of whether or not role-related identities are observed. Indeed, recent scholars typically examine role-based identities without offering any explanation for the probable mechanism that links structural location with personal identity (e.g., Burke & Reitzes, 1991; Gecas & Seff, 1989; Wiltfang & Scarbeez, 1990). Obviously, this is ignoring rather than solving the problem. Evidence that roles are associated with identity will be of limited value unless and until social scientists can provide compelling theory and research findings that identify the mechanisms or processes that explain such relationships.

THE INTERACTIONIST/PROACTIVE PARADIGM

Advocates of the interactionist/proactive paradigm subscribe to a view of people as architects of their lives, who experience and act upon a sense of agency, and who proactively seek to impose their identities and preferences on the social world (e.g., Rosenberg, 1981; Ryff, 1986; Turner, 1962; Zurcher, 1977). A corollary proposition of this perspective is that the self is based on the interpretations and meanings that individuals use in processing social interactions. Obviously, individuals differ in interpretations of and the meanings attached to social interactions. For this reason, as well as others not covered here, advocates of interactionist perspectives view the self as less "determined" by the social environment than those who use a more structural orientation. Thus, the proactive nature of the self reflects not only the effects of human agency on social structure, but also the power of the individual in creating the self upon which human agency rests.

From the interactionist perspective, one of the primary motives of social behavior is the desire to protect and nurture the self—at minimum to avoid situations and environments that are at odds with the self (e.g., Lewicki, 1983; Mehlman & Snyder, 1985; Rosenberg, 1979). Previous research suggests two major ways that the self plays an active, initiating role: (1) as a mediator of the impact of social structure on individual outcomes and (2) as a determinant of behavior that, in turn, changes or develops social structure.

Considerable research indicates that individual outcomes—both attitudinal and behavioral—can be better explained by examining the mediating effects of self-perceptions as well as the exogenous effects of social structure. For example, both self-esteem and perceptions of control have been observed to mediate the impact of stressful life events on depression (e.g., Ensel, 1991; Essex & Klein, 1989; Holahan & Moos, 1991; Krause, 1987). Investigators interpret the mediating role of the self in two primary ways (George, 1990). Though the two modes of interpretation differ only subtly, they represent implicit theories about the nature and power of the self. Some scholars appear to view the self as simply one step in a causal chain that begins with social structure and ends with individual outcomes.

From this perspective, social structure is the "engine" that drives the process under observation, and self-perceptions are simply intermediate outcomes generated by social structure. Other investigators view the self as more independent and powerful. From this perspective, self-perceptions are a kind of "gatekeeper" that determines the degree to which social structure is able to influence individual outcomes.

Another tradition in the interactionist/proactive paradigm suggests that the self can play an even more active role by generating the development of or changes in social structure. From this perspective, the self not only reacts to social structure, but shapes and creates it. Several important qualitative studies highlight the role of the self as an active protagonist during later life (e.g., Hochschild, 1973; Matthews, 1979; Unruh, 1983). As a whole, these studies suggest that, despite disease, economic deprivation, and ageism, older adults create supportive and viable communities in which their physical, emotional, and social needs are met in ways compatible with their views of self and society. And, although this research is based largely on qualitative studies, other scholars have recognized the initiating role of the self and advised their colleagues to pay more attention to it (e.g. , Thoits, 1994). Matilda White Riley, for example, reminds us that cohorts change history, just as history changes cohorts (M. W. Riley, 1994; M. W. Riley & J. W. Riley, 1994).

The interactionist/proactive research tradition also has problems and limitations, however. First, compared to research in the structural/deterministic tradition, the research base is very small. Consequently, even major propositions in the interactionist paradigm continue to have too little empirical support to permit comfortable generalizations. In addition, the lack of an extensive research base means that this paradigm is not enriched by information about major contingencies and complexities which undoubtedly require articulation.

Second, it is difficult to compare findings and generalize conclusions across studies in this tradition. This in part reflects the well-known problems associated with the samples typically used in qualitative studies (e.g., small numbers of participants, lack of representative samples). But even more important, I think, is the fact that researchers performing qualitative studies typically do not share a common set of concepts and coding categories. Instead, investigators typically use a "grounded theory" approach, creating categories and concepts de novo. Although this approach results in rich narratives that are closely tied to participants' personal vocabularies and interpretations, it is difficult to compare findings across studies— or even determine whether authors are describing the same social phenomena.

Third, some of the most valued assumptions of the interactive/proactive perspective have been difficult to test. For example, in the observational studies that dominate this tradition, it is difficult for investigators to forge any measurable links between behavior and the self. Researchers typically assume that behavior observed in natural settings is triggered by self-perceptions and self-related motives, but that view remains more assumption or interpretation than documented fact.

Finally, although short-term longitudinal studies are very common in the symbolic interactionist tradition that underlies most previous studies of the initiating role of the self, longer-term longitudinal studies are virtually absent. Consequently, this tradition has not contributed much to our understanding of self and identity across the life course. Nor do we have much evidence about the long-term effects of human agency on social structure.

INTEGRATING STRUCTURAL AND INTERACTIONIST PARADIGMS

Hopefully, these brief summaries of the structural and interactionist paradigms used in understanding and studying self and identity have portrayed both as attractive and enlightening. One of the primary contentions of this chapter is that both paradigms offer important and valid insights about the complex relationships between people and the social structures in which they are embedded. Given that, we need to better integrate both perspectives into our research designs and interpretations of empirical findings. To date, there has been far too little effort devoted to such integration.

I do not want to do a disservice to these two important research traditions. Certainly we should not assume that there is a war going on in which one side is trying to exterminate the other. Indeed, it is my sense that most scholars whose work relies on a single paradigm would nonetheless acknowledge the importance of both. That is, scholars whose research rests on structural models of the self would probably agree that interactionist perspectives are valuable—and vice-versa. My discomfort is with leaving this "live and let live" attitude as the final resolution. It seems to me that by failing to better integrate the two paradigms, we miss the opportunity to observe the fundamental dynamics of self and society—the dialectic rhythm in which the self cannot be divorced from social context and social structure cannot be severed from its inhabitants.

But how might we accomplish the goal of better integrating these two views of the self? In my opinion, the best way of accomplishing this is to challenge both research traditions to incorporate questions and interpretations of the other into their empirical inquiries. I think it unlikely that efforts to theoretically integrate these paradigms will have much payoff. It is clear that both paradigms have solid theoretical foundations, and supporting empirical evidence. And the utility of both demonstrates that the two paradigms are not inherently contradictory. In contrast, there seems to be considerable potential for incorporating elements of both paradigms into the kinds of research generally pursued using only one of the paradigms. The rest of this chapter addresses four areas in which I see immediate opportunities for such integration.

PRIORITY AREAS FOR INTEGRATING STRUCTURAL AND INTERACTIONIST PERSPECTIVES

I. Self-Selection Into Social Environments

Selection effects are important issues in examining the self in social context, both empirically and conceptually. "Selection effects" are used broadly here to refer to the situation in which observations taken at a given point in time are partially a function of factors that took place prior to those observations.

Cross-sectional correlations fail to tell us anything about causal direction. Many cross-sectional studies report substantial relationships between social location or social roles and self-perceptions. These studies cannot determine, however, whether self-perceptions are a result of social location (including roles), or whether the dominant causal direction is from self- perceptions to social location, which is what one would expect if individuals proactively select their social environments. Longitudinal data have the potential to clarify causal direction, but only if both possibilities are empirically tested. Unfortunately, in the vast majority of longitudinal studies to date, only the structural/deterministic hypothesis is tested. Thus, tests of the relative importance of social determinism versus self-selection are largely unavailable (for an excellent discussion of how selection effects may be operating in a wide variety of studies, see Elder & O'Rand, 1995). In line with earlier comments about the complementary nature of structural and interactionist perspectives, I would expect empirical findings to support both causal directions. But much could be learned about the contingencies and conditions under which each direction is dominant.

Distinct from the empirical testing for selection effects is the question of how they are interpreted. Evidence of selection effects can be interpreted very differently, depending on the theoretical allegiances of the investigator. Advocates of structural/deterministic perspectives interpret selection effects as evidence of the persisting effects of structural processes that allocate roles, resources, and responsibilities to societal members. Life course scholars view selection effects as evidence that early transitions and experiences exert enduring effects. The cumulative advantage/disadvantage hypothesis, which is currently popular among life course scholars, is an illustration of the "mainstreaming" of selection effects into social science theory (e.g., Crystal, 1995; O'Rand, 1996). Advocates of the interactionist paradigm view selection effects as evidence that individuals proactively choose their social environments—and often assume that the self is a critical factor in those choices. Unfortunately, scholars often ignore the fact that there are competing explanations for selection effects. In particular, researchers relying on structural theories rarely acknowledge the possibility that selection effects may represent proactive personal efforts to engage in certain social environments, to avoid other social environments, and to modify social structure itself.

For purposes of illustrating the potential importance of self-selection, let's consider one of the most thoroughly investigated issues in aging research in the social sciences: age differences in life satisfaction or subjective well-being. Despite the crisis orientation that historically dominated gerontological research, there is no evidence that older adults experience lower levels of subjective well-being than their younger peers (e.g. Campbell, Converse, & Rodgers, 1976; George, Okun, & Landerman, 1985; Rodgers, 1982). Indeed, a majority of studies suggest that most older adults are more satisfied than both young adults and, especially middle-aged persons. Age patterns of subjective well-being are frequently described as paradoxical. Although objective life conditions—including health, social bonds, and economic resources—are related to subjective well-being for adults of all ages, those relationships are weakest for older adults in both bivariate and multivariate analyses (e.g., Campbell et al., 1976; George, Okun, & Landerman, 1985; Liang, Dvorkin, Kahana, & Mazian, 1980). And, on average, of course, older adults are less advantaged in objective life circumstances than young and middle-aged adults.

An important question is why the relative disadvantages experienced by older adults do not more greatly dampen their sense of life quality—or, conversely, why levels of subjective well-being among young and middle-aged adults are not higher than they are. Some research has focused on age differences in the ways that adults of various ages cognitively and emotionally process concepts such as aspirations and equity (e.g., Carp & Carp, 1982; George & Clipp, 1991; Liang & Fairchild, 1979). Overall, these studies report that subjective well-being is higher when (1) life conditions are congruent with personal aspirations and (2) life conditions are viewed as equitable. These processes partially explain age differences in subjective well-being because older adults are more likely than their younger peers to view their life conditions as congruent with their aspirations and as equitable—despite being, on average, less advantaged in objective life circumstances. I am confident that these social-psychological processes provide a partial answer to these paradoxical research findings.

It also is likely, however, that self-selection into preferred environments partially accounts for these age differences. One of the psychosocial factors for which age may serve as a rough proxy is one's history of searching for preferred environments, finding them, and becoming embedded comfortably in them. Identifying the occupational environment, community roles, and social relationships that best serve us may require a long-term process of trial and error, combined with growth in self-knowledge. Thus, subjective well-being may be especially high in late life because it takes us years to sort out and maximize the match between self and social structure.

I am not aware of research that has explicitly tested this proposition. But there seem to be strong clues to such self-selection in several areas, three of which I will mention briefly. First, there is consistent evidence that most adults change jobs several times before making long-term occupational commitments (e.g., Howard & Bray, 1988; Miller, 1988). Most job changes take place during early adulthood. It has been observed for more than 30 years that persons age 45 and older are more satisfied, on average, with their jobs than are younger workers (e.g., Glenn, 1985; Kalleberg & Loscocco, 1983; Mortimer, Finch, & Maruyama, 1988). The time required to find an optimal fit between self and job is the most common and best supported explanation for this age pattern (e.g., Caston & Braito, 1985; Kalleberg & Loscocco, 1983; Wright & Hamilton, 1978).

Second, age and marital satisfaction exhibit a similar pattern. Marital satisfaction is higher among older adults than among young and middle-aged adults (e.g., Reedy, Birren, & Schaie, 1981; Sweet & Bumpass, 1987).

Although part of this increase appears to reflect relief from childrearing responsibilities in late middle age (e.g., Spanier, Lewis, & Coles, 1975), it also is clear that a strong selection process underlies age differences in marital quality. Unsatisfying marriages tend to end in divorce, leaving satisfying marriages as the norm in late middle age and old age (e.g., Lauer & Lauer, 1986; Lupri & Frideres, 1981).

Third and finally, consider the research base on "religious switchers"—persons who, as adults, commit themselves to religious affiliations other than those in which they were socialized as children and/or participated during early adulthood. Research to date suggests that decisions to switch religious denominations are as much a function of comfort with the characteristics of religious members as of religious beliefs in the "adopted" denomination (e.g., Kluegel, 1980; Roof & Hadaway, 1979; Roof & McKinney, 1987; Sandomirsky & Wilson, 1990). Again, it appears that people frequently seek social environments compatible with their self-perceptions.

If it were taken seriously, the hypothesis of self-selection into social environments would have substantial implications for research design and analysis of data, as well as interpretation of findings. Clearly, more emphasis would be placed on collecting longitudinal data that permit examination of both the impact of self-perceptions on selection of social environments and the effects of exposure to social environments on self-perceptions. It also would be useful to compare the effects of self-selected and imposed environments on self-perceptions. For example, let's assume for the moment that self-selection of social environments is a prerogative that most of us exercise most of the time. Under these conditions, movement into a new social context may have little potential to change self-perceptions (although there might well be strong correlations between self-perceptions and the characteristics of the new environment). When we enter new social environments not of our own choosing, however, the potential for changes in self-perceptions may be considerably higher. Similarly, the effects of length of exposure to social environments on self-perceptions may differ for self-selected and imposed social contexts. When social environments are self-selected, stability of self-perceptions is likely, in both the short and the long term. When social environments are imposed on individuals, length of exposure to those environments may be a critical factor in the extent to which changes in self-perceptions are observed. If empirically observed, these patterns would support both the structural and interactionist paradigms, as well as identifying some of the conditions under which each is likely to be supported.

II. Assessing Environments for Self-Direction

Several scholars have described the historical emergence of the modern sense of self. Robert Jay Lifton (1993) describes what he terms the "Protean Self" as flexible, autonomous, and, most importantly, capable of dramatic transformations across time, space, and experience. John Meyer (1986) credits the social differentiation resulting from industrialization, urbanization, and the rise of the modern nation state with generating a sense of self based on the individual rather than the collectivity and on a temporalized view of life that facilitated social construction of concepts such as life course, personal biography, and social clocks. The terms autonomy and self-direction are prominent in the modern sense of self described by these and other scholars. If these historical interpretations are valid, the desire for self-direction should be a conspicuous component of modern identity, albeit with variability within populations.

Social scientists have examined self-direction in only rudimentary ways to date. Most relevant is research on internal versus external locus of control (see Burger, 1992 for a general review and Baltes & Baltes, 1986 for the most thorough discussion of aging and locus of control). Despite an impressive volume of studies, this research tradition is limited in a number of ways. Let me insert a note of caution, however. I am not convinced that locus of control is synonymous with self-direction, although I would expect them to be significantly correlated. There may be meaningful, but subtle differences between these social-psychological phenomena. For example, a sense of control may be broader than self-direction. Sense of control often includes not only control of self, but also some level of control of the environment and/or other people. Self-direction, in contrast, may be more narrowly restricted to the ability to be the primary architect of one's life. There are other social-psychological states, with separate research traditions, that also might be examined in relation to control and self-direction. Primary examples include self-efficacy and mastery (e.g., Bandura, 1982; Gecas, 1991). Thus, an important conceptual task is sorting out the similarities and differences among the set of concepts that seem closely related to self-direction.

Another limitation of locus of control research is that it has focused primary attention on a narrow range of potential outcomes. The vast majority of investigations of locus of control focus on its relationships with and effects on mental health and subjective well-being. A smaller number of studies examine the links between locus of control and physical health and health behaviors. Without question, these studies have been important in understanding the role of psychosocial factors in health and well-being. If, however, locus of control is a pervasive and consequential facet of the self, we remain relatively ignorant of its broader effects.

One research tradition focuses directly on self-direction rather than locus of control: studies of the impact of self-direction in the workplace. Investigators in this field have developed rather sophisticated measures of occupational self-direction (e.g., multidimensional instruments of established validity and reliability). Analogous to research on locus of control, there is strong evidence that high levels of occupational self-direction help protect individuals from job stress, psychological distress, and, physical health problems. But researchers also have demonstrated that occupational self-direction is related to a variety of outcomes other than health/well-being. Among these are job satisfaction, absenteeism at work, job turnover, and even childrearing practices (e.g., Belanger, 1989; Halaby & Weakliem, 1989; James & Jones, 1980; Kohn & Schooler, 1983; Shore, Thornton, & Shore, 1990). Additional research is needed outside the workplace that examines self-direction in relation to a broad range of outcomes.

In the remainder of this section, I will describe three opportunities for bridging structural and interactionist paradigms via research on self-direction. A first window of opportunity is examining the antecedents of self-direction. Surprisingly, little research has focused on the social determinants of a sense of control or self-direction. Mirowsky and Ross (1989) performed perhaps the best research to date on this topic. They found robust relationships between feelings of control, on the one hand, and demographic characteristics (e.g., age, sex, race) and fundamental social resources, especially socioeconomic status, on the other hand. But these relationships cannot tell us the whole story. These predictors of a sense of control are largely ascribed statuses or relatively stable social characteristics, such as social class. As such, they cannot explain intraindividual changes in self-determination that are experienced in relation to aging or other biographical or social dynamics. Thus, additional research on this topic is badly needed.

Second, and as emphasized throughout this chapter, one method for integrating structural and interactionist perspectives is to consider both paradigms as possible explanations for observed empirical findings. An example may help to illustrate the potential of this strategy. A life-course issue that has received substantial attention in the last two decades is the transition to adulthood. Structural theories have served as the conceptual underpinnings for virtually all of this research. In brief, investigators viewed the transition to adulthood as a strategic site for examining the effects of norms on behavior and the negative effects of violating those norms. The "normative" or "orderly" sequence in the transition to adulthood consists of completing school, followed by first full-time job, followed by first marriage. (The transition to parenthood was also examined in some studies; normatively, it should occur after first marriage.) Any deviation from this sequence is viewed as "non-normative" or "disorderly." There is now a large research base testing these propositions, including data from varied cohorts, men and women, Whites and racial/ethnic minorities, and multiple societies. Findings have been remarkably consistent across studies. Young adults exhibit an enormous array of sequence patterns, the majority of them exhibit non-normative patterns, and the consequences of disorderly sequences are modest (e.g., Hogan, 1978; 1981; Marini, 1984; Rindfuss, Swicegood, & Rosenfeld, 1987). The outcomes examined include educational attainment, occupational prestige, income, marital stability, and subjective well-being. Advocates of the structural paradigm were surprised to observe the negligible price one pays for violating widespread social norms.

There are several possible explanations for the above findings. One which has been ignored by these investigators is the issue of self-direction or, more broadly, the interactionist view of individuals as proactive initiators of their lives. In the absence of rare and powerful external forces, I believe that most people experience the transitions that they desire at the time and in the order that they prefer. Under these conditions, a variety of sequences might be expected to perform equally well (George, 1996). As an interactionist, I would argue that the ability to self-direct one's life may be more important than living up to social norms. Clearly, there are numerous research topics for which interactionist perspectives provide plausible alternatives to structural theories.

A third opportunity to bridge structural and interactionist paradigms would be to examine both objective and subjective components of self-direction and the relationships between objective and subjective components. Conceptually, the subjective component of self-direction is individuals' perceptions of their ability to direct or control their lives. In fact, available research, even that based on structural theories, has relied exclusively on subjective perceptions of self-direction. But surely environments also differ in the opportunities and constraints that they pose for self-direction. The development of techniques for assessing the self-direction potential of various social environments would be a major contribution to the field. Especially relevant for our purposes, there may be age or life course differences in the extent to which social environments promote or discourage self-direction. Part of the social and psychological cost of nursing home residence, for example, is substantial loss of self-direction. But that is probably the most obvious and extreme example. I recall talking to a woman, providing home care to her demented husband, who decided not to use respite care services offered by our Aging Center and to stick with paid sitters instead (despite the fact that our respite care was less expensive). Her rationale was that respite workers reported to us, whereas the sitters were hired by and reported to her. In her words, "I just feel like I'll be more in charge if I hire the person who stays with my husband." That sounds like concern about self-direction or control to me—and yet we probably pay insufficient attention to the ways in which use of social and health services are perceived as threats to self-direction (but see Saup, 1986; Streib, Folts, & LaGreca, 1985). Space limitations preclude discussing them, but it is likely that sub-texts in self-care, patient-physician interaction, and intergenerational social support raise issues of self-direction. And, of course, if we can demonstrate how characteristics of social environments facilitate and impede self-direction, it may be possible to structure environments such that loss of self-direction is minimized.

III. Persuading Structuralists to Take a Broader View of the Self

Most advocates of structural perspectives on the self view social roles as proximate determinants of self or identity. Indeed, the terms "self-in-role" and "role identity" are common in this research tradition (e.g., Burke & Tully, 1997; Stryker & Serpe, 1982). There is no question that social roles often have strong effects on personal identity and self-concept. Nonetheless, the interactionist perspective reminds us that (1) people are more than the roles they enact and (2) some components of the self are not based on conventional social roles. Use of techniques such as the "Who Are You?" (Kuhn & McPartland, 1954) for eliciting individuals' self-perceptions document that, although social roles are important components of identity, they are equaled in importance by characteristics unrelated to social roles. Examples of such characteristics include personality traits, physical appearance, and health (e.g., Bond & Cheung, 1983; Gordon, 1968; Kuhn & McPartland, 1954).

Distinct from the issue of social roles, investigators using structural theories as the foundation for research on the self also tend to focus on discrete, narrowly defined elements of the self. Examples of such elements include self-consciousness, gender identity, and identification with work and family roles. Many measures of discrete elements of the self are sophisticated and of documented psychometric adequacy. Moreover, research based on discrete elements of the self has generated important results concerning the links between social structures and personal identity (e.g., Burke, 1989; Burke & Reitzes, 1981; Eagly, 1987; Katz, 1986).

From an interactionist perspective, however, both an exclusive reliance on role-based identities and the use of discrete elements of the self are problematic. As previously noted, many components of the self are not role-based—and to dismiss other sources of identity does not do justice to the complexity and richness of the self. Similarly, reliance on discrete elements of the self (especially research based on a single element of the self—which is common) fails to capture the complexity of the self. In essence, interactionists might argue, investigators in the structural tradition may have excellent views of selected trees, but seem unaware of or unconcerned about the larger forest.

It also may be dangerous to make conclusions based on investigation of very discrete elements of the self and/or identities related only to social roles. Precisely because the self is complex, investigators need to be aware of issues such as the individual's salience hierarchy of personal identities, desired as well as achieved dimensions of the self, and whether the individual's identities are internally consistent. These and other concepts that relate to the organization and structure of the self are important in understanding the impact of the self on behavior. For example, whether an individual performs well at work will depend not only on his or her work-based identity, but also on the importance of that identity relative to others and the worker's desire to excel on the job.

It is doubtful that advocates of the structural paradigm will ever take on the task of developing and using comprehensive measures of self and identity. They could, however, cast a wider net than is typical in research to date. A few examples will help to illustrate the potential of this strategy. First, although comprehensive measures of identity may be unreasonable, investigators could routinely measure multiple elements of the self. Obviously, selection of specific elements would depend on the research question. But inclusion of multiple components of the self would allow investigators to determine whether observed relationships between structural variables and self-perceptions are consistent or inconsistent across relevant elements of the self.

Second, scholars using the structural paradigm could use the measurement skills that generated measures of role-based identities to develop measures of important aspects of the self that are not role-based. It should be possible, for example, to develop measures of identity elements such as self-perceptions of health, likability, and physical attractiveness. I would expect these identity elements to be related to social structural variables, just as role-based identities are. Thus, development of non-role based elements of the self would enhance our appreciation for the strong and pervasive links between self and social context.

Finally, there is increasing evidence that the desired or aspired self is a strong motivational factor in human behavior. Scholars of the self have long recognized the importance of the distinction between the actual and desired self (e.g., Higgins, 1987; Rosenberg, 1979). But conceptualization and measurement of "possible selves," as developed by Hazel Markus and her colleagues (e.g., Markus & Nurius, 1986; Markus & Wurf, 1987; Nurius, 1991) has generated new excitement about the desired self as a cognitive structure and motivational factor. Recent work on possible selves has been conducted almost exclusively by psychologists. Consequently, we know very little about the links between the desired self and social environments. Scholars relying on structural perspectives on the self are ideally positioned to address this issue—and by doing so would help to integrate structural and interactionist paradigms.

IV. Persuading Interactionists to Take Social Structure Seriously

Thus far, most of my discussion has addressed the need to infuse research based on the structural paradigm with interactionist perspectives. The reverse of that is also needed; that is, we need to note the ways in which interactionist research would be enhanced by attention to social structure. It is ironic that social structure has been so widely ignored in interactionist research. The theories upon which the interactionist paradigm rests, especially the classic and pioneering work of scholars such as Cooley (1902/1964) and Mead (1934), forcefully assert that the self emerges in social context, is shaped by the social environment, and cannot be understood outside of social context. Thus, neglect of social structure in research based on the interactionist paradigm results from the procedures used to select samples and collect data, rather than from limitations in theory.

Many of the contributions of research based on the interactionist paradigm rest on qualitative, ethnographic studies. In general, the proactive and initiating components of the self have been best and most richly portrayed in ethnographic studies. But those studies typically ignore social structure. A major reason for this neglect is use of samples that are homogeneous with regard to social structure, thus making structural factors constants. For example, many of the most compelling qualitative studies in aging research have relied on observations of and/or in-depth interviews with people residing in settings such as nursing homes, retirement communities, and SRO hotels; with persons receiving specific types of services (e.g., home care); or participating in specific organizations such as senior centers (e.g., Gubrium, 1975; Hochschild, 1973; Marshall, 1975; Matthews, 1979; Myerhoff, 1978; Unruh, 1983). These environments are not only homogeneous in social structure; they also tend to recruit (self-selection) residents/participants who are socially homogeneous (e.g., in socioeconomic status and health).

There are at least three ways in which studies based on the interactionist paradigm could usefully incorporate attention to social structure. First, interactionists should develop hypotheses that link social structure and personal identity. Hypotheses, in the positivistic sense, are rather rare in interactionist research using qualitative methods. (This is not true of survey research based on the interactionist paradigm—e.g., Burke & Reitzes, 1991; Gecas & Schwalbe, 1983; Schafer & Keith, 1985). But interactionist scholars could develop general hypotheses, sufficient for guiding research design, without losing the richness of experience that is the hallmark of qualitative research. For example, the self-protective mechanisms that older adults develop to sustain a positive sense of self have been identified in multiple qualitative studies (e.g., Hochschild, 1973; Matthews, 1979). It would be relatively easy to develop hypotheses about how the structural characteristics of various social environments (1) make it more or less difficult to use or develop such mechanisms and (2) are associated with the specific self-protection strategies developed and employed. Interactionists also need to recognize that social structure includes more than very broad concepts such as socioeconomic status. Age and gender composition are examples of structural factors that can be studied at the micro level.

Second, scholars using the interactionist paradigm are in an ideal position to examine both objective environmental characteristics and subjective perceptions of the environment, the relationships between them, and their joint and separate effects on self-perceptions. Such studies have the potential to be far more than an "accounting" procedure in which facets of the self are sorted on the basis of whether they are more strongly related to objective or subjective parameters of social environment. Research along these lines would highlight the dialectic nature of the self, capturing both the ways in which the self is shaped by social structure and, conversely, what I have previously called the "gatekeeping" function of the self (George, 1990), in which the self literally determines the degree to which social structure (or other external factors) are permitted to affect self-perceptions.

Third, and a potentially powerful method of integrating structural and interactionist perspectives, is the use of explicit comparisons of the self across social environments that are structurally diverse. It is ironic that social structure has largely been ignored by researchers using qualitative methods. Given the tradition of selecting specific environments for their studies, it should be relatively simple to add structural comparisons to qualitative research. One can imagine studies that compare subjective experiences generally and self-perceptions in particular across structurally heterogeneous environments. For example, self-perceptions could be compared between older adults living in age-heterogeneous and age-homogeneous residential settings. Similarly, identities could be compared in environments that vary by socioeconomic status or that are heterogeneous versus homogeneous with regard to the social class of persons in those environments. In general, scholars using the interactionist paradigm, especially those performing qualitative research, are well-positioned to sample social environments, thus generating important knowledge about the links between social structure and the life of the self.

FINAL THOUGHTS

The theme of this chapter is that integrating social structural and interactionist perspectives has the potential to further our understanding of the self in social context. I have attempted to identify specific issues relevant to this theme and suggest useful directions for future research. But the underlying theme, throughout, was the need for integration of paradigms and the advantages of viewing them as complementary rather than competing views of social reality.

It is worth noting that this theme—variously termed integration, synthesis, and cross-fertilization—is emerging throughout science. There is now a strong emphasis on viewing the mind and the body as inexorably linked—which is a reversal of scientific thinking for most of this century. Multidisciplinary research, though still the exception rather than the rule, is increasingly common and is a priority for many research-funding agencies (e.g., the National Institutes of Health). Within disciplines, tight theoretical boundaries and rigid methodologic allegiances are breaking down, and being replaced by efforts to integrate, synthesize, and broaden—at any rate, that is the trend in my discipline, sociology.

I applaud this movement toward integration and inclusiveness rather than separation and exclusion. As I've tried to demonstrate, integration will have significant scientific payoff. In addition, this attitude of inclusiveness, in which social phenomena are examined using multiple theoretical and methodologic perspectives, seems to me to be the only defensible stance for scholars and scientists. If the scientific community is not able to tolerate diversity in viewpoints and bridge that diversity in ways that creates a sum that is greater than the sum of its parts, who will?

REFERENCES

Baltes, M. M., & Baltes, P. B. (Eds.) (1986). *The psychology of control and aging.* Hillsdale, NJ: Lawrence Erlbaum.

Bandura, A. (1982). Self-efficacy mechanisms in human agency. *American Psychologist, 37,* 122–147.

Belanger, J. (1989). Job control and productivity: New evidence from Canada. *British Journal of Industrial Relations, 27,* 347–364.

Bond, M. H., & Cheung, T. S. (1983). College students' spontaneous self-concept: The effect of culture among respondents in Hong Kong, Japan, and the United States. *Journal of Cross-Cultural Psychology, 14,* 153–171.

Brim, O. G., Jr. & Wheeler, S. A. (1966). *Socialization after childhood: Two essays.* New York: Wiley.

Burger, J. M. (1992). *Desire for control: Personality, social, and clinical perspectives.* New York: Plenum.

Burke, P. J. (1989). Gender identity, sex, and school performance. *Social Psychology Quarterly, 52,* 159–169.

Burke, P. J., & Reitzes, D. C. (1981). The link between identity and role performance. *Social Psychology Quarterly, 44,* 83–92.

Burke, P. J., & Reitzes, D. C. (1991). An identity theory approach to commitment. *Social Psychology Quarterly, 54,* 280–286.

Burke, P. J., & Tully, J. (1977). The measurement of role/identity. *Social Forces, 55,* 880–897.

Campbell, A., Converse, P. E., & Rodgers, W. L. (1976). *The quality of American life.* New York: Russell Sage Foundation.

Carp, F. M., & Carp, A. (1982). Test of a model of domain satisfactions and well-being: Equity considerations. *Research on Aging, 4,* 503–522.

Caston, R. J., & Braito, R. (1985). The worker-to-job "fit" hypothesis: Further evidence. *Work and Occupations, 12*, 269–284.

Cooley, C. H. (1964). *Human nature and the social order.* New York: Scribners (Originally published 1902).

Corsaro, W. A., & Eder, D. (1995). Development and socialization of children and adolescents. In K. S. Cook, G. A. Fine, & J. S. House (Eds.), *Sociological perspectives on social psychology* (pp. 421–451). Boston: Allyn and Bacon.

Crystal, S. (1995). Economic status of the elderly. In R. H. Binstock & L. K. George (Eds.), *Handbook of aging and the social sciences* (4th ed.) (pp. 388–411). San Diego: Academic Press.

Demo, D. H., & Savin-Williams, R. C. (1983). Early adolescent self-esteem as a function of social class: Rosenberg and Pearlin revisited. *American Journal of Sociology, 88*, 763–774.

Dion, K. K. (1985). Socialization in adulthood. In G. Lindzey & E. Aronson (Eds.), *Handbook of social psychology: Volume 2. Special fields and applications* (pp. 123–147). New York: Random House.

Eagly, A. H. (1987). *Sex differences in social behavior: A social-role interpretation.* Hillsdale, NJ: Erlbaum.

Ebaugh, H. R. F. (1988). *Becoming an ex: The process of role exit.* Chicago: University of Chicago Press.

Elder, G. H., Jr., & O'Rand, A. M. (1995). Adult lives in a changing society. In K. S. Cook, G. A. Fine, & J. S. House (Eds.), *Sociological perspectives on social psychology* (pp. 452–477). Boston: Allyn and Bacon.

Ensel, W. M. (1991). "Important" life events and depression among older adults: The role of psychological and social resources. *Journal of Aging and Health, 3*, 546–566.

Essex, M. J., & Klein, M.H. (1989). The importance of self-concept and coping responses in explaining physical health status and depression among older women. *Journal of Aging and Health, 1*, 327–348.

Gecas, V. (1982). The self-concept. *Annual Review of Sociology, 8*, 1–33.

Gecas, V. (1991). The self-concept as a basis for a theory of motivation. In J.A. Howard & P. L. Callero (Eds.), *The self-society dynamic: Cognition, emotion, and action* (pp. 171–188). Cambridge: Cambridge University Press.

Gecas, V., & Burke, P. J. (1995). Self and identity. In K. S. Cook, G. A. Fine, & J. S. House (Eds.), *Sociological perspectives on social psychology* (pp. 41–67). Boston: Allyn and Bacon.

Gecas, V., & Schwalbe, M. L. (1983). Beyond the looking-glass self: Social structure and efficacy-based self-esteem. *Social Psychology Quarterly, 46*, 77–88.

Gecas, V., & Seff, M. A. (1990). Social class and self-esteem: Psychological centrality, compensation, and the relative effects of work and home. *Social Psychology Quarterly, 53*, 165–173.

George, L. K. (1980). *Role transitions in later life.* Monterey, CA: Brooks/Cole.

George, L. K. (1983). Socialization, roles, and identity in later life. In A. C. Kerckhoff (Ed.), *Research in the sociology of education and socialization. Volume 4. Personal change over the life course* (pp. 235–263). Greenwich, CT: JAI Press.

George, L. K. (1985). Socialization to old age: A path analytic model. In E. Palmore, J. Nowlin, E. W. Busse, I. C. Siegler, & G. L. Maddox (Eds.), *Normal Aging III* (pp. 326–335). Durham, NC: Duke University Press.

George, L. K. (1990). Social structure, social processes, and social psychological states. In R. H. Binstock & L. K. George (Eds.), *Handbook of aging and the social sciences* (3rd ed.) (pp. 186–204). San Diego: Academic Press.

George, L. K. (1996). Missing links: The case for a social psychology of the life course. *The Gerontologist, 36,* 248–255.

George, L. K., & Clipp, E. C. (1991). Subjective components of aging well. *Generations, 15,* 57–60.

George, L. K., Okun, M. A., & Landerman, R. (1985). Age as a moderator of the determinants of life satisfaction. *Research on Aging, 7,* 209–233.

Glenn, N. D. (1985). Age, cohort, and reported job satisfaction in the United States. In Z. S. Blau (Ed.), *Current perspectives on aging and the life cycle.* (Vol. 1). Greenwich, CT: JAI Press.

Goldberg, E. L., Comstock, G. W., & Sioban, D. H. (1988). Emotional problems and widowhood. *Journal of Gerontology, 43,* 206–218.

Gordon, C. (1968). Self-conceptions: Configurations of content. In C. Gordon & K. J. Gergen (Eds.), *The self in social interaction* (pp. 115–136). New York: Wiley.

Gubrium, J. F. (1975). *Living and dying at Murray Manor.* New York: St. Martin's Press.

Halaby, C. N., & Weakliem, D. L. (1989). Worker control and attachment to the firm. *American Journal of Sociology, 95,* 549–591.

Higgins, E. T. (1987). Self-discrepancy: A theory relating self and affect. *Psychological Review, 94,* 319–340.

Hochschild, A. R. (1973). *The unexpected community.* Berkeley, CA: University of California Press.

Hogan, D. P. (1978). The variable order of events in the life course. *American Sociological Review, 43,* 573–586.

Hogan, D. P. (1981). *Transitions and social change: The early lives of American men.* New York: Academic Press.

Holahan, C. J., & Moos, R. H. (1991). Life stressors, personal and social resources, and depression: A 4-year structural model. *Journal of Abnormal Psychology, 100,* 31–38.

House, J. S. (1977). The three faces of social psychology. *Sociometry, 40,* 161–177.

Howard, A., & Bray, D. W. (1988). *Managerial lives in transition: Advancing age and changing times.* New York: Guilford.

James, L. R., & Jones, A. P. (1980). Perceived job characteristics and job satisfaction: An examination of reciprocal causation. *Personnel Psychology, 33*, 97–135.

Kalleberg, A. L., & Loscocco, K. A. (1983). Aging, values, and rewards: Explaining age differences in job satisfaction. *American Sociological Review, 48*, 78–90.

Katz, P. A. (1986). Gender identity: Development and consequences. In R. D. Ashmore & F. K. Del Boca (Eds.), *The social psychology of male-female relations* (pp. 21–67). New York: Academic Press.

Kluegel, J. (1980). Denominational mobility: Current patterns and recent trends. *Journal for the Scientific Study of Religion, 19*, 26–39.

Kohn, M. L. (1977). *Class and conformity: A study in values.* Chicago: University of Chicago Press.

Kohn, M. L., & Schooler, C. (1983). *Work and personality: An inquiry into the impact of social stratification.* Norwood, NJ: Ablex.

Krause, N. (1987). Chronic strain, locus of control, and distress in older adults. *Psychology and Aging, 2*, 375–382.

Kuhn, M. H., & McPartland, T. S. (1954). An empirical investigation of self-atttitudes. *American Sociological Review, 19*, 68–76.

Lauer, R. H., & Lauer, J. C. (1986). Factors in long-term marriages. *Journal of Family Issues, 7*, 382–390.

Lewicki, P. (1983). Self-image bias in person perception. *Journal of Personality and Social Psychology, 45*, 384–393.

Liang, J., Dvorkin, L., Kahana, E., & Mazian, F. (1980). Social integration and morale: A re-examination. *Journal of Gerontology, 35*, 746–757.

Liang, J., & Fairchild, T. (1979). Relative deprivation and perception of financial adequacy among the aged. *Journal of Gerontology, 34*, 746–759.

Lifton, R. J. (1993). *The protean self.* New York: Basic Books.

Lupri, E., & Frideres, J. (1981). The quality of marriage and the passage of time: Marital satisfaction over the family life cycle. *Canadian Journal of Sociology, 6*, 283–305.

Marini, M. M. (1984). Age and sequencing norms in the transition to adulthood. *Social Forces, 63*, 229–244.

Markus, H., & Nurius, P. (1986). Possible selves: The interface between motivation and the self-concept. In K. Yardley & T. Honess (Eds.), *Self and identity: Psychosocial perspectives* (pp. 213–232). New York: Wiley.

Markus, H., & Wurf, E. (1987). The dynamic self-concept: A social-psychological perspective. *Annual Review of Psychology, 38*, 299–337.

Marshall, V. W. (1975). Socialization for impending death in a retirement village. *American Journal of Sociology, 80*, 1124–1144.

Matthews, S. H. (1979). *The social world of older women.* Beverly Hills, CA: Sage.

Mead, G. H. (1934). *Mind, self, and society.* Chicago: University of Chicago Press.

Mehlman, R. C., & Snyder, C. R. (1985). Excuse theory: A test of the self-protective role of attributions. *Journal of Personality and Social Psychology, 49*, 994–1001.

Meyer, J. W. (1986). The institutionalization of the life course and its effects on the self. In A. B. Sorensen, F. E. Weinert, & L. R. Sherrod (Eds.), *Human development and the life course: Multidisciplinary perspectives* (pp. 199–216). Hillsdale, NJ: Lawrence Erlbaum.

Miller, J. (1988). Jobs and work. In N. J. Smelser (Ed.), *Handbook of sociology* (pp. 327–359). Newbury Park, CA: Sage.

Mirowsky, J., & Ross, C. E. (1989). *Social causes of psychological distress*. New York: Aldine de Gruyter.

Mortimer, J. T., Finch, M. D., & Maruyama, G. (1988). Work experience and job satisfaction: Variation by age and gender. In J. T. Mortimer & K.M. Borman (Eds.), *Work experience and psychological development through the life span* (pp. 109–155). Boulder, CO: Westview.

Mortimer, J. T., & Lorence, J. (1979). Occupational experience and the self-concept: A longitudinal study. *Social Psychology Quarterly, 42*, 307–323.

Mutran, E., & Reitzes, D. C. (1981). Retirement, identity, and well-being: Realignment of role relationships. *Journal of Gerontology, 36*, 134–143.

Myerhoff, B. (1978). *Number our days*. New York: Simon and Schuster.

Nurius, P. (1991). Possible selves and social support: Social cognitive resources for coping and striving. In J. A. Howard & P. L. Callero (Eds.), *The self-society interface: Cognition, emotion, and action* (pp. 239–258). New York: Cambridge University Press.

O'Rand, A. M. (1996). The precious and the precocious: Understanding cumulative disadvantage and cumulative advantage over the life course. *The Gerontologist, 36*, 230–238.

Reedy, M. N., Birren, J. E., & Schaie, K. W. (1981). Age and sex differences in satisfying love relationships across the adult life span. *Human Development, 38*, 52–66.

Riley, M. W. (1994). Aging and society: Past, present, and future. *The Gerontologist, 34*, 436–446.

Riley, M. W., & Riley, J. W., Jr. (1994). Structural lag: Past and future. In M. W. Riley, R. L. Kahn, & A. Foner (Eds.), *Age and structural lag* (pp. 15–36). New York: Wiley.

Rindfuss, R. R., Swicegood, C. G., & Rosenfeld, R. A. (1987). Disorder in the life course: How common and does it matter? *American Sociological Review, 52*, 785–801.

Rodgers, W. L. (1982). Trends in reported happiness within demographically defined subgroups, 1957–78. *Social Forces, 60*, 826–842.

Roof, W. C., & Hadaway, C. K. (1979). Denominational switching in the seventies. *Journal for the Scientific Study of Religion, 18*, 363–378.

Roof, W. C., & McKinney, W. (1987). *American mainline religion: Its changing shape and future*. Rutgers, NJ: Rutgers University Press.

Rosenberg, M. (1965). *Society and the adolescent self-image*. Princeton, NJ: Princeton University Press.

Rosenberg, M. (1979). *Conceiving the self*. New York: Basic Books.

Rosenberg, M. (1981). The self-concept: Social product and social force. In M. Rosenberg & R. Turner (Eds.), *Social psychology: Sociological perspectives* (pp. 593–624). New York: Basic Books.

Rosenberg, M., & Pearlin, L. I. (1978). Social class and self-esteem among children and adults. *American Journal of Sociology, 84*, 53–77.

Rosow, I. (1965). Forms and functions of adult socialization. *Social Forces, 44*, 35–45.

Rosow, I. (1985). Status and role change through the life cycle. In R. H. Binstock & E. Shanas (Eds.), *Handbook of aging and the social sciences* (1st ed.) (pp. 62–93). New York: Van Nostrand Reinhold.

Ryff, C. D. (1986). The subjective construction of self and society: An agenda for life-span research. In V. W. Marshall (Ed.), *Later life: The social psychology of aging* (pp. 33–74). Beverly Hills, CA: Sage.

Sandomirsky, S., & Wilson, J. (1990). Processes of disaffiliation: Religious mobility among men and women. *Social Forces, 68*, 1211–1230.

Saup, W. (1986). Lack of autonomy in old age homes: A stress and coping study. *Journal of Housing for the Elderly, 4*, 21–36.

Schafer, R. B., & Keith, P. M. (1985). A causal model approach to the symbolic interactionist view of the self-concept. *Journal of Personality and Social Psychology, 49*, 963–969.

Schuster, T. L., & Butler, E. W. (1989). Bereavement, social networks, social support, and mental health. In D. A. Lund (Ed.), *Older bereaved spouses* (pp. 55–68). New York: Hemisphere.

Shore, T. H., Thornton, G. C., III, & Shore, L. M. (1990). Distinctiveness of three work attitudes: Job involvement, occupational commitment, and career salience. *Psychological Reports, 67*, 851–858.

Smith, M. B. (1968). Competence and socialization. In J. Clausen (Ed.), *Socialization and society* (pp. 117–149). Boston: Little, Brown.

Spanier, G. B., Lewis, R. A., & Coles, C. L. (1975). Marital adjustment over the family life cycle: The issue of curvilinearity. *Journal of Marriage and the Family, 37*, 263–275.

Spenner, K. I., & Rosenfeld, R. A. (1990). Women, work, and identities. *Social Science Research, 19*, 266–299.

Streib, G. F., Folts, N. E., & LaGreca, A. J. (1985). Autonomy, power, and decision-making in 36 retirement communities. *The Gerontologist, 25*, 403–409.

Stryker, S. (1980). *Symbolic interactionism:: A social structural version*. Menlo Park, CA: Benjamin Cummings.

Stryker, S., & Serpe, R. T. (1982). Commitment, identity salience, and role behavior. In W. Ickes & E. Knowles (Eds.), *Personality, roles, and social behavior* (pp. 199–218). New York: Springer Verlag.

Sweet, J. A., & Bumpass, L. L. (1987). *American families and households*. New York: Russell Sage Foundation.

Thoits, P. A. (1994). Stressors and problem-solving: The individual as psychological activist. *Journal of Health and Social Behavior, 35*, 143–160.

Turner, R. H. (1962). Role-taking: Process versus conformity. In A. M. Rose (Ed.), *Human behavior and social processes* (pp. 20–41). Boston: Houghton Mifflin.

Unruh, D. R. (1983). *Invisible lives*. Beverly Hills, CA: Sage.

Wiltfang, G. L., & Scarbeez, M. (1990). Social class and adolescents' self-esteem: Another look. *Social Psychology Quarterly, 53*, 174–183.

Wortman, C. B., & Silver, R. C. (1990). Successful mastery of bereavement and widowhood: A life-course perspective. In P. B. Baltes & M. M. Baltes (Eds.), *Successful aging: Perspectives from the behavioral sciences* (pp. 225–264). New York: Cambridge University Press.

Wright, J. D., & Hamilton, R. F. (1978). Work satisfaction and age: Some evidence for the "job change" hypothesis. *Social Forces, 56*, 1140–1158.

Zurcher, L. A., Jr. (1977). *The mutable self*. Beverly Hills, CA: Sage.

CHAPTER 3

Neoteny, Naturalization, and Other Constituents of Human Development

Dale Dannefer

INDIVIDUAL AND SOCIAL:
DICHOTOMOUS OR DIALECTICAL?

The zoologist Stephen Austad (1992) has shown that opossums living on Sapelo Island, off the coast of the Carolinas, age differently than do American mainland opossums. The mainland opossums live only 2–3 years; they begin reproducing at only 6 to 8 months of age, bear two litters over the next year and age quickly. Most die by age three. By contrast, island opossums can live more than 4 years, and half of the females reproduce for 2 years—although they have smaller litters. The apparent reason is natural selection: Predators that kill defenseless opossums pervade the mainland environment, and therefore it has selected those that quickly produce large litters. There are no predators on Sapelo Island, and thus it favors those reproduce longer, produce more litters, and age more slowly.

The author thanks Gerald Coles, Elaine Dannefer, Katherine Douthit, and Peter Uhlenberg for critical comments on an earlier draft. Special thanks to Victor Marshall and Carol Ryff for their comments and constructive criticism.

This is an example of a differential aging pattern that results from selection creating a change in the genome: Two different environments produce distinct patterns of aging by modifying the gene pool of the population. Notice that this explanation of differential reproduction does not entail any consideration of the environmental regulation of gene expression or of biological mechanisms of homeostasis—factors which combine to produce individual phenotypes and actual living opossum organisms.

This account of opossum aging serves to dramatize two fundamentally different ways of conceiving relations between the individual organism and the environment that are not always clearly distinguished in the study of human aging and development. The first can be called *parallel* or *dichotomous*: An organism is born into a pregiven environment, and its success is based on its capabilities to survive to reproduction in that environment.

The second approach focuses on how discrete organisms and discrete environments influence each other in the patterned interactions of everyday life. This approach can be called *interactive* or *dialectical* because it centers on the dynamics between an actual individual and the immediate environment. The individual is shaped to varying degrees by its exchanges with the environment, and these exchanges also affect the environment itself. Note that this approach does not include genotypic change as either cause or effect, as in the opossum case.

In the parallel model, individual and environment are largely prestructured entities that engage in a matching game (a game in which natural selection plays a central role); in the dialectical model, individual and environment are not fixed entities to be "matched", but are continuously being reconstituted in everyday interaction. These two conceptions, which imply fundamentally different dynamics, are often confused in both theory and research in development and aging.

Most research on development and aging in the social and behavioral sciences is concerned with change in actual individuals, entailing a combination of phenotypic expression and organism-environment interaction. Nevertheless, researchers often rely on a biological framework that was forged primarily in an effort to deal with evolutionary change, and hence with changes in the genotype (cf. Dannefer, 1989; Morss, 1990, 1996). For example, terms such as adaptation, selection, adjustment, goodness-of-fit, and "ecological niche" are drawn from an evolutionary paradigm. They bring with them an often implicit presumption of fixed, prestructured entities, e.g., the "person", the "social environment", the "psyche", and the "family." *Adaptation* and *adjustment* imply the existence of a natural environment that imposes fixed requirements on the individuals that inhabit it (e.g., Barkow, Cosmides, & Tooby, 1992). *Selection* (cf. Baltes, 1987; Marsiske, Lang, Baltes, & Baltes, 1995) implies the existence of stable individuals who may differ in their adaptive potential for a given environment, and of behavior routines that can be selected by an individual. *Goodness-of-fit* (e.g., Lerner, Lerner, & Zabski, 1985) also implies a fixed environmental structure, a *niche*, perhaps, for which a properly suited individual can be selected; *optimization*" reflects the view that people engage in behaviors to enrich and augment their general reserves and to maximize their chosen life courses . . ." (Baltes & Baltes, 1990, p. 22) and "means that—within the framework provided by the genome and society—individual competencies, existing goal-directed means, and outcomes are acquired and maintained at levels as well as in directions desirable for a person" (Marsiske et al., 1995, p. 48).

Applied to individual aging, such terms extend the concept of selection beyond its evolutionary significance in reproduction to phenotypic adaptation. Society, no less than the genome, is seen as posing a fixed set of constraints. Thus, whether referring to genotype or phenotype, these concepts belong to a discourse of parallel levels of reality that interact in limited ways, and in which one level shapes the other only indirectly, through the mechanism of selection—the individual is seen as selecting activities to engage in and contexts to which she can adapt. The notion of an interaction in which the person is *constituted*, and in which the social context is *constituted*, is absent. Thus, the reliance on the concept of selection implies an assumption of largely independent processes at work at levels of human development and of the constitution of society. For purposes of the present discussion, I will call this approach a parallel process model, because there is a parallel movement through time of individual and environment, but no identifiable influence upon the constitution of one by the other. The most interesting and important interface is in processes of selection.

DISTINCTIVES OF HUMAN DEVELOPMENT
AND THE ROLE OF THE SOCIAL

For studying the development of many species, the parallel process model is entirely appropriate. It is inappropriate for studying human development, however, despite its popularity. This section attempts to clarify the importance of this discontinuity by asserting three anthropological principles that are distinctives of human development and aging: *Extero-gestation, neoteny, and world-construction.* The first two of these features describe the human organism's exceptional predisposition for responsiveness to the environment; the third involves human agency, and the complex of uniquely human processes involved in world-building—in building, sustaining, and reproducing human relationships and human systems of interaction.

Exterogestation

Exterogestation (Montagu, 1989) refers to the uniquely "unfinished" or "embryonic" condition of the human infant (Gould, 1977b, 1977c; Montagu, 1989). Exterogestation means that "important organismic developments, which for animals are completed in the mother's body, take place in the human infant after its separation from the womb" (Berger & Luckmann, 1967, p. 48). Despite the length of human gestation in chronological time, the rate of development of humans is the slowest of any primate species (Gould, 1977c, pp. 365–369). The maturity evidenced by newborns of other primate species is evidenced by humans at about 21 months after conception (Gould, 1977b, 1977c, Montagu, 1961). A result is that, relative to the overall pace of development, the time spent in utero "is truncated and abbreviated" (Gould, 1977b, p. 72). Because of this condition, Adolf Portmann claimed that the human infant experiences an "extrauterine *fruhjahr*" (early-year), a concept virtually synonymous with exterogestation (Portmann, 1956; cf. Berger & Luckmann, 1967). Human infants are unusually helpless and unformed (digits and the ends of limb bones lack ossification at birth; Schultz, 1949); the brain has attained only about 40% of its final size, compared, e.g., to 70% for chimpanzees (Holt, Cheek, Mellits & Hill, 1975; Passingham, 1975; see also Gould, 1977b). The concept of exterogestation is not a mere dramatization of infant dependency: For most species, physical birth is a marker of discontinuity in developmental rates. For humans, however, the natal discontinuity in developmental rate does not occur at 9 months, but at about 21 months (Gould, 1977c).

Exterogestation means that humans experience a long period of embyronic growth responding directly to a historically and culturally specific social context. Not only habits and perceptions, but the structuring of the body (including, e.g., posture, gait, perception, and larynx development) and capabilities of movement (e.g., the development of physical characteristics that facilitate culture-specific dance or gymnastic or athletic abilities) are formed in social interaction. Thus, the human infant is beginning to witness and practice the motions and rhythms of parents and society at a point in maturation long after which other primates would still be snuggled in the womb.

This relatively premature period of extrauterine development would not carry the significance it does if it were not for the specially evolved capability of human infants to capitalize on this circumstance with a mind that is simultaneously undergoing continued rapid growth, and becoming organized in response to experience; a mind that is preprogrammed for flexibility and learning through experimentation and interaction, rather than one that is preprogrammed by instincts that would restrict activity to specialized patterns of behavior.

Neoteny

Neoteny refers to the retention of juvenile characteristics into adulthood through the deceleration of physical development (Gould, 1977c; Montagu, 1989). Just as in the case of exterogestation, humans also differ dramatically from other primates with respect to neoteny (Krogman, 1972). It has both physiological and psychological aspects. Its physiological aspect is reflected in how unusually childlike the adult human is in overall shape, compared to other species (Lorenz, 1971; Montagu, 1989; Gould, 1977c). Neoteny underlies human abilities for responsiveness and change, even in physical characteristics, that have been observed in later life. Characteristics observed to respond to contextual change have included not only gait and posture, but also aspects of structural anatomy, including facial shape, which can be structurally altered by factors such as respiratory difficulties (Champagne, 1991; Tourne, 1990) and length of fingers, which Langer found to increase under experimental conditions of experiential juvenescence (1989). Of much greater significance, of course, are the distinctly human capabilities, retained throughout the life course, for learning, change and ". . . the maintenance of an active, creative interaction with the environment" (Lorenz, 1971, p. 180; cf. Perlmutter, 1990). It is possible for humans of every age—even centenarians—to learn new languages and develop new relationships, new practices, and new technologies.

Both the extrauterine *fruhjahr* and neoteny point to the profound level of interaction that characterizes the species-being of homo sapiens, a level of interaction that is constitutive of the phenotype on an ongoing basis, as human individuals develop and age over the life course. Although built on a base of organismic developmental processes, what distinguishes human beings is an openness and responsiveness to the environment that is necessary for human development to occur.

While these principles mean that there is a level of indeterminacy and contingency in human development, they do not mean that human developmental outcomes are unpredictable. Rather, they suggest that it will be fruitful to look to factors in the environment, rather than to the internal programming of the organism itself (as expressed in ideas like "stages", "normal aging" or "internal clocks") in order to find the ordering principles that account for age-related outcomes. As I discuss further below, these internal processes are regulated, in part, by both micro- and macro-level social forces.

The importance of culture must be acknowledged early in a discussion of this issue, because members of different societies differ not only in aspects of their physical development and health, but also in the conceptualization of physical conditions and changes that are offered to them by their societies. For example, the physical symptoms most often reported by Japanese women during the midlife years appear to be quite different than those reported in the U.S.; in fact, the Japanese have no concept equivalent to Western menopause (Lock, 1993). This finding illustrates the extent to which aspects of social organization and culture interact with changes in physical conditions over the life course. It raises important questions, as yet unanswered, concerning the extent to which organic change occurs differentially as the organism responds to different cultures.

As a footnote to the discussion of neoteny and exterogestation, it is worth noting that these features make humans especially responsive and susceptible to the sorts of effects of experience upon development, and upon physiological functioning and well-being, that have been observed for other animals as well as humans. Enriched experience has a positive effect on brain growth in birds and rats (Diamond, 1988) as well as in humans. Seratonin levels have been shown to shift dramatically within the same individual as a function of one's position in a group—a finding that appears quite well established for Vervet monkeys; some evidence exists for a similar pattern among college males (McGuire & Raleigh, 1985; Raleigh & McGuire, 1990; Raleigh, Brammer, McGuire, & Yuwiler, 1985). The field of psychoneuroimmunology is demonstrating how mood affects immune-system functioning (Ader, Cohen, & Felten, 1995), and of course, mood is related to experience and social context. Interestingly, such effects have recently been demonstrated for adult female family caregivers—a difference attributed to the stress of caregiving (Kiecolt-Glaser, Glaser, Gravenstein, Malarkey, & Sheridan, 1996).

In some cases, it appears that such experience-based effects are broadly misinterpreted as biogenetic effects, especially when they are organized in a population by major axes of social structure such as age. This may be the case with midlife women's experience of depression in the contemporary U.S., which some important evidence suggests is related only to role over-load, rather than to the hormonal changes to which it has frequently been attributed (McKinlay, McKinlay & Bambrilla, 1987).

Occupational and educational differentials in the risk of Alzheimer's disease demonstrate that the social organization of organismic physical change extends to later life (Stern, Gurland, Tatemichi, Tang, Wilder, & Mayeux, 1994). Two hypotheses have been debated about the reason for the inverse correlation: 1) That educational and occupational levels are correlated with more varied and demanding cognitive activities (cf. Kohn & Slomczynski, 1990), increasing the complexity of the neural structures of the brain, thus providing a compensatory reserve in the cognitive appa-ratus (Powell et al., 1994; Stern et al., 1994); 2) that the adverse effects of many kinds of low-status work take a toll on the overall integrity of the organism, including the mind (Cohen, 1994). Although the importance of social forces in explaining individual differences in the potential to resist Alzheimer's disease is present in both hypotheses, the first hypothesis is especially consistent with the concept of neoteny, since it implies that learning continues to shape neural structures in the brain over the life course.

In any case, these examples suggest that a broad array of effects are at least partly regulated, and others created, by social forces. The flexible and responsive character of the human organism may make such effects even more powerful in the case of humans. The parameters of such responsive-ness are set by the fundamental and constitutive interactive dynamics that are both afforded and required by exterogestation and neoteny. These devel-opmental characteristics set the stage for a third distinctive of human devel-opment, and one that is so essential that human development will not occur without it: The uniquely human social process of world construction.

World-Construction

A third distinctive of human development engages more directly the social constituents of development because it entails a direct and proactive link-age of the individual to social systems: The fact that human behavior is *purposeful*; it is not guided by instincts but by *intentions* (Weber, 1978). Human activity externalizes intentions and in so doing reproduces or gen-erates social relationships, and as these become institutionalized, they comprise various forms of social structure (Berger & Luckmann, 1967; Dannefer & Perlmutter, 1990). Thus, while engaging in purposeful activity, human beings co-constitute the social systems they live within at the same time that each person's own being, self, and personhood is being constituted in social interaction. The essence of self-society relations is an irreducible reciprocity through which both human development and social systems are constituted in the course of social interaction. It is important to add that both human development and social systems are constituted *only* in the course of social interaction; without social interaction, no learning of language and self-development of the young occurs, and without social interaction, social systems cannot exist. Thus, although the focus of this chapter is the self and human development, not social systems, a brief discussion of how human activity generates social systems is warranted.

THE CO-CONSTITUTION OF SOCIAL RELATIONS AND HUMAN DEVELOPMENT

A social system is a stable set of interdependent entities; at the micro level, these entities are individual human actors and the dyads, triads, and small face-to-face groups they form. Typically, newborns enter pre-existing social systems into which they are integrated over time. Thus, the character of the systems or groups in which each actor participates initially is not a matter of choice, and for many individuals, this never becomes a matter of choice. Those groups are constituted and governed by social system processes. At least two basic types of social processes are relevant to human development: *social reality production* and *social allocation* (Dannefer & Perlmutter, 1990). The following sections will discuss each of these types of processes, and then will focus on the specific aspects of systems which tend to ensure their own legitimation—processes in which knowledge and, therefore, science play strategic roles.

Social Reality Production

A fundamental premise of social reality production (SRP) is the fact that human beings must externalize their intentions in action in order for society to happen. Externalizing thought in action is necessary to communicate, and communication of some sort is necessary to create and sustain relations with others. If members of a social system stop interacting, society breaks down. In acts that are so familiar that they occur without aware-ness, humans constantly produce and reproduce social relations while enacting the routines of everyday life, and those relations comprise social systems. Fundamentally, those relations depend on purposeful human action and communication, and will not be sustained without it. Popular acknowledgments of this fundamental principle can be seen in the frequent allusions to the importance of continuous communication in maintaining relationships such as friendship or marriage.

The ongoing process of SRP in which human actors are typically deeply enmeshed is to a large extent a massive enterprise of self-fulfilling prophecies: One's action conveys an expectation for the other, and the other responds in a way that reinforces the expectations. Habitualized pat-terns of interaction develop, and when these are broadly shared and regu-larly reproduced, we can say they have been institutionalized (Berger & Luckmann, 1967).

It is easiest to see the operation of SRP at the level of face-to-face inter-action. There, it is possible to trace the formation and disintegration of the power of groups through the structure and content of members' interac-tions. Both family therapists and organizational consultants are analysts and facilitators of such micro-level SRP. But it is not only the social sys-tem itself that is shaped through the interaction process; it is also the indi-vidual developmental trajectories of system members. Whether or not by intent, other group members unavoidably make appraisals of each mem-ber's characteristics and abilities; inclusion or exclusion from activities or future opportunities may be based on those appraisals; and the self-appraisal of every aspect of the member in question is likely to be influ-enced by the informal and formal messages offered by the other members.

Systematic observation of micro-interaction has yielded many accounts, from nursery schools to nursing homes and many settings in between, of how the processes of aging and development of individuals are caught and distorted in the dynamics of social reality producing processes in every-day life.

For example, consider the following sequence of events occurring in an all-Black urban Midwestern school, reported in Gubrium, Holstein and Buckholdt's recent work (1994). Since this account will also be used to discuss social allocation and power in subsequent sections, I quote at some length.

Very early in the school year, children within classrooms had been placed in three different ability groups. According to the teacher in the episode reproduced here, criteria for group placement included kindergarten teachers' reports, a group intelligence test, and this teacher's own observations and evaluation during the first 2 weeks. When asked about the placement rationale for a particular student named Terry, the teacher responded:

> "Ha! That's an easy one. Look at what . . . [kindergarten teacher] said about him. He should have stayed in kindergarten if there weren't so many new kids this year. And his IQ, 57 . . . I know his parents, both winos and poor. His brother was here last year but we had to send him to "special". Terry's a sure candidate, too . . . you've seen how he acts . . . he just sits there and stares into space . . . I haven't heard him say one intelligible word since school started."
>
> . . . At the end of February, a series of events caused the teacher to reconsider briefly her evaluation of Terry. (As an experiment, learning dyads were constructed by pairing) . . . children from the "advanced" group with the "slow" children for about twenty minutes each day. The pairs of children were taken from the room and allowed to work together in the privacy of a small office . . .
>
> One day shortly after this experiment begain, the observer, who was listening outside the room, could not recognize the voice of the student who was serving as instructor. When he entered the room, he found Terry helping the supposedly more advanced child with letter recognition. Terry continued to switch . . . roles with his partner for several days, until they both knew all the letter(s) . . . At first, the teacher did not believe the reports about Terry. Finally, she came to see for herself and found that it was true. She asked Terry and his partner to give a demonstration to the other children . . . and invited the principal and several other teachers . . .
>
> Terry made many other unexpected advances during the remainder of the semester. He became a leader in spelling, reading and arithmetic . . . at the end of the year (his IQ score was) 131. Yet ironically the teacher kept him in the slow group . . ." (1994, pp. 92–93)

The authors go on to explain that in second grade, Terry moved from the area, but returned late in the year, resuming his original pattern:

> Once again, he appeared sullen and unresponsive . . . He did not read, nor would he identify letter names or sounds . . .
>
> The second-grade teacher was aware of Terry's progress during the last part of his first-grade year. Still, she dismissed this as unimportant because

. . . he had received so much personal attention. "He won't make it in a regular classroom," she asserted. "We can't give special attention to so many kids." (1994, p. 94)

Although documentation of actual interaction sequences involving Terry could provide more detail about the processes of SRP, this account nevertheless reveals key aspects of SRP processes. The social system of the traditional classroom is, by definition, a hierarchical structure in which the teacher is the central power figure. It is part of the teacher's role to create and sustain the school day as an orderly and predictable sequence of avtivities. As the order and structure of the classroom becomes established and realized as routine, the lives of class members are also being defined and realized in particular ways that also tend to fit the routine. In many kinds of systems, including institutionalized systems like schools, the routine is shaped by pre-existing assumptions and parameters of the social system in question.

The case of Terry illustrates how SRP creates "self-fulfilling prophecies" by objectifying teacher appraisals of student potentials, by directing student opportunities, and by neutralizing and rejecting counter-evidence. Stability is thus achieved partly through the maintenance of individuals' positions in the group largely intact. Individual identities are also thereby maintained—in ways that are consistent with the established structure of pre-existing assumptions and constraints, but that do not necessarily reflect their academic capabilities. SRP in the culture of this school occurs in a pre-existing culture that assumes a) that students have relatively fixed academic potentials; b) that these differences are measurable and accurately known by teachers; c) that the differences form a basis for a stratified classroom organization; d) that student potentials are stable over time. Once the system is up and running with these and related premises as elements of the underlying culture, counter-evidence can readily be neutralized.

This case illustrates a set of dynamics that were identified and formalized in labelling theory (Lemert, 1951), which has also been applied to similar institutional regulation of individual opportunities at other points in the life course, including nursing home life (e.g. Dannefer, Stein & Gelein, 1998; Gubrium, 1975; Kuypers & Bengtson, 1984). Although the case of Terry illustrates an unfortunate consequence of social system operation, the system dynamics of labelling processes inevitably create positive spirals of self-fulfilling prophecy, as well as negative ones. Children initially defined as bright are off to a running start in their relation with their teachers, and may enjoy an enduring advantage over their classmates in their teachers' eyes. Unformed abilities and potentials are thereby created or destroyed through an interaction-amplifying or "deviation-amplification" process (Maruyama, 1968). The effects of such class-room processes—both positive and negative—have been documented experimentally in the classic tradition of the Pygmalion research (cf. Rosenthal & Jacobsen, 1968).

Even when the outcome is positive, however, what is being described here is a social system process in which the labelled individual partici-pates in a subordinate manner. Thus, the agentic force of the individuals in question, including the positively labelled individual is, in principle, no more in evidence in the case of positive than negative labelling. This raises the question of whether and how genuine human agency might be augmented—a question that, in any domain, is ultimately political. To a limited degree, this can be addressed structurally (e.g., reducing the macro-level pressures upon schools and other institutions for special diag-noses, or for invidious categorization more generally); more profoundly, it can be done educationally (through creating more insight, awareness, and self-reflexivity on the part of teachers and other professional gate-keepers regarding the socially generative consequences of their actions) (cf. Schon, 1984). Of course, utilizing the insights gained from increased understanding of self-perpetuating social cycles is independent of the insights themselves.

Social Structure and Allocation

A system is, by definition, a set of interrelated parts. When the processes of SRP become habitualized and institutionalized in interdependent roles, and a ready supply of people to serve as role incumbents is available, the resulting social system can be readily seen to exist independently of the actors who occupy the roles. In modern, bureaucratized societies, many such roles are age-graded. Again, school provides an obvious example: The number of age-specific roles for students and teachers remains more or less stable over time, while the actors occupying these roles regularly change position. When the number of people changes dramatically while the number of roles remains the same, or vice versa, the result, obviously, is a quantitative mismatch between people and roles that causes strain (cf. Riley, Kahn, & Foner, 1994).

The mechanisms surrounding the problem of fitting people to roles are called processes of social allocation (Dannefer & Perlmutter, 1990; Riley,

Johnson, & Foner, 1972). As has been widely publicized, the strains created by the baby boom cohorts illustrates the seriousness of the problem of fitting a finite number of individuals to a finite but different number of socially established roles (which can be seen, e.g., in desks in schoolrooms; spaces in college classes; and entry-level and senior jobs). Applying the logic of a "seller's market", some scholars (Easterlin, 1980; Waring, 1976) have argued that small cohorts have some advantages over large ones.

As a general rule, the greater the specificity of qualification for role incumbents, the more difficult the problems of allocation. When age is a criterion of role incumbency, fewer people are eligible, and their tenure in the role temporally circumscribed. Thus, the "age-irrelevant society" (cf. Neugarten, 1996), "Society for all ages" (Hagestad, 1998), or "age-integrated" (Riley et al., 1994) society offer obvious advantages in reducing potential strains on a social system because it eliminates the strains imposed by the movement of cohorts of widely varying sizes through an age-stratified system of roles.

However, allocation also occurs within age strata, as age peers are stratified within the same organization. Research on career mobility in one large corporation indicated that entry-level white-collar workers confront a process of tournament mobility (Rosenbaum, 1984). As one ascended the corporate ladder and succeeding levels generally had fewer slots, not everyone could move at the same rate, and substantial advantage accrued to the "fast trackers" who began to move first. Some became sidelined and immobile (cf. Kanter, 1977, Ch. 6).

Such allocation processes are manifest in the account of Terry. Allocation arises as an issue with one of the teacher's first statements: "He should have stayed in kindergarten if there weren't so many new kids this year." (Gubrium et al., 1994, p. 92). Terry's presence in the first grade is, then, partly a function of available space. Other allocation processes may be present in the special education program. Schools—or individual teachers charged with establishing or protecting a program—may experience budgetary and other pressures to create and justify the existence of a special education program, and to find students to populate special education classrooms. Thus, the funding available for "special ed" and related programs has sometimes produced a motive for classifying children as needing special education, independent of their actual needs.

In addition, the teachers also have a systemic view of the allocation of attention to Terry. He cannot develop normally, they say, because they don't have the time to devote to him. This implies a specific set of organizational rules for the allocation of teachers' attention—a scarce resource in classrooms.

SRP, Allocation and the Micro-Macro Link

Social reality production prototypically occurs on the micro level of face-to-face interaction, in situations such as the classroom where Terry and his peers and their teacher were all thrown together. Social allocation also occurs in micro-level as well as larger systems, and is especially visible in a formally organized system, such as a school class. However, the intentions of the teacher or even the principal are not sufficient to explain the content of the agenda that organizes the everyday routines and activity patterns and issues of allocation that comprise the social reality of the school. Terry's teacher and school officials are enacting practices and creating structures dictated by policymakers, administrators, educational and developmental experts, and legislators whose collective intent imposed an answer—arguably political more than humanistic—to the question of what young children should be doing with their time.

In enacting policy directives from above and deploying their students through experiences defined by categories imposed from above (contact hours, age grading, "special"), the teachers and counselors are applying to the local situation a generalized cultural definition of the reality of schoolchildren.

Despite the manifest power of macro level institutions, it is important to note that micro level forces are perhaps even more resistant to intervention, because they are fundamental features of all human interaction. Even if these centralized, macro-structural imperatives were absent, it is in the nature of social processes that the ongoing reproductive cycle of habitualized micro-interaction will tend to generate social order, and will simultaneously attribute gratuitous and sometimes destructive labels to individuals. Young individuals are generally especially vulnerable to these forces, since they cannot control many aspects of their daily routines, and yet their potentials are regularly assessed and defined by others in the course of everday interaction. Such social processes remain a barrier between the strongest and purest of good intentions of educators, and their potential to act in a way that maximizes the developmental potential of students.

These are hardly unfamiliar points in many areas of sociological discourse. In developmental theory and in life-course theory, however, SRP and social allocation processes are both virtually invisible. This point is the more remarkable when one considers that neoteny—the basis of the unique flexibility of human development—has also been also been almost completely ignored. Clearly, in both of these areas—social processes no less than distinct features of human development—warrant theoretical attention. In a complex and centralized society, policies developed at the state or national level shape what occurs at the micro level of the classroom or the principal's office by setting the agenda of local situations. Thus, centralized political, economic, and cultural forces regulate the organization of opportunities; opportunities regulate the form and quality of development for individual human beings. The tendency of developmental theory to ignore these systematic connections between levels of organization must be corrected if theory is to avoid the fallacy of "naturalization"—of treating phenomena as though they were part of nature and hence inevitable, when they are really the products of human activity.

The rendering invisible of the organization means that it is invisible to the researcher. When this is the case, the researcher no less than Terry's teacher is vulnerable to a naturalization of structure; to an attribution to nature of aspects of the dialectic of development that are social in origin.

Naturalization is a highly effective mechanism of social legitimation because it is difficult to oppose that which is seen as natural. When the combination of the power and invisibility of macro-structures shapes human development trajectories and outcomes in decisive ways, and yet remain unacknowledged in scientific discourse, science is itself engaged in the legitimation of prevailing social arrangements. I turn now to a more detailed examination of naturalization and legitimation as forces that impact human development.

SOCIAL LEGITIMATION AND HUMAN DEVELOPMENT

From the standpoint of participants in a social system, both the constitution of social reality in interaction and the operation of larger social systems are typically oblique if not invisible. Those aspects of everyday life that are unnoticed and taken for granted are inevitably assumed to be normal and, perhaps, natural. Taken-for-granted social practices and conditions that are embedded in cultural assumptions and hence widely regarded as natural pervade the relevant institutional domains of contemporary society: In school, age-grading and ability grouping; in work, notions of a single career and of upward mobility beliefs that the individual controls the pace of his/her career progress; and that older workers are less open to new ideas and generally less capable; in the case of family, traditional sex-role expectations and the assumed normality of dramatic resource inequalities between families.

In the study of development, examples of both inter-age and intra-age processes of naturalization can readily be found. I conclude with examples of each.

Naturalization of Inter-Age Differences

Consider the widespread assumption of the "three boxes of life" (education, work/childrearing, and retirement) as comprising the stage sequence of a natural life course. The proliferation of stage theories in adult development and in the career development field as well can be seen as expansions of this theme; such theories usually include an claim of universality, implying that the stage pattern is nothing less than the realization of human nature (e.g., Cumming & Henry, 1961; Gutmann, 1987; Levinson, 1978, 1994).

A sociohistorical analysis provides a plausible explanation both for the emergence of the "three boxes of life" and for the popularity of stage theories. With modernization, many aspects of human development have been centrally organized by cultural, economic, and political circumstances, resulting in the institutionalization of the life course (e.g., Kohli & Meyer, 1986), an increasing standardization of role sequences over the life course, and an increasing uniformity of role configurations at each age (Hogan, 1981). As the development of modernity has progressed, succeeding cohorts have moved through life-course stages increasingly in lockstep, creating the age-related cleavages in activity routines (studentry [Parsons, 1972, Parsons & Platt, 1973]; adulthood; retirement) that provide a broad social appearance of age-graded stages. Other researchers have described similar patterns in Europe (e.g., Kohli, Rein, Guillemard, & van Gunsteren, 1991) and corresponding patterns of change have also been reported for the marital life course in the USA (Buchmann, 1989; Uhlenberg, 1977).

Historians of adolescence (Gillis, 1977; Katz & Davey, 1978; Kett, 1977) and aging (Achenbaum, 1979; Chudacoff, 1989) have detailed the technical, political, and cultural transformations from which these changes in the configuration of the life course have resulted, and also how changes in life-course patterns affected general cultural ideas about development and aging. When culturally recognized patterns of development and aging form the basis for theory without being critically scrutinized, theory participates in naturalization, and becomes a legitimator of existing social arrangements. Kett (1977) argues that the institutionalization of schooling in the 19th century provided the necessary conditions for the concept of adolescence to become plausible, but there is nothing in the theory of adolescence about its sociohistorical specificity and its dependence upon modernization (cf. Lichtman, 1987). Rather, the explanation for the origin of such stages is sought in evolutionary principles, especially in the prereproductive and reproductive life course (Morss, 1990): again, in terms of detached processes operating in parallel at individual and environmental levels, rather than in the mutually constitutive interactions between levels. Applied to human development, the parallel processing model is a mechanism of naturalization that helps to legitimate social arrangements by securing their invisibility.

The interactive model proposes, by contrast, that the psychosocial complex that regularly emerges in the early teenage years in modern societies is formed by the interaction of organismic maturation with sociohistorically specific family forms, societal expectations for individual mobility and for social change, and institutionalized reward structures. The hardwiring of universal patterns of physical growth and puberty is not denied, but these processes are always culturally interpreted, and where cultural definitions are relatively strong, they are inevitably internalized in ways that regulate emotion, activity, and self-definition; these internalizations do exert an influence upon the body itself.

Naturalization of Intra-Age/Intracohort Differences

Studies of learning disabilities (Coles, 1987; Roush, 1995) and school performance more generally have documented the tendency to treat socially generated processes that have their output at the individual level as individual pathologies. Because naturalization in such instances entails reduction to the individual level, inevitably it encourages one to look for explanations and solutions at the level of the individual student. Because individuals are assumed to vary inherently in socially valued abilities, the concepts such as goodness-of-fit and selection fit quite readily in this situation.

Guided by such assumptions, and without a framework for conceptualizing humans and social systems as mutually co-constituting, it is only reasonable to assume a "parallel processing" vocabulary. Here the tendency toward naturalization employs the concepts drawn from evolutionary theory discussed above, concepts that reinforce the invisibility of the social arrangements. It would be said, for example, that Terry is not *adapting* to the school. Terry's *niche* is in special education, so he is being *selected* for it. Here, he should *adjust*. This discussion assumes parallel process-ing—an individual with fixed characteristics who is having trouble deal-ing with a social order that is assumed to be natural, but which is rendered invisible by the concepts used—to Terry's considerable devel-opmental detriment.

The significance of naturalization is in its effect as a legitimator of existing arrangements. If a social practice is rooted in nature, its legitimacy can scarcely be questioned, even if it does not always seem entirely benef-icent or fair. It is viewed simply as an inevitable part of the teaching and evaluating of children.

The current popularity of terms like "context" and "interaction" has been sustained largely through their cooptation by the evolutionary and organismic logic of "parallel processing." The resurgence of interest in sociobiology has generated a new flurry of arguments that view the inter-action between individual and society as governed by selection pressure. For example, in an impressive attempt to integrate both social and organ-ismic processes, Belsky, Steinberg and Draper (1991) propose the evolu-tionary notion of "reproductive fitness" as a central concept. Human reproductive fitness is, like that of other species, maintained by either "quantity" or "quality" patterns of mating and rearing—the former entail-ing rapid maturation, early puberty and pregnancy, high numbers of off-spring and high mortality; the latter entailing slower maturation, fewer offspring handled with relatively great care, and low mortality. Although they allow for a partial role of experience in shaping individual "types", they propose integrating genetic variation with empirical established social effects

> via the notion of differential susceptibility to environmental experience: Whereas some individuals may be genetically predisposed to respond to contextual stress and insensitive rearing by maturing early and engaging in relatively indiscriminate sexual behavior, others may be genetically predis-posed to respond to sensitive rearing by deferring sexual behavior and establishing enduring pair bonds in adulthood. Thus . . . nature may deter-mine the likelihood that, and the extent to which, an individual will be influ-enced by a particular set of environmental conditions. (1991, p. 650)

In real-life terms, the difference they postulate obviously is correlated with the contrasting contemporary U.S. lifestyles of impoverished (notably urban) subpopulations characterized by early fecundity, and by relatively high mortality rates; and the middle-class subpopulations, which experience later age at first birth, and where age-specific mortality rates are relatively low and life expectancy higher. Thus, different adaptive strategies are hypothesized to flow from differential genetic predispositions, maximizing the reproductive fitness of different subpopulations (1991). It is an argument that is consistent, elegant, and as dazzling in its sweep across disciplines and populations as it is in its connection to urgent social problems. It is also an argument detached from evidence (as the authors themselves acknowledge), and from the perspective of the present paper, their argument is itself a prime examplar of the social process of naturalization at work.

Indeed, Belsky et al. (1991) return us to almost precisely where we began: they propose an explanation of differences across human society that is the precise equivalent to the differences Austad (1992) reports in mainland and island opossums: Early fecundity and pregnancy followed by early and high rates of mortality in one case, and the opposites in the other, with each seen as an adaptive strategy of evolution that maximizes reproductive fitness. The difference is that the criterion of reproductive fitness appears reasonable in the opossum case, but cannot be justified in the human case on either theoretical or empirical grounds. The theoretical reasons are provided in the general facts regarding the life of the human species emphasized earlier in this paper: The flexibility of development, and the central role of culture, in defining the significance of sexuality and reproductive activity in individual's lives. The empirical reasons are grounded in the robust findings regarding intracohort diversity: The range of variation in first pregnancy and childbirth within a cohort is of a greater order of magnitude than the onset of fertility, and exhibits dramatic intracohort fluctuations that cannot be explained by historical changes in age at menarche, and that could have nothing to do with reproductive fitness.[1]

It is not news to point out that the explanation for human behavioral differences with respect to the onset of fecundity and the commencement of sexual activity can be adequately explained with no allusion to differential

---

1. One important study reports that, among unmarried 15–19 year-olds, 13.8 births occurred for each 1000 White females, while 90.3 births occurred for each 1000 Black females (Dryfoos & Bourque-Scholl, 1981). Between 1965 and 1978, the proportion of births to Chicago teenagers who were unmarried mothers increased by 80%—a dramatic trend which, according to Hogan and Kitagawa (1985), is typical for the U.S. as a whole. It is difficult to see how such dramatic historical and cultural variation in human reproductive practices can be predicted from the gradual downward trend of change in age of menarche (from 13.3 in 1940 to about 12.5 in the 1970s [Malina, 1979]) or modest intergroup differences in age at menarche (Steinberg, 1988; Wierson, Long, & Forehand, 1993).

genetic predisposition: The onset of fecundity is known to be associated with stress-related factors, something that an emphasis on the responsiveness of the organism to the environment would prepare one to expect. At the same time, intergroup differences in the age of menarche are small (Jones, Leeton, Mcleod, & Wood, 1972; Steinberg, 1988.) Thus, they cannot account for the magnitude of differences in the probability of pregnancy and childbirth, which are related to conditions of girls' lives that are fully defined by cultural (e.g., meaning of relationships; social understanding of sexuality, contraception, parenting, etc.; valuation of priorities) and social-structural (e.g., relationship options; perceived future opportunities) factors.

The importance of such factors is recognized by Belsky et al., which makes their commitment to the genetic argument—an easy target for Occam's razor—difficult to understand or to justify. The presumption of a genetic contribution is ultimately untested in their model (as they acknowledge), and adds no explanatory power to it (cf. Dannefer, 1993; Maccoby, 1991). Given that discernible changes in the genome require differential survival to reproduction, it is clear that the empirical quantity-quality distinction described by Belsky and associates has emerged mainly in the 20th-century U.S. (the late 20th century, some would claim—cf. Wilson, 1987, 1996) cannot reasonably account for the selection of differential genetic predispositions in the two groups.

Indeed, this spurious theoretical commitment to an unneeded and unfounded principle is itself an empirical phenomenon in need of explanation. While the development of such an explanation must lie beyond the scope of the present discussion, what can be readily and unequivocally said is that the effect of such an argument is the naturalization of social processes, and therewith the simultaneous legitimation of prevailing social arrangements and the deflection of attention from urgent social problems. For, if a significant part of the explanation for the behavior of humans who pursue high-fertility/high-mortality strategies is that they are simply implementing a genetic predispostion that assures the survival of the genome, the policy implications are much less complex than if such humans are creating relationships and planning their actions in response to destructive and exploitative economic and political forces. To the extent that emphasis is placed on the former, the latter can be allowed to become increasingly invisible.

Because of such dynamics, the constituent social processes of human development include not only allocation and the micro-interactional level of social reality production, but must also include the production of knowledge (including naturalization and other legitimating knowledge), and in modern societies this is a centrally regulated process that requires macro-level analyses. In irreducible ways, culture and politics are thus consituents of human development.

SUMMARY, AND SOME IMPLICATIONS FOR RESEARCH

Based on the premise that a theory of human development requires consideration of the interaction of both individual and social constituents from the earliest periods of growth, I have suggested that the widespread reliance on evolutionary concepts in developmental thinking has impeded an adequate theoretical formulation. The unique features of human development (exterogestation, neoteny, world-production) are the proper foundation of theorizing about human development, the life course, and aging. Given the flexible potentials of the human organism, the character of development is constituted and shaped by social and cultural forces, through processes of social reality production and social allocation. I discussed one kind of macro-level social-reality producing process, naturalization, in order to show its relevance to social policy and practices that may affect developmental outcomes.

The discussion emphasizes the importance for theory, as well as for policy and practice, of extending research on how social variation may regulate health and age, and how social change may extend healthy life and postpone disability. The practical value and, indeed, the urgency of such research increases with the graying of the population. The discussion also carries some general implications for conceptualizing such research. First, that flexibility of developmental potentials means that intra-age and intra-cohort variability is to be expected, and that accounting for such variability is no less important than general inter-age and intercohort comparisons.

Second, whether the source of influence is most usefully conceptualized as micro or macro (that is, seated on mother's lap, or seated in front of a computer connected to NBC's website), actual development is itself "locally" situated. It occurs irrepressibly in everyday life, within and between human actors in the immediacy of individual experience and face-to-face interaction. Because of the flexibity of the human organism, manifested in neoteny and world-openness, micro-interaction is inevitably constitutive of development. At the same time, and especially in modern and postmodern societies, key parameters of micro-interaction are unavoidably and, indeed, increasingly shaped by much broader political and cultural forces, including centralized and imposed state practices.

Third, because social relations, or social systems, comprise a major and important component of the social context in which development occurs, actual social systems—rather than "context" as a variable removed from social systems, deserve to be studied (Dannefer, 1992; Riley, 1963). And fourth, the role of culturally embedded assumptions and language regarding age and development has been particularly neglected, and may be a fruitful approach to identifying, clarifying, and mapping how the macro becomes instantiated in microinteraction. Social systems are constituted linguistically, and then regulate access to language and information. Social systems organize individual acticitiy patterns which in turn have an influence on physical and mental health (e.g., the education-Alzheimer's link); the definition and understanding of bodily change processes are also properties of social systems, and require analysis in contextualized terms (e.g., the example of menopause as a culture-specific concept).

Were the indications of the limited body of research amassed thus far borne out and extended in larger and more generalized studies, the payoff would not only be a more comprehensive and integrated theoretical understanding, but some tangible gains in the practical area of, as Riley has put it, "postponing the onset of disability" through institutional and educational changes. Given that such changes may have significant potential to reduce disability at a time when the population is graying at a dramatic rate, investment in such research can only be regarded as a priority of some urgency.

REFERENCES

Achenbaum, A. (1979). *Old age in the New Land*. Baltimore: Johns Hopkins.

Ader, R., Cohen, N., & Felten, D. (1995). Psychoneuroimmunology: Interactions between the nervous system and the immune system. *Lancet, 345*, 99–103.

Austad, S. (1992). On the nature of aging. *Natural History, 102*, 25–52.

Austad, S. N., & Fischer, K. E. (1991). Mammalian aging, metabolism and ecology: Evidence from bats and marsupials. *Journal of Gerontology, Biological Sciences, 46*, B47–B53.

Baltes, P. B. (1987). Theoretical propositions of life-span developmental psychology: On the dynamics between growth and decline. *Developmental Psychology, 23*, 611–626.

Baltes, P. B., & Baltes, M. M. (1990). Psychological perspectives on successful aging: The model of selective optimization with compensation. In P. B. Baltes & M. M. Baltes (Eds.), *Successful aging: Perspectives from the behavioral sciences* (pp. 1–34). New York: Cambridge University Press.

Barkow, J. H., Cosmides, L. & Tooby, J. (Eds.). (1992). *The adapted mind: Evolutionary psychology and the generation of culture*. New York: Oxford University Press.

Belsky, J., Steinberg, L. & Draper, P. (1991). Childhood experience, interpersonal development and reproductive strategy: An evolutionary theory of socialization. *Child Development, 62*, 647–670.

Berger, P. L., & Luckmann, T. (1967). *The social construction of reality*. New York: Anchor.

Buchmann, M. (1989). *The script of the life course: Entry into adulthood in a changing world*. Chicago: University of Chicago Press.

Caspi, A., & Moffitt, T. E. (1993). When do individual differences matter? A paradoxical theory of personality coherence. *Psychological Inquiry, 4*, 247–271.

Champagne, M. (1991). Upper airway compromise and the long face syndrome. *Journal of General Orthodontics, 2*, 18–25.

Chudacoff, H. (1989). *How old are you? Age consciousness in American culture*. Princeton, NJ: Princeton University Press.

Cohen, C. I. (1994). [Letter to the editor]. *JAMA, 272*, 1405.

Coles, G. (1987). *The learning mystique*. New York: Fawcett.

Cumming, E. & Henry, W. (1961). *Growing old*. New York: Basic.

Dannefer, D. (1989). Human action and its place in theories of aging. *Journal of Aging Studies, 3*, 1–20.

Dannefer, D. (1992). On the concept of context in developmental discourse: Four meanings of context and their implications. In D. L. Featherman, R. M. Lerner, & M. Perlmutter (Eds.), *Life-span development and behavior* (Vol. 11, pp. 83–110). . Hillsdale, NJ: Erlbaum.

Dannefer, D. (1993). When does society matter for individual differences? Implications of a counterpart paradox. *Psychological Inquiry, 4*, 281–284.

Dannefer, D., & Perlmutter, M. (1990). Development as a multi-dimensional process: Individual and social constituents. *Human Development, 33*, 108–137.

Dannefer, D., Stein, P. & Gelein, J. (1998). Microtemporal and macrotemporal linkages in life-course institutionalization: The case of the resident career in long-term care. Paper presented at the XIV World Congress of Sociology, Montreal (July).

Diamond, M. (1988). *Enriching heredity*. New York: Fress Press.

Dryfoos, J. G., & Bourque-Scholl, N. (1981). *Factbook on teenage pregnancy*. New York: Guttmacher Institute.

Easterlin, R. (1980). *Birth and fortune*. Chicago: University of Chicago Press.

Fiatarone, M. A., Marks, E. C., Meredith, C. N., Lipsitz, L. A., & Evans, W. J.

(1990). High intensity strength training in nonagenarians: Effects on skeletal muscle. *JAMA, 263,* 3029–3034.

Gillis, J. (1977). *Youth and history: Tradition and change in European age relations 1770–present.* New York: Academic.

Gould, S. J. (1977a). The child as man's real father. In S. J. Gould (Ed.), *Ever since Darwin: Reflections on natural history* (pp. 63–69). New York: Norton.

Gould, S. J. (1977b). Human babies as embryos. In S. J. Gould (Ed.), Ever since Darwin: Reflections on natural history (pp. 70–75). New York: Norton.

Gould, S. J. (1977c). *Ontogeny and phylogeny.* Cambridge, MA: Belknap Harvard.

Gubrium, J. F. (1975). *Living and dying at Murray Manor.* New York: St. Martins.

Gubrium, J. F., Holstein, J., & Buckholdt, D. R. (1994). *Constructing the life course.* Dix Hills, NY: General Hall.

Gutmann, D. (1987). *Reclaimed powers: Toward a new psychology of men and women in later life.* New York: Basic.

Hagestad, G. (1998). Toward a Society for All Ages: New Thinking, New Language, New Conversations, Keynote Address, The United Nations (October).

Hogan, D. (1981). *Transitions and social change: The early lives of American men.* New York: Academic.

Hogan, D., & Kitagawa, E. M. (1985). The impact of social status, family structure and neighborhood on the fertility of black adolescents. *American Journal of Sociology, 90,* 825–855.

Holt, A. B., Cheek, D. B., Mellits, E. D., & Hill, D. E. (1975). Brain size and the relation of the primate to the nonprimate. In D. B. Cheek (Ed.), *Fetal and postnatal cellular growth: Hormones and nutrition* (pp. 23–44). New York: Wiley.

Jones, B., Leeton, J., McLeod, I., & Wood, C. (1972). Factors influencing the age of menarche in a lower socioeconomic group in Melbourne. *Medical Journal of Australia, 21,* 533–535.

Kanter, R. M. (1977). *Men and women of the corporation.* New York: Basic.

Katz, M. B., & Davey, I. E. (1978). Youth and early industrialization in a Canadian city. *American Journal of Sociology, 84,* S81–119.

Kett, J. (1977). *Rites of passage: Adolescence in America 1790–1920.* New York: Basic.

Kiecolt-Glaser, J. K., Glaser, Gravenstein, S., Malarkey, W. B., & Sheridan, J. (1996). Chronic stress alters the immune response to influenza virus vaccine in older adults. *Proceedings of the National Academy of Science USA, 93,* 3043–3047.

Kohli, M., & Meyer, J. W. (1986). Social structure and the construction of life stages. *Human Development, 29,* 145–180.

Kohli, M., Rein, M., Guillemard, A., & van Gunsteren, H. (1991). *Time for retirement.* New York: Cambridge.

Kohn, M. L., & Slomczynski, K. M. (1990). *Social structure and self-direction: A comparative analysis of the United States and Poland.* Cambridge, MA: Basil Blackwell.

Krogman, W. M. (1972). *Child growth.* Ann Arbor: University of Michigan Press.

Kuypers, J., & Bengtson, V. L. (1984). Perspectives on the older family. In W. H. Quinn & G. A. Houghston (Eds.), *Independent aging: Family and social systems perspectives.* Rockville, MD: Aspen.

Langer, E. (1989). *Mindfulness.* Reading, MA: Addison-Wesley.

Lemert, E. (1951). *Social pathology.* New York: McGraw-Hill.

Lerner, J. V., Lerner, R. M., & Zabski, S. (1985). Temperament and elementary school children's actual and rated academic performance: A test of a "goodness-of-fit" model. *Journal of Child Psychology and Psychiatry, 26,* 125–136.

Levinson, D., Darrow, C. N., Klein, E. B., Levinson, M. H., & McKee, B. (1978). *Seasons of a man's life.* New York: Knopf.

Levinson, D., & Levinson, M. (1994). *Seasons of a woman's life.* New York: Knopf.

Lichtman, R. (1987). The illusion of maturation in an age of decline. In J. M. Broughton (Ed.), Critical theories of psychological development (pp. 127–148). New York: Plenum.

Lock, M. (1993). *Encounters with aging: Mythologies of menopause in Japan and America.* Berkeley, CA: University of California Press.

Lorenz, K. (1971). *Studies in animal and human behaviour (Vol. II).* Cambridge, MA: Harvard.

Maccoby, E. E. (1991). Differential reproductive strategies in males and females. *Child Development, 62,* 676–681.

Malina, R. M. (1979). Secular changes in size and maturity: Causes and effects. In A. F. Roche (Ed.), *Secular trends in human growth, maturation and development* (Monographs for the Society for Research in Child Development), Vol. 44, pp. 59–102.

Marsiske, M., Lang, F. R., Baltes, P. B., & Baltes, M. M. (1995). Selective optimization with compensation: Life-span perspectives on successful human development. In R. A. Dixon & L. Backman (Eds.), *Compensating for psychological deficits and declines: Managing losses and promoting gains* (pp. 35–79). Mahwah, NJ: Erlbaum.

Maruyama, M. (1968). The second cybernetics: Deviation-amplifying mutual causal processes. In W. Buckley (Ed.), *Modern systems research for the behavioral scientist* (pp. 304–313). Chicago: Aldine.

McGuire, M. T., & Raleigh, M. J. (1985). Serotonin-behavior interactions in vervet monkeys. *Psychopharmacology Bulletin, 21,* 458–463.

Mckinlay, J. B., McKinlay, S. M., & Bambrilla, D. (1987). The relative contributions of endocrine change and social circumstances to depression in mid-aged women. *Journal of Health and Social Behavior, 28,* 345–363.

Modell, J., Furstenberg, F. F., Jr., & Strong, D. (1978). The timing of marriage in the transition to adulthood: Continuity and change, 1860–1975. *American Journal of Sociology, 84,* S120–S150.

Montagu, A. (1961). Neonatal and infant immaturity in man. *JAMA, 178,* 56–57.

Montagu, A. (1989). Growing young (2nd. ed.). Granby, MA: Bergin & Garvey.

Morss, J. (1990). *The biologising of childhood*. Hillsdale, NJ: Erlbaum.

Morss, J. (1996). *Critical developments*. London: Routledge.

Neugarten, B. (1996). *The meaning of age: selected papers of Bernice L. Neugarten*. Edited and with foreword by D. A. Neugarten. Chicago: University of Chicago Press.

Parsons, T. (1972). Higher education and changing socialization. In M. W. Riley, M. Johnson & A. Foner (Eds.), *Aging and society*, Vol. III: *A sociology of age stratification* (pp. 236–291). New York: Russell Sage Foundation.

Parsons, T., & Platt, G. (1973). The American univeristy. Cambridge, MA: Harvard University Press.

Passingham, R. E. (1975). The organization of the brain in man and his ancestors. *Brain, behavior and evolution, 11*, 73–90.

Perlmutter, M. (1990). *Late life potential*. Washington, DC: Gerontological Society of America.

Portmann, A. (1956). Zoologie und das neue Bild vom Menschen. Hamburg: Rowohlt. As cited in Berger and Luckmann, p. 195.

Powell, A. L., Brooks, J., Zahner, D. A., Zhang, Z. M., Akay, Y. M., & Micheli-Tzanakou, E. (1994). [Letter to the editor]. *JAMA, 272*, 1405–1406.

Raleigh, M. J., Brammer, G. L., McGuire, M. T., & Yuwiler, A. (1985). Dominant social status facilitates the behavioral effects of serotonergic agonists. *Brain Research, 348*, 274–282.

Raleigh, M. J., & McGuire, M. T. (1990). Social influences on endocrine function in male vervet monkeys. In T. E. Ziegler & F. B. Bercovitch (Eds.), *Monographs in Primatology 13: Socioendocrinology of primate reproduction* (pp. 95–112) . New York: Wiley-Liss.

Riley, M. W. (1963). *Sociological research. Vol. I: A case approach*. New York: Harcourt Brace.

Riley, M. W., Foner, A., & Kahn, R. (1994). *Age and structural lag: Society's failure to provide meaningful opportunities in work, family, and leisure*. New York: Wiley-Interscience.

Riley, M. W., Johnson, M. E., & Foner, A. (1972). *Aging and society: Vol. 3. A sociology of age stratification*. New York: Russell Sage.

Rosenbaum, J. (1984). *Career mobility in a corporate hierarchy*. New York: Academic.

Roush, R. (1995). Arguing over why Johnny can't read. *Science, 247*, 1896–1898.

Rosenthal, R., & Jacobsen, L. (1968). Pygmalion in the Classroom.

Schon, D. (1984). *The reflective practitioner: How professionals think in action*. New York: Basic.

Schultz, A. H. (1949). Ontogenetic specializations of man. *Archiv Julins Klaus-Stiftung, 24*, 197–216.

Steinberg, L. (1988). Reciprocal relation between parent-child distance and pubertal maturation. *Developmental Psychology*, 122–128.

Stern, Y., Gurland, B., Tatemichi, T. T., Tang, M. X., Wilder, D., & Mayeux, R. (1994). Infuence of education and occupation on the incidence of Alzheimers' disease. *JAMA, 271*, 1010.

Tourne, L. P. (1990). The long face syndrome and impairment of the nasopharyngal airway. *Angle Orthodontist, 60*, 167–76.

Uhlenberg, P. (1977). Changing configurations of the life course. In T. K. Hareven (Ed.), *Transitions: The family and the life course in historical perspective* (pp. 65–97). New York: Academic.

Waring, J. (1976). Social replenishment and social change: The problem of disordered cohort flow. *American Behavioral Scientist, 19*, 237–256.

Weber, M. (1978). *Economy and Society, Vol I: An Outline of Interpretive Sociology*. Edited by G. Roth and C. Wirth. Berkeley: University of California Press.

Wierson, M., Long, P. J., & Forehand, R. L. (1993). Toward a new understanding of early menarche: The role of environmental stress in pubertal timing. *Adolescence, 28*(112), 913–924.

Wilson, W. J. (1987). *The truly disadvantaged: The inner city, the underclass, and public policy*. Chicago: University of Chicago Press.

Wilson, W. J. (1996). *When work disappears*. Chicago: University of Chicago Press.

CHAPTER 4

Continuity Theory, Self, and Social Structure

Robert C. Atchley

INTRODUCTION

This chapter deals with continuity theory and its potential for helping us understand the relationship between aging, self, and social structure. Continuity theory is a theory of continuous adult development and adaptation. Adult development and aging, including the evolution of various components of the self, occur in the context of particular social structures. Social structure can be defined in two ways: as the organized interrelation of social roles, and as the use of hierarchies of ascribed social attributes to condition individuals' access and allocation to social roles (Theodorson & Theodorson, 1969).

Social structure is thus not only an "enduring, orderly, and patterned relationship between elements of a society" (Abercrombie, Hill & Turner, 1988, p. 228), but it also involves the mechanisms used to assign categories of people to various sociocultural niches. Social attributes themselves are part of social structure because social attributes are arranged in hierarchies of relative social desirability and people are assigned to these categories in a universalistic, impersonal manner. Thus, men are preferred to women; young adults are preferred over older adults; Whites are preferred over other races; Anglos are preferred over Hispanics, and so on. For example, gender and age are important determinants of who is selected for desirable jobs and for less desirable jobs. Sight unseen, women and older adults are often relegated to the region of less desirable jobs. Any personnel placement agency will verify this fact. In this way, social attributes are very much related to where individuals are located in social and economic organizations. Position in the social structure thus results from the interaction of two types of social structures: the hierarchies of preferred social attributes and the hierarchies of organizational positions.

But a word of caution is in order here. Abercrombie et al. (1988) pointed out that difficulties can potentially arise when we use social structure as a causal concept. Social structures are not readily observable and are quite susceptible to reification.

The emphasis in this chapter is on how structured social attributes influence where individuals fit into the social and economic structure of the society and, in turn, how both aspects influence conceptions of the self. While it may be true that society is organized into age strata that interact politically based on differences in life-stage role definitions (Riley, 1995), for individuals, age is most often used to determine role eligibility, role appropriateness, or role modifications that attempt to take age into account. In this context, older age results in structured inequality in ways comparable to gender, racial, or social class inequality. But just as the self is constantly developing, so too are our ideas about how we should use age to condition what we expect of ourselves and others in our social relationships. Thus, self and social structure are interrelated and both are constantly evolving.

The main goals of the chapter are to describe how continuity theory was created to identify important processes underlying adult development in middle and later life; discuss basic aspects of continuity theory as theory; outline the basic elements used to study continuity, especially as they apply to the study of the self; show how continuity theory might be used in relating the self to social structure; and give research examples of how continuity theory can be used to study the relation of individuals' social structural attributes to various components of the self.

HOW DID CONTINUITY THEORY ARISE?

Continuity theory originated from the observation that despite widespread changes in health, functioning, and social circumstances, a large proportion of older adults showed considerable consistency over time in their terns of thinking, activity profiles, and social relationships. But the long-term consistency that became the foundation of continuity theory was not the homeostatic equilibrium predicted by activity theory (Rosow, 1963). Instead, continuity was conceived of more flexibly, as strong probabilistic relationships between past, present, and anticipated patterns of thought, behavior, and social arrangements.

Although this paper deals with my rendition of continuity theory (Atchley, 1971, 1989, 1993, 1995, 1998), I was by no means the first to articulate the principle that humans tend use well-established habits of mind to make sense out of their world and choose courses of action (e.g., James, 1890). I believe that Maddox (1968) was first to apply this principle in gerontology. Based on data from the Duke Longitudinal Study, Maddox observed that over time, people tended to maintain their customary lifestyle patterns of activity as they aged. In my 1971 article, I too found that elders tended to maintain patterns of leisure participation across the retirement transition. I also observed that many elders carried their occupational identities with them into retirement. The apparent contradiction between what the conventional academic wisdom of the day said ought to be the relation between identity and behavior—retirement should result in a loss of an occupational identity—and what I and others observed—a carry-over of occupational identity into retirement—intrigued and stimulated me to look for underlying mechanisms. How was it possible that elders were able to maintain a strong and consistent sense of self, high morale, and consistent lifestyle structures despite presumably major social changes such as retirement, widowhood, or disability?

A high prevalence of continuity in attitudes, beliefs, and values; self-conceptions; social relationships; lifestyles; and environments has been observed by a number of investigators (e.g., Antonucci, 1990; and Atchley, 1994, 1998; Bengtson, Reedy, & Gordon, 1985; Cohler, 1993; Fiske & Chiriboga, 1990; Troll, 1982), so we can be reasonably confident that continuity is a common empirical outcome. Continuity theory takes this empirical finding one step further to attempt to explain why consistency occurs in such a large proportion of cases, sometimes even to the detriment of individual adaptation. Unlike most other theories of adult development, which were extensions of child development theories (e.g., Erikson, 1963; Levinson, 1978), continuity theory was constructed from studies of adaptation in middle-aged and older adults.

That aging brings change is undeniable; so how can we say that continuity is the most prevalent form of adaptation to aging? The key is to use a concept of continuity as the persistence of general patterns, rather than a more static concept of continuity as sameness in the details contained within those patterns. Thus, an artist who has spent years drawing and who takes up printmaking is making a change in the details of his or her life as an artist, but is showing continuity of commitment to art as an element of self and lifestyle. In this sense, continuity and change are not mutually exclusive categories that cannot exist simultaneously within an individual self and/or lifestyle. Rather, continuity and change are themes that usually exist simultaneously in people's lives, and our job as researchers is to assess the relative balance between continuity and change at various points in time, over time, and across various life transitions. We should avoid trying to categorize later life as either having continuity or not; both continuity and change are matters of degree, and they coexist. We also need to assess the extent to which people are drawn toward continuity in making decisions related to goal-seeking and adaptation to life changes, including aging-related changes.

CONTINUITY THEORY AS THEORY

As theory, continuity theory is a feedback systems theory (Bailey, 1994; Buckley, 1967). Feedback systems theories are theories of continuous evolution. Feedback systems theories of adult development assume that people need mental structures in order to organize and interpret their life experiences (Levinson, 1990). Over time, adults develop considerable investment in their conceptions of themselves and the world around them. Individuals are presumed to be dynamic, self-aware entities who use patterns of thought created out of a lifetime of experience to describe, analyze, evaluate, decide, act, pursue goals, and interpret input and feedback. Through their own personal conceptions of how the world is and how it works, their personal strengths and weaknesses, what they are capable of, and what they prefer or dislike, individuals can make effective decisions and thus acquire a sense of personal agency. These conceptions are all present in Buckley's (1967) groundbreaking application of feedback systems theory to social psychology. Continuity theory extends these concepts and applies them to adaptation in middle and later life.

Continuity theory assumes that the primary goal of adult development is adaptive change, not homeostatic equilibrium. It assumes that adults' patterns of adaptive thought continue to develop through learning across the lifespan and that the goal is not to remain the same, but to adapt longstanding individual values and preferences to new situations as adults experience life course changes, aging, and social change.

Continuity theory is constructionist. It assumes that in response to their life experiences, people actively develop individualized personal constructs (Kelly, 1955), ideas of what is going on in the world and why. Some of our most important personal constructs concern ideas about the self and our personal lifestyles. Continuity theory posits that our personal constructs are influenced by the social constructions of reality we learn from those around us and from the mass media, but are not determined by them. No matter how strong society's efforts to influence personal constructs, individuals ultimately are free to decide for themselves how to construe their personal reality. An important implication of this aspect of the theory is that subjective perceptions of continuity become more theoretically relevant than researchers' perceptions of objective continuity.

Continuity theory assumes that patterns of thought and behavior that endure over time are a result of selective investments of time and energy. It posits that people make decisions, based on feedback from experience, about where it is best to focus their efforts to develop skills and knowledge. People select and develop ideas, relationships, environments, and patterns of activity based on their personal constructs of desired developmental direction and of available opportunity. Individuals invest themselves in the internal and external frameworks of their lives, and these relatively robust frameworks allow individuals to accommodate a considerable amount of evolutionary change without experiencing crisis.

Continuity theory is about adaptation. It presumes that individual choices are made not only to achieve goals, but to adapt to constantly changing circumstances, as the individual sees them. Accordingly, continuity theory deals with the development and maintenance of adaptive capacity.

Continuity theory is based on observations of adults in middle age and later life, but it may also apply to the development and maintenance of adaptive capacity in young adulthood as well. Once individuals have developed a strong sense of self, close personal relationships, and a relatively durable lifestyle, continuity theory could be expected to come into play in explaining their decision making processes concerning adaptation to life.

If we assume that a primary motive people have for creating their mental and lifestyle structures is to allow them to adapt to life circumstances and to pursue life satisfaction, then we would expect individuals to use these highly personalized adaptive structures to make decisions about the future, which if effective could be expected to reinforce through positive feedback the value of continuity in decision making strategies. One mechanism behind this process is the observation that within most personality types and lifestyle patterns, most people manage to adapt successfully. For example, Williams and Wirths (1965) looked at successful adaptation to aging within several lifestyle types. They found that most elders were able to adapt successfully in most lifestyle types. There was no single lifestyle pattern that was clearly better in terms of leading to successful aging. One interpretation of these findings is that their respondents had selected lifestyles that fit their individual personalities and life goals.

It is also important to acknowledge that continuity theory is not a theory of successful aging, nor is it a deterministic theory that predicts specific outcomes of adaptation. Instead, continuity theory is a theory of how people attempt to adapt and the mental frameworks they can be expected to use in doing so.

Continuity theory does not predict that using a continuity strategy for decision making will lead to successful adaptation; it simply predicts that most people will try continuity as their first adaptive strategy. Continuity theory does not assume that the results of continuity are necessarily positive. The evidence indicates that even those with low self-esteem, abusive relationships, and poor social adaptation resist the idea of abandoning their internal and external frameworks. Apparently, firm ground to stand on, even if it predicts a miserable future, is for some people preferable to an unknown future. Similarly, although positive feedback loops may produce positive change, negative feedback loops can increase disorder.

Continuity theory provides a conceptual way of organizing the search for coherence in life stories and of understanding the dynamics that produce basic story lines, but continuity theory has no ideology concerning which stories are "right" or "successful." However, through its diagnostic concepts, continuity theory can help us understand why particular people have developed in the way they have.

Continuity strategies seem to be adaptive for a majority of elders, in that continuity strategies result in maintenance of life satisfaction in most cases, even among those who experience disability (Atchley, 1998). However, an unyielding desire for continuity can also be maladaptive for individuals who face life changes that cannot be assimilated within what seems to them to be continuity of self and lifestyle.

Continuity theory is not deterministic. It does not predict specific self or lifestyle content as a result of aging or adaptation. Instead, it tells us where to look to find the internal and external elements people use in adapting to various life circumstances, including aging-related changes. Inter-individual comparability is in the general form and processes of adaptation, not in the specific outcomes, which are contingent for each individual on his or her specific personal constructs. Similar types of social psychological structures and processes are presumed to be at work, even though they may produce widely varying individual results. The heart of continuity theory is the presumption that people are motivated to continue to use the adaptive apparatuses they have constructed throughout adulthood to diagnose situations, chart future courses and to adapt to change. Table 4.1 presents examples of assumptions and propositions extracted from this discussion of continuity theory.

ELEMENTS OF CONTINUITY THEORY

To use continuity theory requires information on four dimensions of an individual over time: idea structures, lifestyle, personal goals, and adaptive capacity. Internal continuity is assessed in terms of the maintenance of a consistent structure of ideas about the self and the phenomenal world. External continuity is assessed in terms of consistency over time in the social roles, activities, and relationships that make up lifestyle. Personal goals tell us the values the individual wants to actualize as he or she develops. They define an ideal self and an ideal lifestyle that constitute the benchmark for assessing the results of adaptation. Adaptive capacity can be assessed by the extent to which the person is able to maintain morale in the face of change.

Internal Structure

The ideas, mental skills, and information stored in the mind are organized into loose structures such as self-concept, personal goals, world-view, philosophy of life, moral framework, attitudes, values, beliefs, knowledge, skills, temperament, preferences, and coping strategies. Note that each of these constructs is a general label under which a large number of specific thoughts and feelings could be subsumed. These general structures represent different dimensions that, when combined, form a unique whole that distinguishes one person from another. In making life choices and in adapting to change, people are motivated to maintain the inner structures that represent a lifetime of selective investment. Ongoing consistency of

Table 4.1 Continuity Theory: Assumptions and Propositions

Continuity Theory

Assumptions

- Continuity means evolutionary consistency and linkage over time. Stability or equilibrium is a type of continuity, but evolutionary forms of continuity are more common.
- Continuity over time is commonly observed in the psychological, behavioral, and social patterns of aging individuals.
- Continuity usually coexists with discontinuity.
- Continuity is more evident in general patterns than in the specifics subsumed under general patterns.
- Individual perceptions of reality consist of personal constructs individuals actively develop by learning from life experience. Culture and socialization influence personal constructs but do not determine them.
- Internal and external patterns of continuity are highly individuated.
- To each individual, what constitutes continuity is highly subjective.
- Individual patterns of adaptive thought continue to develop throughout life.
- Using continuity strategies to pursue goals or adapt to change does not necessarily lead to successful results.

Propositions

- General patterns of thought, behavior, and relationship are robust and can accommodate considerable change in detailed patterns without triggering a sense of discontinuity.
- Through decision making about self-concept, life course, and lifestyle, and experiencing the consequences, individuals acquire a sense of personal agency.
- Enduring general patterns of thought, behavior, and relationship are the result of selective investments of time and attention made by individuals over a period of many years. People are motivated to protect these investments.
- Continuity of general patterns of thought, behavior, and relationship is the first strategy people usually attempt to use to achieve their goals or adapt to changing circumstances.
- Continuity of personal goals provides individuals with an enduring sense of developmental direction.

psychological structures is viewed by individuals as an important prerequisite for psychological security.

In the context of the present chapter, we are interested particularly in looking at continuity in the self. A difficulty in studying continuity in the structure and functioning of the self stems from a lack of agreement on salient dimensions of the self. Each person has literally hundreds of self-referent ideas. Scholars who study the self thus need to find ways to organize self-referent conceptions into meaningful categories that can be used to aggregate and communicate research results as well as to build theory. Atchley (1982) organized the self into *self-concept* (objective characteristics of the self); *ideal self* (hoped-for self); *self-values* (personal goals); *self-esteem* (self-liking); and *self-evaluation* (moral self-assessment). Bengtson et al. (1985) added *self-striving* (behavior aimed at creating hoped-for selves and avoiding feared or disvalued selves). Markus and Nurius (1986) introduced the concepts of past, present and future or *possible selves*, and Rodin and Langer (1980) stressed the importance of *self-agency*, one's perceived capacity to make things happen, as an important support for self-esteem.

Atchley (1982, 1991) and Markus and Herzog (1991) both conceived of individuals as being active participants in the creation, development, and perpetuation of the structure and dynamics of the self. Markus and Herzog (1991) theorized that individuals develop self-schemas that summarize self-referential experience. Examples might include "I can do just about anything I set my mind to" or "I take things hard" or "Having a satisfying job is important to me." These self-schema help the individual interpret and integrate self-referential experience, promote and defend the self, and develop motivation and a sense of developmental direction. Markus and Herzog theorized that self-schema could be influenced by social structural antecedents such as occupation, marital status, race, or gender, as well as by life events, social role changes, and changes in health. Markus and Herzog also theorized that psychological well-being and activity patterns could both be seen as results of the structure and dynamics of the self.

External Structure

Ideas about social roles, activities, relationships, living environments, and geographic locations are also organized in a person's mind. As a result of priority setting and selective investment throughout adulthood, by middle age most adults have unique and well-mapped external life structures or lifestyles that differentiate each person from others. Most people attempt to set priorities and make selective investments that will produce the greatest possible satisfaction for them given their constraints. As a result, they see their evolving life structure as an important source of social security.

Also, continuity of activities and environments concentrates people's energies in familiar domains where practice can often prevent or minimize the social, psychological, and physical losses that cultural concepts of aging might lead us to expect. Continuity of relationships preserves the network of social support that is important for creating and maintaining solid concepts of self and lifestyle.

Continuity of activities, relationships, and environments has obvious practical advantages, but continuity theory would lead us to expect psychic payoffs as well, because external continuity usually involves the actualization of a hoped-for self and avoidance of feared or disvalued selves.

Goal Setting

Continuity theory assumes that adults have goals for developmental direction: ideals about themselves, their activities, their relationships, and their environments toward which they want to evolve. These personal goals are the focus of self-striving.

Specific developmental goals, even whether people have such goals, are influenced by both socialization and location in the social structure—family ties, gender, social class, organizational environment, and so forth. But these goals can also be profoundly affected by life experience. Adults use life experiences to make decisions about selective investments: which aspects of themselves to focus their attention on, which activities to engage in, which careers to pursue, which groups to join, what community to be part of, and so on.

Maintaining Adaptive Capacity

As they continue to evolve, adults also have increasingly clear ideas about what produces effective decisions and what gives them satisfaction in life, and they aim to fashion and refine an external life structure that complements their internal structures and delivers the maximum life satisfaction possible given their circumstances. The ideas aging adults have about adaptation to life are results of a lifetime of learning, adapting, personal evolution, and selective investment, all in interaction or negotiation with their external social and physical environments. It should not be surprising, then, that in adapting to change, including changes in social structure, adults are motivated to continue to use the internal and external patterns they have spent so much time and energy developing.

CONTINUITY THEORY, SELF, AND SOCIAL STRUCTURE

The relation between social structure and the self has been addressed primarily by social psychologists working in a sociological tradition. In this tradition, the focus has been on the influence of individual differences in location within social structures on individual differences in various dimensions of the self. For example, in his groundbreaking work on adolescent self-images, Rosenberg (1965) looked at how such disparate social structural factors such as religious dissonance within the family, parental divorce, and birth order influenced self-esteem. In most cases, he found substantially lower self-esteem among students with less advantaged social structural characteristics.

In the sociology of aging, the argument relating social structure to advantage or disadvantage in access to resources for the development of the self has been made eloquently by Dannefer (1992). He argued that the people-sorting functions of social institutions such as schools have lasting influences on life chances, and that structural characteristics such as gender, race, and social class exert major influences on the allocation decisions made by these institutions. Thus, a person's economic situation in later life can in many cases be traced directly back to school decisions concerning that person's ability, which in turn were conditioned by factors such as gender, race, ethnicity, or social class.

In their theory of the dynamics of the self in later life, Markus and Herzog (1991) posited that social structural factors such as employment, marital status, race, and gender constituted antecedents of the self, which in turn was conceived of as an amalgam of remembered past, current, and perceived possible self conceptions. Bengtson et al., (1985) looked at age itself as a social structural variable that could presumably have an effect on self-conceptions. Despite the widespread expectation of a negative effect of aging on self-esteem, Bengtson et al., found in most cross-sectional studies of age and self-esteem that there was either no correlation, or self-esteem was higher for the older respondents.

Theoretically, there has been only crude mapping of how social structure might be expected to influence the relation between aging and the self. In this regard, continuity theory may be helpful. As social structural variables, gender, socioeconomic status, and age[1] have all been shown to be powerful influences on life circumstances. Being female, being of lower socioeconomic status, and being older would seem to independently increase the odds of facing life changes under which continuity strategies might be less applicable. For example, many women who become divorced or widowed in midlife or later find that remarriage is not a viable option, so they cannot apply a continuity lifestyle strategy based on being part of a heterosexual couple. Likewise, people of lower socioeconomic status have a much higher probability of severe disability compared with those of middle or upper socioeconomic status. Even with gender and social class controlled, being in an older age category means higher risk of lifestyle changes or physical changes that would seem to increase the difficulty of using continuity as an adaptive strategy.

The challenge of linking social structure with individual outcomes is always to identify the mechanisms through which the social structural variables operate. The hypothesis here is that social structural attributes may significantly influence the odds of being able to use continuity strategies in adapting to aging, and when continuity cannot be applied as a result of involuntary factors, the result for the self could be expected to be negative.

STUDYING CONTINUITY, SELF, AND SOCIAL STRUCTURE

How can continuity theory be tested? First, continuity is most likely to occur in generalized social psychological constructs, such as the hierarchy of personal goals, general activity preferences, or networks of social relationships, rather than in perceptions and memories of very specific ideas, behaviors, or relationships. This conception deals effectively with the apparent paradox that continuity and change usually coexist within indi-

---

1. In the general social science literature, age is seldom included along with gender, race, or social class as a major social structural attribute. But the widespread existence of age discrimination and the fact that legislation to reduce age discrimination was patterned after laws designed to cope with gender and racial discrimination, both support the conception that older age is a disadvantaging social structural characteristic (Riley, 1995).

vidual lives. Continuity is seen by individuals in terms of general themes running through their lives (Fiske and Chiriboga, 1990; Kaufman, 1986), even though there may be substantial changes in the specifics surrounding those themes.

How much relatedness is needed over time in order to qualify as continuity? By tracing individual patterns in attitudes, behavior, and relationships over multiple points in time, researchers usually can easily distinguish consistency from sudden change and from chaos. Such objective measures are useful for determining the prevalence of continuity. Here it is important to emphasize substantively meaningful similarities and differences over time, rather than simply statistically significant differences, which are often quite small in practical terms.

Theories of the relation between aging and the self are best tested using longitudinal panel data. Some often-cited studies have relied on retrospection to look at the relation of aging to the self (Kaufman, 1986), but retrospection has significant drawbacks if we accept the notion that the self may be a highly revisionist reporter of personal history (Greenwald, 1980). Longitudinal panel data have the advantage of providing data on changes over time in actual self-reports, rather than reconstructions of changes in the self.

The difference between objective and subjective assessmentsô of continuity has important implications for research. When it occurs, objective continuity in ideas, behavior, or relationships can usually be assumed to result, at least in part, from individuals' choices. However, it is also important to study subjective continuity—the individual's perceptions of the relative amount of continuity and change over time. Subjective continuity also includes the extent to which individuals express a preference for continuity as a strategy for planning, making decisions, or adapting to change.

Research results generally suggest that subjective continuity is indeed both a goal and an outcome for most aging individuals and that objective continuity of ideas, behavior and relationships is the most prevalent outcome among aging individuals over time.

RESEARCH EXAMPLES

In this section of the chapter, we look at two research examples that take us from the abstract, theoretical level to the process of answering specific research questions. We consider two research questions: 1) To what extent do social structural factors influence aging individuals' perceptions of their personal agency? and 2) How does functional disability, as a social structural factor, influence various components of the self: personal agency, emotional resilience, and personal goals?

Data to address these questions are drawn from the Ohio Longitudinal Study of Aging and Adaptation. This study collected survey data over a 16-year period from a population of 1,274 small-town residents who were age 50 or over at the beginning of the study (Atchley, 1994). Deaths and panel attrition reduced the number remaining in the panel to 474 in 1991. Unlike many panel studies of aging, this study included a large number of self-referent conceptions. Table 4.2 shows items selected as indicators of three general self-referent categories: personal agency, emotional resilience, and personal goals. Using factor analysis, the specific items included as indicators were selected from larger sets of measures for each category. Data for these items were available from surveys conducted in 1975, 1977, 1979, 1981, and 1991. In addition to the self-referent data, data were collected on age, gender, education, functional disabilities, and causes of functional disabilities as well as timing of retirement or widowhood, activity participation, subjective well-being, and numerous other variables.

Because continuity theory is about long-term patterns of thought and behavior, the analyses presented here emphasize long time intervals. Let us first look at the relationships between antecedent and current social structural variables and perceived personal agency.

SOCIAL STRUCTURAL ATTRIBUTES AND PERSONAL AGENCY

As shown in Table 4.2, respondents who were scored high in personal agency were those who strongly agreed that they could do just about anything they put their mind to, could be called a go-getter, and if they wanted something, went out and got it. We use path analysis to look at age, gender, and education (as antecedent structural variables) and functional disability (as a current, intervening social-structural variable) as influences on perceptions of personal agency. We also included a baseline measure of personal agency.

Figure 4.1 shows the basic logic of the two-stage multiple regression analysis used to generate the path coefficients. In stage one, gender, age and education were treated as exogenous social structural variables and

Table 4.2 Indicators of Self-Referent Dimensions

Self-Referent Dimensions	*Specific Statements Used as Indicators*
Personal Agency	Indicate how much you agree or disagree with each of the following statements as they apply to you now.
	• I can do just about anything I put my mind to. (agree)
	• I am a go-getter. (agree)
	• If I want something, I go out and get it. (agree)
Emotional Resilience	Next is a series of items about how life has been for you recently. Indicate how much you agree or disagree with each item.
	• Things keep getting worse as I get older. (disagree)
	• Little things bother me more this year. (disagree)
	• I sometimes think that life isn't worth living. (disagree)
	• I am as happy now as when I was younger. (agree)
	• I have a lot to be sad about. (disagree)
	• I am afraid of a lot of things. (disagree)
	• I get mad more than I used to. (disagree)
	• I take things hard. (disagree)
Personal Goals	Rate how important or unimportant each goal is in your life:
	• Being well-informed
	• Having close ties with my family
	• Being prominent in community affairs
	• Having a substantial income
	• Having a satisfying job
	• Forming a close, long-lasting friendships
	• Being self-reliant
	• Seeking new experiences and opportunities
	• Having a comfortable place to live
	• Being seen as a good person by others
	• Being dependable and reliable
	• Being a religious person

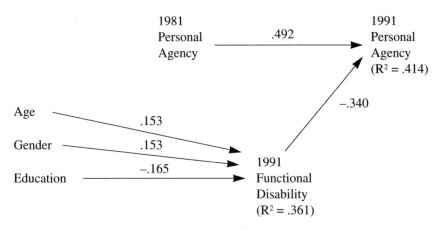

Figure 4.1 shows 1981 Personal Agency connected by .492 to 1991 Personal Agency (R² = .414). Age connects by .153, Gender by .153, and Education by −.165 to 1991 Functional Disability (R² = .361), which connects by −.340 to 1991 Personal Agency.

N = 277

Figure 4.1 Path analysis of social-structural predictors of perceptions of personal agency.

used to predict functional disability (adjusted R^2 for this stage of the model was .361), with age, gender and education all contributing to the prediction of 1991 functional disability. This analysis provides an assessment of the indirect effects of social structural variables on personal agency through their effects on functional disability. In stage two, the direct effects of age, gender, and education on personal agency in 1991 were assessed. Baseline personal agency in 1981 was also included in the regression analysis. Functional disability score in 1991 was taken as a concurrent social structural variable.[2] Functional disability score was the number of everyday activities, such as working at a full-time job, walking a half-mile, doing heavy work around the house (such as shoveling snow or washing walls), walking up and down stairs, doing light housework, and getting out into the community, that the respondent reported being unable to do.[3] The influence of antecedent social structural vari-

---

2. Ordinarily, functional disability is considered a personal attribute. But a case can be made that movement from the able-bodied segment of the population to the disabled segment means a revolutionary change in access to social opportunity structures. Indeed, the disability rights movement is based in large part on the argument that disability is an important social-structural disadvantage that must be neutralized by law if disabled people are to have equal access to opportunities for self-determination.

3. This definition of functional disability is less severe than the often-used Activities of Daily Living scale, which measures basic tasks of self-care. In fact, although many had functional disabilities, none of the respondents in this study reported ADL impairments.

ables was evaluated in two ways: direct effects on 1991 personal agency scores, and indirect effects through the impact of antecedent social structural characteristics on 1991 functional disability. The numbers by the lines in figure 4.1 are the standardized regression coefficients for each link. For more straightforward presentation, statistically nonsignificant paths were omitted from Figure 4.1.

The results of this modest path analysis are interesting. First, continuity of personal agency is the most powerful factor operating in the model (beta = .492). Such stability of indicators over time is not unusual in gerontological research, which in itself could be taken as support for continuity theory. But note that the association of 1981 and 1991 personal agency scores is far from perfect. Continuity was the most powerful factor, but other factors operated as well. Second, neither age, nor education, nor gender had direct effect on personal agency, either in 1981 or in 1991. This finding is certainly contrary to the conventional wisdom, which would lead us to expect lower personal agency scores from the older, the less educated and the female respondents. Third, age, education, and gender all had significant indirect effects on personal agency through their influence on functional disability. This finding supports the notion that antecedent social-structural attributes have their impact indirectly, through their influence on the more immediate conditions confronting the aging self. Fourth, among social-structural characteristics, functional disability was the only one that had a significant direct impact on personal agency (beta = −.340). This finding suggests that, compared with general social-structural factors, socially conditioned physical constraints have a more powerful effect on personal agency. We will return to this theme when we look in more detail at the effect of functional disability on various components of the self. The overall adjusted R^2 for the model predicting 1991 personal agency was .414, a respectable level of explanation from just two direct independent variables.

Theoretically, this analysis supports the idea that continuity in the personal agency component of the self is prevalent across a large variety of social structural subgroups within the aging population. But this correlation-based operational definition of continuity is unsatisfying because it does not get at the individual balance of continuity and change. To illustrate how this concern can be addressed, the next example looks at a small subsample in much greater detail.

FUNCTIONAL DISABILITY AND
COMPONENTS OF THE SELF

Our second research example looks separately at the effects of aging on the self compared with effects of functional disability on the self. Following continuity theory, the hypothesis is that people who age without disability show continuity in all three dimensions of the self, even though they might experience social structural changes such as retirement or widowhood. Following Atchley's (1991) argument on the potential negative effects of disability on the self, the hypothesis is that development of disability has negative effects on various dimensions of the self. The rationale is that the development of disability alters the individual's social-structural location in ways that introduce physical and lifestyle constraints on action, which in turn negatively influence people's perceptions of their personal agency, reduce their conceptions of themselves as emotionally resilient, and cause them to abandon some of their personal goals.

To adequately assess the effects of both aging and disability, it was desirable to be able to begin with a population that had no functional disabilities and then to compare continuity and change in self-conceptions over time for two groups: those who experienced aging as a gentle slope, and those who developed several functional disabilities during the study. The disability group consisted of 29 respondents who reported no functional disabilities in 1975, but who had developed 3 or more functional disabilities by 1991. Again, functional disability was defined as inability to do three or more of the following: work at a full-time job, heavy work around the house, ordinary work around the house, walk half a mile, walk up and down stairs, and go out to a movie, to church, to a meeting or to visit. A control group was constructed from among those who had no functional disabilities at any time during the study by matching respondents in the disability group with those in the control pool on age, gender, and education. This matching strategy was used because these social structural variables indirectly influenced personal agency in the earlier analysis. Controlling for them allows us to compare the disability and control groups without the muddying indirect effects of age, gender, and education. The final groups consisted of 29 respondents each—17 women and 12 men in each group. Table 4.3 shows the age distribution of all respondents in both groups in 1991, by gender.

It is a difficult task to trace patterns of response on multiple indicators over five waves of data. The standard computer data analysis packages do

Table 4.3 Age and Gender of Disability and Control Group Respondents in 1991

	Total	Female	Male
65–69	8	2	6
70–74	12	8	4
75–79	20	12	8
80–84	14	8	6
85–89	2	2	
90–94	2	2	
Total	**58**	**34**	**24**

not provide an option for displaying data this way, and there are no statistical procedures that allow what is in effect a multivariate time series analysis. Instead, worksheets were constructed that portrayed individual survey items or scale scores in each column and the rows were the five survey waves. The investigator could then look down the columns and highlight the magnitude and direction of change that occurred over time for each item or scale score. Positive and negative changes were separately color-coded. In addition to charting all of the self-referent items listed in Table 4.2, the worksheets included data over time on functional disabilities or lack of them, marital status, the interval in which retirement and or widowhood occurred (if applicable), level of participation over time in each of 16 types of activities, and overall activity level scores over time. Overall morale or life satisfaction was not included because nearly half of the morale scale items were used for the self-referent category of emotional resilience.

To aggregate data on personal agency, emotional resilience, and personal goals and to assess continuity and change within cases required the development of decision rules. For example, data on personal agency came from three indicators. If at least two of the three showed improvement over time and the other was consistent, then the case was classified as "positive change." If two of the three remained consistent over time and one improved, the case was classified as "continuity with positive change." If all indicators were consistent over time, the case was categorized as "continuity." If two indicators showed consistency over time and one showed negative change, then the case was classified as "continuity with negative change." If two or more indicators showed negative change over time and the other indicator showed continuity, then the case was classified as "negative change." Table 4.4 shows the decision rules used to classify cases

Table 4.4 Decision Criteria for Classifying Cases in Terms of Degree and Direction of Continuity and Change, by Self-Referent Dimension

Degree & Direction of Continuity & Change	Self-Referent Dimensions		
	Personal Agency	Emotional Resilience	Personal Goals
Positive Change	2+ increased 1 or fewer consistent	4+ increased 4 or fewer consistent	6+ increased 6 or fewer consistent
Continuity with Positive Change	1/3 increased 2/3 consistent	2–3 increased 5–6 consistent	3–5 increased 7–9 consistent
Continuity	3/3 consistent	7+ consistent	10+ consistent
Continuity with Negative Change	1/3 declined 2/3 consistent	2–3 declined 5–6 consistent	3–5 declined 7–9 consistent
Negative Change	2+ declined 1 or fewer consistent	4+ declined 4 or fewer consistent	6+ declined 6 or fewer consistent

into the three multiple-item self-referent categories by degree and direction of change or continuity.

To employ the scheme shown in Table 4.4 also required decision rules in terms of what constituted continuity. Obviously, continuity or consistency could be defined as having the exact same score over time, and many respondents showed this pattern on several items. However, the items all used a Likert format, so that a more conceptual definition of continuity could be easily adopted. For example, for the item "I can do just about anything I put my mind to," a respondent might score strongly agree, agree, strongly agree, strongly agree, and agree over the five waves of the study. Is this change or continuity? There is fluctuation among the responses, but they remain in the agree category, so an argument could be made for consistency or continuity, but not absolute stability. On the other hand, suppose another respondent to that same item checked strongly agree, agree, strongly agree, strongly agree, and then disagree. This latter respondent not only made a shift in magnitude of response from time 4 to time 5, but also switched from feeling able to "do just about anything I put my mind to" to not feeling that way. This is a clear-cut case of discontinuity or change. This approach was used to score the individual items in terms of continuity or change over time. When respondents switched from agree to disagree or vice versa from time to time over the study, they were classified as reporting change. Fluctuations within the agree or disagree category were classified as continuity. For the personal goals items, the major categories were important and unimportant, with the strongest responses being labeled very.

Table 4.5 shows the degree and direction of change and continuity for the three dimensions of the self, by disability status.[4] Perhaps the most striking finding is that unadulterated continuity accounted for a majority of the cases for both the disability and control groups in five of the six analyses. Only personal agency for those who developed disability showed less than a majority (41%) in the continuity category. This is strong support for continuity theory's assertion that people are predisposed to continue their patterns of thinking about themselves as they adapt to aging. Note that these findings span multiple data points over a period of 16 years, and remember that disability and control group differences are not influenced by age, gender, or education, because the groups were matched on these characteristics.

A second important finding is that development of disability influenced some self-referent dimensions, but not others. Personal agency for those who developed disability is the only situation in which a substantial proportion (28%) experienced negative change. In addition, for emotional resilience, "continuity with negative change" is more prevalent in the disability group compared to the control group (38% compared to 21%). On the other hand, the self-values that comprise personal goals are completely dominated by unadulterated continuity for both disability and control groups.

We expected that the activity constraints of disability would reduce people's perceptions of personal agency. This expectation is partially borne out, but only in comparison to the very low prevalence of negative change in the control group, which again supports the idea that aging in itself seldom has an effect on perceptions of personal agency. Only 28% of those who became disabled experienced negative change. A majority of those who developed disability showed either continuity or improvement in their sense of personal agency. The disability and control groups are not very different in terms of the proportions who experienced "continuity with negative change" in their perceptions of personal agency over time. This means, of course, that some negative change occurred even among those

---

4. Remember, we are looking at functional disabilities that are limiting but not as devastating as ADL disabilities.

Table 4.5 Longitudinal Continuity and Change in Dimensions of the Self, by Disability Status

	Self-Referent Dimensions											
	Personal Agency				Emotional Resilience				Personal Goals			
Degree and Direction of Continuity and Change	No Disability		Developed Disability		No Disability		Developed Disability		No Disability		Developed Disability	
	N	%	N	%	N	%	N	%	N	%	N	%
Positive Change	1	3	1	3	1	3	—	—	—	—		
Continuity with Positive Change	4	14	2	7	2	7	1	3	—	—	3	10
Continuity	15	52	12	41	20	66	15	52	28	97	24	83
Continuity with Native Change	7	24	6	21	6	21	11	38	1	3	2	7
Negative Change	2	7	8	28*	1	3	2	7	—	—	—	—
Total	29	100	29	100	29	100	29	100	29	100	29	100

* Group difference significant at the .05 level, using chi-square.

who experience physical aging as a gentle slope. Positive change in personal agency is rare for either group.

We expected that the frustrations of disability would result in decreased emotional resilience, but a very large majority of both groups experienced continuity or positive change in perceived emotional resilience.

We expected that the realities of functional disability would cause the individuals in the disability group to downgrade the importance of some personal goals, but personal goals showed a very high prevalence of continuity. Regardless of disability status, people tended to maintain their personal goals over time. The individuals in this study had very different priorities in terms of their ratings of their personal goals. For example, 37 respondents thought "being a religious person" was important; 21 thought this goal was unimportant. There was considerable variety among individuals in value profiles, but there was very little intra-individual change in values over time.

To get a sense of the dynamics of negative change in self-perceptions, we looked closely at the cases in which such changes occurred. In the cases that involved disability, the dynamics of declining perceptions of personal agency were straightforward. In nearly all of the 8 cases of negative change in personal agency following disability, the respondents had experienced profound lifestyle changes as a result of their underlying disability. For example, these respondents reported the onset of serious and highly constraining underlying conditions such as emphysema, severe asthma, chronic bronchitis, acute leukemia, Parkinson's disease, and paralysis. Their negative views of their personal agency were highly realistic in view of the activity restrictions imposed on them by their chronic conditions.

The two control-group respondents who showed negative change in their perceptions of personal agency were men in their early 80s who experienced dramatic activity losses in key activities. Specifically, having given up long-time participation in sports characterized both of the respondents in the control group who had negative change in their perceptions of personal agency. One also reported a substantial reduction in his frequency of church attendance. Thus, substantial reductions in specific role-related activity, not generalized changes such as retirement, were associated with negative changes in personal agency for the two control-group men who reported negative change in the absence of functional disability.

This second research example has several implications for the study of the self. While the small size of the samples poses a serious limit on the generalizability of the findings, the results do suggest several theoretical and methodological points that might be worth taking into account in future research on the aging self.

First, personal agency, emotional resilience, and personal goals appear to be separate dimensions of the self, and these separate dimensions showed different patterns of continuity and change over time. Personal goals fluctuated very little over time and, contrary to expectations, did not shift to accommodate disability or decline in frequency of specific day-to-day activities. Another way of saying this is that although middle-aged and older individuals vary considerably in terms of what they think is important, once they develop a personal value system, they tend to retain that value system, even in the face of substantial external change.

Emotional resilience also showed a high degree of continuity over time, but disability introduced negative elements into that continuity much more frequently than mere aging did. Finally, among elders who developed disability, a substantial minority experienced negative change in their perceptions of their personal agency. Disabled elders who showed a declining sense of agency were quite likely to be dealing with very limiting underlying conditions such as breathing disorders, paralysis, leukemia or Parkinson's disease; whereas elders whose disabilities consisted of less profoundly disabling conditions such as arthritis, musculoskeletal problems, or even low vision were more likely to report continuity in their sense of personal agency.

At least for the dimensions of the self reported here, there was much more continuity than change in self-referent conceptions over a considerable length of time. These findings suggest that the internal desire for continuity overrides external, situational pressures to change, at least for these three elements of the self. Thus, the propensity toward continuity might be seen as establishing a threshold that could be used to identify when Markus and Herzog's (1991) dynamic model of the self might be mobilized into action. In other words, continuity could be expected to be the general rule, but when change exceeds a subjectively defined threshold, then changes in the self might be expected.

In the absence of seriously limiting disability, aging people achieve continuity across various dimensions of the self, which supports continuity theory. Seriously limiting disability tended to supersede the continuity principle for a small minority of respondents, but only for personal agency. Less serious disability and reductions in long-standing activities can bring a negative tone to continuity without neutralizing the value of continuity as a concept that describes the patterns of self-perception over time.

The methods used in our research examples show that continuity theory can indeed be used to generate and test hypotheses about the self. Continuity can be conceptually and operationally differentiated both from absolute stability in item scores and from change. The methods used to assess the degree and direction of continuity and change are labor-intensive, but they produce a high degree of inter-rater reliability because they are based on decision rules for integrating a mass of quantitative data. The Likert scale format especially lends itself to this technique, but it can be used with other scale formats as well. These techniques can be used to study continuity in a variety of individual characteristics.

SUMMARY AND CONCLUSIONS

The basic logic of treating social attributes such as age, gender, education, and disability status as social structural characteristics presumes that these attributes are used to allocate individuals to different regions of the sociocultural environment. Older people do live in different social worlds compared with the young. Women live in different social regions than men. Educated people experience different social environments than the uneducated. The able-bodied experience different social worlds than the physically disabled. These differences extend to existential, subjective experiences of life as well as to objective opportunity structures, especially in the economy. That older age, being female, having lower education, and being disabled independently result in greater social disadvantage is well documented. But it is also well documented that most aging people are somehow able to neutralize the effects of these disadvantages for the self. Despite numerous disadvantages, adults are able to maintain consistent and satisfying lifestyles and positive and enduring self-conceptions.

Continuity theory contends that most aging adults are able to achieve these positive results because over their adult lives they have developed robust frameworks of ideas, adaptive skills, relationships, and activities that create internal and external environments—lifeworlds—that insulate most of them from the ageism of our culture and that allow them to adapt effectively to changes associated with aging. Continuity of values, activities, and relationships is a preferred adaptive strategy because for most aging adults the consistent self-schema that underlie internal and external continuity have stood the test of time and continuity of self and behavior has consistently delivered a significant measure of psychological and social security.

Our research examples looked at patterns of self-conception in a panel of respondents over periods of 10 and 16 years. The results showed that continuity of the self was indeed the most common outcome over extended time periods. This was true for all three components of the self we examined: personal agency, emotional resilience, and personal goals. The results also showed that general social attributes such as age, gender, and education did not directly relate to individual differences in self-perceptions of personal agency in later life. These latter findings suggest that for most people the aging self had long ago adapted positively to whatever structural disadvantages these factors may have had for this dimension of the self. However, age, gender and education all had a bearing on which people experienced functional disability, which in turn was significantly related to perceiving the self as having less agency.

We argued that functional disability is a social-structural attribute that has more immediate implications for the self than antecedent structural attributes. However, we found that functional disability had its negative effects primarily on perceived personal agency, and then only in a minority of cases. Emotional resilience showed an even milder effect of functional disability, and personal goals were not affected by functional disability at all. These findings suggest that continuity is an extremely powerful influence on values, but that as ideas become more directly related to immediate experience, extreme changes have greater potential effects for the self. Our findings suggested that for most adults, the threshold of change required to activate a reorganization in the long-standing structure of the self is quite high indeed.

In an analysis reported elsewhere (Atchley, 1998), we looked at patterns of activity over the 16 years of the study and found that for all but the most serious disabilities, panel members were able to adapt to various life changes in ways that maintained their customary pattern of activities, albeit often at a lower frequency of participation. Continuity of pattern was strongly related to maintaining a high degree of subjective well-being. This same relationship was observed in the current study for various elements of the self. Thus, continuity means being able to maintain familiar and preferred patterns of thought and behavior. It does not mean that nothing changes. Many respondents experienced declines in activity level, but if they could maintain their pattern of activities, then life remained satisfying and their sense of personal agency was maintained as well.

The research illustrations in this chapter showed that continuity theory can be effectively used to develop and test hypotheses concerning the relation between age, other ascribed social attributes, and the self. The results also showed that continuity can indeed be measured and operationally differentiated from both sameness and change.

REFERENCES

Abercrombie, N., Hill, S., & Turner, B. S. (1988). *Dictionary of sociology (*2nd ed.*).* London: Penguin.

Antonucci, T. C. (1990). Social supports and social relationships. In R. H. Binstock & L. K. George (Eds.), *Handbook of aging and the social sciences* (3rd ed., pp. 205–226). New York: Academic Press.

Atchley, R. C. (1971). Aging and leisure participation: Continuity or crisis? *The Gerontologist, 11*, 13–17.

Atchley, R. C. (1982). The aging self. *Psychotherapy: Theory, Research, and Practice, 19*, 388–396.

Atchley, R. C. (1989). A continuity theory of normal aging. *The Gerontologist, 29*, 183–190.

Atchley, R. C. (1991). The influence of aging and frailty on perceptions and expressions of the self. In J. E. Birren, J. E. Lubben, J. C. Rowe, & D. E. Deutschman (Eds.), *The concept and measurement of quality of life in the late years* (pp. 209–225). New York: Academic Press.

Atchley, R. C. (1993). Continuity theory and the evolution of activity in later life. In J. R. Kelly (Ed.), *Activity and aging* (pp. 5–16). Newbury Park, CA: Sage.

Atchley, R. C. (1994, November). *Is there life between life course transitions?* Paper presented at the Annual Meeting of Gerontological Society of America, New Orleans.

Atchley, R. C. (1995). Continuity theory. In G. L. Maddox R. C. Atchley, J. G. Evans, C. E. Finch, D. F. Hultsch, R. A. Kane, M. D. Mezay, & I. C. Siegler (Eds.), *The encyclopedia of aging* (2nd ed., pp. 227–230). New York: Springer.

Atchley, R. C. (1998). Activity adaptations to the development of functional limitations and results for subjective well-being in later adulthood. *Journal of Aging Studies, 12*, 1, 19–38.

Bailey, K. D. (1994). *Sociology and the new systems theory*. Albany: State University of New York Press.

Bengtson, V. L., Reedy, M. N., & Gordon, C. (1985). Aging and self-conceptions: Personality processes and social contexts. In J. E. Birren & K. W. Schaie (Eds.), *Handbook of the psychology of aging* (2nd ed., pp. 544–593). New York: Van Nostrand Reinhold.

Buckley, W. F. (1967). *Sociology and modern systems theory*. Englewood Cliffs, NJ: Prentice-Hall.

Cohler, B. J. (1993). Aging, morale, and meaning: The nexus of narrative. In T. R. Cole, W. A. Achenbaum, P. L. Jakobi, & R. Kastenbaum (Eds.), *Voices and visions of aging*. New York: Springer Publishing Co.

Dannefer, D. (1992). On the conceptualization of content in developmental discourse: Four meanings of context and their implications. In D. L. Featherman, R. M. Lerner, & M. Perlmutter (Eds.), *Lifespan development and behavior* (Vol. 11, pp. 84–110). Hillsdale, NJ: Erlbaum.

Erikson, E. H. (1963). *Childhood and society*. New York: MacMillan.

Fiske, M., & Chiriboga, D. A. (1990). *Change and continuity in adult life*. San Francisco: Jossey-Bass.

Greenwald, A. (1980). The totalitarian ego. *The American Psychologist, 35*, 603–618.

James, W. (1890). *Principles of psychology*. Vol. 1. New York: Holt.

Kaufman, S. R. (1986). *The ageless self*. Madison: University of Wisconsin Press.

Kelly, G. (1955). *The psychology of personal constructs*. New York: Norton.

Levinson, D. J. (1978). *Seasons of a man's life*. New York: Alfred A. Knopf.

Levinson, D. J. (1990). A theory of life structure development in adulthood. In C. N. Alexander & E. J. Langer (Eds.), *Higher stages of human development* (pp. 35–53). New York: Oxford University Press.

Maddox, G. L. (1968). Persistence of life style among the elderly: A longitudinal study of patterns of social activity in relation to life satisfaction. In B. L. Neugarten (Ed.), *Middle age and aging* (pp. 181–183). Chicago: University of Chicago Press.

Markus, H., & Herzog, A. R. (1991). The role of the self-concept in aging. *Annual Review of Gerontology and Geriatrics, 11*, 110–143.

Markus, H., & Nurius, P. (1986). Possible selves. *The American Psychologist, 41*, 954–969.

Riley, M. W. (1995). Age stratification. In G. L. Maddox (Eds.), *Encyclopedia of aging* (2nd ed., pp. 42–45). New York: Springer.

Rodin, J., & Langer, E. (1980). Aging labels: The decline of control and the fall of self-esteem. *Journal of Social Issues, 36*, 12–29.

Rosenberg, M. (1965). *Society and the adolescent self-image*. New York: Basic.

Rosow, I. (1963). Adjustment of the normal aged. In R. H. Williams, C. Tibbitts, & W. Donohue (Eds.), *Processes of aging: Social and psychological perspectives* (Vol. 2, pp. 195–223). New York: Atherton.

Theodorson, G. A., & Theodorson, A. G. (1969). *Modern dictionary of sociology*. New York: Thomas Y. Crowell.

Troll, L. (1982). *Continuations: Adult development and aging*. Monterey, CA: Brooks/Cole.

Williams, R. H., & Wirths, C. (1965). *Lives through the years*. New York: Atherton.

CHAPTER 5

Identity and Adaptation to the Aging Process

Susan Krauss Whitbourne

T he concept of identity provides a rich theoretical framework from which to view the psychological development of the individual in the context of a social-structural perspective. In this chapter, I will explore a set of concepts related to identity that have proven useful in understanding the ways that individuals confront and react to their own aging within the framework of the larger society. Following a general orientation to life course themes and issues, I will describe the model of identity on which these concepts are based, and then indicate how identity relates to the individual's adaptation to life events, and to a multiple threshold model of physical and psychological aspects of the aging process. The relationship between identity and related concepts of coping and control will also be explored, with predictions for age variations in behaviors related to adaptation to aging in the later adult years. Although the focus of the present chapter is on intraindividual processes, the relationship of these processes to social and contextual factors forms an integral theme. Preliminary data will also be presented along with recommendations for future qualitative and quantitative research relating self to society from the standpoint of the model.

LIFE COURSE THEMES AND ISSUES
IN THE AGING OF THE SELF

The aging of the individual occurs in a context of a long adaptational history, in which the individual has confronted numerous physiological, psychological, and contextual challenges. From the perspective of the aging individual, this theme of the continuity of the self over time is of particular salience. Although many changes occur in the later years of life, these changes are interpreted by the individual against a backdrop of both successful and unsuccessful adaptations to previous gains and losses throughout the earlier years of adulthood.

A second central theme in the psychological study of aging is the need to distinguish between normal aging and disease. It is known that as individuals age, they develop chronic health problems such as arthritis, cardiovascular disease, and diabetes. As prevalent as these problems may be, however, they are not inherent to normal aging and they are not inevitable. A similar observation may be made for psychological difficulties, such as depression or cognitive dysfunction, which are not normal consequences of the aging process. Reinforcing this theme is the fact that variations in susceptibility to physical and psychological health problems occur by the sociodemographic factors of gender, race, and class. These variations are important to understand in their own right, but also highlight the fact that physical health changes in the form of disease are not an inherent part of the aging process.

A third consideration in the study of normal aging is the importance of individual differences. It is a well-established principle in gerontology that as people grow older they become more different. The many and varied experiences that older people have over their lifetimes cause them to become increasingly diverse. Elders who share the same gender, social class, and ethnic background may share certain life experiences, and hence interpretations of events; these are important sources of individual differences. Above and beyond these shared group factors, reactions to experiences associated with aging are likely to reflect the individual's unique psychological and physical capacity to cope with life events.

A fourth point is the extent to which an age-related change can be slowed down, is preventable, or can be compensated. Although the ultimate result of the aging process is a progressive loss of function, there are many steps that individuals can take to slow down the aging process, so that they can prevent deleterious effects of aging before they become apparent. Some of these behaviors fall into the category of the "use it or lose it" (what I shall abbreviate as UIOLI) principle. In other words, exercise and activity can keep a particular physical or psychological function better maintained than inactivity. Conversely, behaviors that fall into the category of "bad habits" are those that are avoided by the individual interested in maintaining positive functioning.

The existence of UIOLIs and bad habits are relevant to the points raised above. Whether individuals take advantage of positive steps to regulate their own aging may be seen as a function of past adaptational strategies to their health and functioning. Secondly, UIOLIs and bad habits may affect the extent to which an individual's normal aging becomes compounded with disease. Third, these behaviors show considerable individual differences, and can themselves compound variations in the genetic vulnerability that a person may have to a particular disease or age-related change. For example, middle-aged individuals who have a familial history of heart disease but who engage in regular aerobic exercise will be less likely to develop serious cardiovascular problems than those who choose not to take advantage of this known health prevention measure. Variations in cultural attitudes toward health and prevention, education, and opportunities to access the health care system can also interact significantly with these individual differences.

Finally, in examining the individual's ability to adapt to the normal aging process, it is essential to keep in mind the resilience that many elders show when faced with the potential stresses associated with the aging process. The study of coping has assumed an increasingly large role in the psychological study of aging, as new evidence continues to be gained about the coping capacities of elders. Not only are older adults seen as able to navigate the often stormy waters of later life, but they are increasingly seen as creating new challenges, goals, and opportunities for themselves. The concept of control has also emerged as a major research focus in psychological gerontology, based on the belief that individuals can, to a certain extent, control their own destinies with regard to the aging process, and through personal effort, creativity, and determination, can manage their own aging, if not actually "beat" it. Again, however, it is important to acknowledge the limitations that may prevent individuals from actualizing this potential due to racial, cultural, educational, and income-related barriers.

APPLICATION OF AN IDENTITY MODEL
TO THE AGING PROCESS

Following from the general themes and issues is a model of the development of the self in adulthood in which identity serves as the major organizing principle within personality, and as the link between the individual and society. In this model (Whitbourne, 1996), identity is theorized to form an organizing schema through which the individual's experiences are interpreted. Identity is conceptualized as a template or set of schemas used as the framework for viewing new events and interactions. Within this model, the content domains of identity are defined as the individual's self-appraisal of personal attributes along the dimensions of biological, psychological, and social qualities. The affective content of identity, for psychologically healthy adults, takes the positive self-referential form encapsulated in the expression "I am a competent, loving, and good person; competent at work, loving in family life, and morally righteous." Conversely, adults suffering from emotional disturbances such as depression are prone to view their worlds through negative self-schemas in which the self, world, and the future are seen as hopeless (Beck, Rush, Shaw & Emery, 1975). The affective content of identity in turn has motivational qualities, as individuals show a preference for viewing themselves and their experiences in a manner that is consistent with their established self-schemas.

Identity Content Domains

The content of identity is proposed to be divided into six portions, interacting in a central core. The central core is theorized to contain those aspects of identity that are most salient to the individual and that represent combinations of qualities from the separate domains. At the central core it is assumed that fundamental self-conceptions derived from early interactions with parents and significant others form the underlying unconscious elements of the self (Whitbourne, 1989). The six identity content domains branching out from this central core each have support within the literature as a separate area or focus within the self. The identity model integrates these separate domains and makes it possible to understand their interrelationships within one overarching framework.

The content of the body, or physical identity, is a major component of identity (Bocknek & Perna, 1994) and can be thought of as incorporating three components (Fox & Corbin, 1989; Hennessy, 1989): the perception of: (1) the appearance of one's own body; (2) competence, or the body's ability to perform tasks needed in daily activities; and (3) one's own health. The area of appearance is regarded as central to the identity of older individuals for both men and women (Harris, 1994; Heidrich & Ryff, 1993a, 1993b). Related to this concept is the notion of social physique anxiety, or the degree to which the individual feels that others are negatively evaluating one's bodily appearance (Hart, Leary, & Rejeski, 1989). The domain of competence has received less attention, but may show up in the form of concern over mobility (the ability to move in the environment), or as concerns about being able to maintain one's independence (Dittman-Kohli, 1990). Interestingly, the desire to have a fit and strong body shows up less often among older adults (Hooker & Kaus, 1994) as a personal goal or desired self-attribute, a concept referred to as the "possible self" (Markus & Nurius, 1986). It is surprising that this is the case, given the prevailing social attitudes toward the importance of fitness, strength, and exercise. However, it might be argued that variations in this component of identity occur along with one's position in the social structure. Those with higher educational levels would be expected to have a stronger desire to maintain bodily fitness, if not attractiveness, and those with higher income levels may be far more conscientious about their appearance.

Health is perhaps one of the strongest components of physical identity, particularly for older adults, as indicated in numerous studies regarding the importance of subjective health to life satisfaction and overall psychological well-being (Ryff, 1989). Comparisons of the self to others are often made on the basis of health (Heidrich & Ryff, 1993b). Most impressively, when asked to describe spontaneously the possible self (Markus & Nurius, 1986) they hope for or fear the most, the majority of older people state that they see themselves in the future in terms of their health (Hooker, 1992). There is also evidence that views about one's health begin to become incorporated into identity in middle age, and, like the possible selves in old age, tend to be negative (Hooker & Kaus, 1994). It is also likely that identity in terms of health has an additional meaning relevant to the role of health and illness in determining the length of one's life. Health, in this regard, may be seen as an index of how far one is in the approach toward the cessation of the body's functions.

In the domain of cognition, there is a growing body of evidence to support the notion that adults are aware of their intellectual skills and incorporate these into their identities. Views of intellectual and memory "self-efficacy," or the ability to succeed at a task, are areas of increasing research interest (Lachman, Bandura, Weaver, & Elliott, 1995). Another area of cognitive identity is the self-attribution of oneself as having intellectual ability (Grover & Hertzog, 1991) or as being "wise" (Staudinger, Smith, & Baltes, 1993). Fear of the loss of intellectual ability is also a significant component of the possible selves of middle-aged and older adults (Hooker & Kaus, 1994). In terms of contributors to feelings of personal well-being, the ability to learn new information appears to play a significant role, particularly as individuals compare themselves to others whom they perceive as less advantaged or suffering from age-related cognitive deterioration (Heidrich & Ryff, 1993b).

The personality domain includes self-attributions of various characteristics relevant to the individual's enduring dispositions. These include emotions (Carstensen & Turk-Charles, 1994), coping and defense styles (Labouvie-Vief, Hakim-Larson, & Hobart, 1987), traits (McCrae & Costa, 1990), values (Ryff, 1989) and interests, hobbies, and beliefs (McCrae & Costa, 1988). Whether or not these dispositions remain stable over time, as is argued by some (McCrae & Costa, 1990), the individual's self-attributions or awareness of personality tendencies may change over the adult years as one becomes more comfortable with "who" one is (McCrae & Costa, 1988).

The next three domains are derived from Erikson's theory (Erikson, 1963) and the assumption that identity is an overarching theme of development in the years of adulthood and old age (Whitbourne & Connolly, 1998). The domain of intimacy refers to the context of close relationships, both with sexual partners and with friends. The domain of generativity includes the extension of the self into the care and well-being of future generations, both through mentoring experiences at work and through parenting or parenting-like roles. The accomplishments of children, in particular, reflect on the individual's identity, although the effects are not unqualifiedly positive. Parents may experience vicarious enjoyment as well as pride regarding their children, but they may also feel some envy and a sense of having missed out on the benefits available to the younger generation (Ryff, Lee, Essex, & Schmutte, 1994). Finally, the domain of ego integrity involves the existential self and the view of oneself as belonging to a certain time and place in history (Erikson, Erikson, & Kivnick, 1986).

Identity Processes

Having defined the contents of identity, it is now possible to elaborate on the model of identity development and its relationship to experiences over the years of adulthood. The individual's experiences, both past and present, are postulated to relate to identity through Piagetian-like processes of assimilation and accommodation, as shown in Figure 5.1. The process of identity assimilation is defined as the interpretation of life events relevant to the self in terms of the cognitive and affective schemas that are incorporated in identity. The events and experiences to which the assimilation function applies can include new aspects of physical or cognitive functioning, major life events, cumulative interactions with the environment over time, or even incidents that take place over the course of daily life. The main criterion for the relevance of an event to identity is that it has some bearing on the individual's self-definition. Thus, the experiences interpreted through identity assimilation can include physical changes associated with the aging process or involvement in a gratifying family role, such as grandparent. Each type of experience can have different meanings across individuals depending on the nature of their current self-conceptualizations in identity.

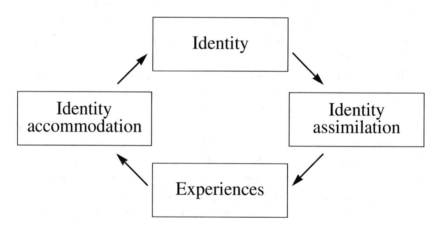

Figure 5.1 Model of adult identity processes.

The process of identity accommodation, by contrast, involves changing one's identity in response to an identity-relevant experience. Identity might change in content in response to one of these events when, for example, an illness or accident causes the individual to acknowledge new health limitations. Again, it is the relevance of the event to the individual's self-definition that determines whether it will be incorporated into identity. According to this model, there are no objective indicators of what events will or will not have the potential to influence the individual's sense of self because their meaning is subjectively determined. A similar argument has been put forth for cognitive models of stress and emotion (Lazarus & Folkman, 1984).

As in Piaget's (Piaget, 1975/1977) discussion of the equilibration process in the development of intelligence, it is assumed that the most desirable state is for the individual's identity to be in a state of dynamic balance with the environment, so that alternation takes place between assimilation and accommodation. In this state, the individual's identity is flexible enough to change when warranted, but not so unstructured so that every new experience causes the person to question fundamental assumptions about the self's integrity and unity. Thus, equilibrium is not a static mode, but involves movement back and forth between assimilation and accommodation. However, it is also assumed that the directionality of processes is, as in Piaget's theory (Piaget, 1975/1977), from assimilation to accommodation, with assimilation being the preferred mode. Psychologically healthy adults prefer and strive to see themselves in relation to events in a positive light and, as discussed above, those who are depressed tend to see themselves in a negative manner. In either case, accommodation is assumed to be prompted when assimilation can no longer fit new events into the individual's existing identity (Kiecolt, 1994).

As applied to the aging process, the mechanisms of assimilation and accommodation are assumed to operate gradually throughout the later years of adulthood and ultimately the individual's identity of the self as "old" emerges from former age-related identities. Although through assimilation individuals may prefer to see themselves as continuous over time and as being stable in their functioning, accommodation eventually alters this sense of self to incorporate a view of the self as aging. More sudden changes in identity are presumed to result from diseases or accidents that cannot be accommodated over a period of time. There may also be class differences in the tendency to use assimilation or accommodation. It is possible to speculate that because opportunities and resources are unequally distributed over the life course, there would be social class differences in the proportional mix of assimilation and accommodation in people's adaptational repertoires (Dowd, 1990). For example, individuals who have limited access to society's resources throughout their lives may be more likely to use accommodation as the preferred mode of adapting to experiences because they have not typically been able to effect change in a desired direction. At this point, however, there are no available data to support such an argument; in earlier research on the identity assimilation and accommodation processes in middle-aged adults, no social class differences were observed in the tendencies toward using either of these processes (Whitbourne, 1986).

Identity in Relation to the Aging Process

The aging process involves a number of inherent changes that can have separate as well as cumulative effects on the individual's identity. The implications for identity of physical and cognitive changes associated with the aging process may be seen as involving both objective and subjective realms. The objective effects of an age-related change on the individual's adaptation involve the real alterations that occur in the individual's everyday life in direct response to a physical or cognitive change. For example, loss of mobility due to changes in the body's joints directly reduces the individual's ability to get to desired locations, both within the home and in travelling outside the home. The individual's adaptation to the environment is reduced in direct proportion to the extent to which loss of mobility has occurred. Relevant to the effects of social class, opportunities for compensation may be seen as varying according to access to resources.

Age-related changes may also influence the individual's adaptation through the subjective or indirect effect of these changes on the individual's identity. Many of these changes have their potential impact through a perceived reduction in feelings of competence. Returning to the example of mobility, reductions in the ability to get around independently reduce the individual's sense of competence—personal power, strength, and effectiveness. To the extent that the individual's identity is altered through this secondary or indirect process, positive adaptation in the sense of well-being and satisfaction is likely to be reduced as well. Again, changes in identity may be seen as dependent on position in the social structure.

An additional factor to consider in this equation is the extent to which an age-related change can be prevented, compensated, or in other ways coped with successfully. In this sense, the relationship between age-related changes and identity may be conceived of as dynamic, reciprocal, and transactional in that individuals may alter the course of their development on the basis of their self-conceptions and ideas about change. Relevant concepts for this analysis are the principles of UIOLIs and bad habits, which play important roles in these dynamic processes. If a UIOLI is available to the individual, that is, if the age-related change can be offset or slowed through behavioral methods, then it is possible for the older person to experience less of a sense of loss or frustration regarding an age-related change, and more of a sense of personal control. Positive adaptation, it would seem, in this case would depend on the individual's willingness to confront the age-related change, look for ways to take advantage of the UIOLI principle, and work to prevent the deleterious effects of this process. On the other hand, a negative outcome will develop if the individual erroneously adopts a fatalistic attitude toward a preventable age-related deficit and lets bad habits take their toll in a free-fall, unabated fashion. Both these attitudes toward change and the behaviors available for compensation may depend on position in society. Those people whose lives have been marked by despondency due to their lack of resources or access to resources may be more likely to adopt such a nihilistic attitude toward the aging process.

It is worth noting that there are some age-related changes that cannot be ameliorated through individual action. In these cases, the individual may experience frustration associated with unsuccessful efforts to adopt the UIOLI principle, particularly if he or she is accustomed to having an impact on life opportunities and outcomes. It actually may be more of a positive adaptation for the individual either to do nothing or to engage in bad habits, because this avoids frustration and at least allows the individual some pleasurable, albeit unhealthy, activities.

Measurement of Identity Processes

Qualitative investigations of the adult identity processes of assimilation and accommodation provided strong evidence for the relationship between the ways that adults incorporate experiences into identity and their psychological adaptation (Whitbourne, 1986b). Interview data with a sample stratified by SES of 94 adults provided initial glimpses into the nature of the identity processes within content areas of work, family, and values. This work was more descriptive in nature, involving qualitative analysis of transcripts based on a semistructured identity interview. Individual differences in identity were not examined specifically; the focus was on outlining the broad picture of the identity processes within these content domains.

Moving from the qualitative level, scales developed to test the relationships between identity assimilation and accommodation and emotional well-being on a broader scale are currently being tested on a larger cross-sectional sample of adults. The "Identity and Experiences Scale- General" (IES-G) assesses the individual's use of identity assimilation and accommodation in a generic sense, with subscales developed on the basis of the semistructured interview responses gathered in the interview study

(Whitbourne, 1986b). Respondents are also asked to choose a significant recent change that has occurred to them (older adults are asked specifically to describe an age-related physical or cognitive change) and then to complete assimilation and accommodation ratings with regard to this particular change (the Identity and Experiences Scale- Specific Aging Form; IES-SA). Currently, data are being gathered to measure the individual's state of balance or equilibrium between assimilation and accommodation. Variations according to gender, socioeconomic status, and race/ethnicity are also being investigated.

A MULTIPLE THRESHOLD MODEL OF AGING AND IDENTITY

Another useful construct that follows from an extension of the identity model to the physical aging process is the multiple threshold model, a model that pertains to the individual's personal awareness of the biological aging process as it impacts on the self. Physical change is the focus of this model, although it also incorporates certain cognitive changes to the extent that they reflect physical changes in the brain.

Definition and Concepts

The multiple threshold model of aging (Whitbourne, 1996) is an attempt to relate age changes in the body to psychological adaptation in a way that integrates the concepts of the nature of aging changes, identity, socialization, and age-related control behaviors. The term "threshold" in this model refers to the individual's point at which an age-related change is recognized. At this point, the individual recognizes the possibility that functions may be lost through aging (or disease), and begins to accommodate to this possibility by changing identity accordingly (see Figure 5.2). Social expectations for one's class, gender, and race/ethnicity may provide input into the level of a threshold. Specific occupational variations can also have an impact on the setting of a threshold, as certain changes may have a great deal more relevance depending on the skills required by one's occupation.

The term "multiple" in this model refers to the fact that the aging process involves potentially every system in the body, so that there is in actuality no single threshold leading into the view of the self as aging. The individual may feel "old" in one domain of functioning, such as in the area

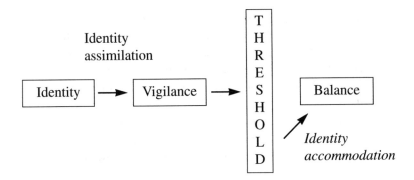

Figure 5.2 Multiple threshold model of aging.

of mobility, but feel "not old," "middle-aged" or possibly "young" in other domains, such as in the area of sensory acuity or intellectual functioning. Whether a threshold is crossed depends in part then on the actual nature of the aging process and whether it has affected a particular area of functioning. However, it is also the case that individuals vary widely in the areas of functioning that they value. It is assumed that changes in areas important to the individual's adaptation and sense of competence will have greater potential for affecting identity than changes in relatively unimportant areas.

Not only are changes in important functions likely to have a greater impact on adaptation and identity, but it is likely that functions most central to identity will be watched for most carefully by the individual. Heightened vigilance to age-related changes in these central aspects of identity can be predicted, then, resulting in the individual's greater sensitivity to noticing early signs of age-related changes in some areas but not others. As a result of the increased vigilance for areas of functioning central to identity, the impact of changes in these areas can be predicted to be even higher than they might otherwise be. On the other hand, with increased vigilance may come increased motivation to take advantage of the UIOLI principle and to avoid bad habits.

The increased vigilance associated with one of these thresholds presents a double-edged sword, in which heightened vigilance leads to behavior that offsets the aging process, thus reducing the dreaded outcomes of loss, but also leads the individual to become acutely sensitive to signs that loss has occurred. It may be in this situation, then, that identity accommodation becomes important. The individual who recognizes that he or she is aging through accommodation is less likely to become discouraged and frustrated at evidence that certain age-related changes cannot be completely reversed. The assimilative individual who desperately attempts to hang onto a youthful identity has the potential be demolished when an event occurs that makes it abundantly clear that the aging process has taken its inevitable toll.

The multiple threshold concept is most easily viewed as a set of linear processes, with the outcome of passing through threshold an alteration in the individual's level of well-being in response to the quality of the individual's coping strategies. The process is not entirely linear, however. Each time a threshold is passed, there is the potential for the individual's identity to be altered through identity accommodation. When this happens, the crossing of the threshold serves as an event relevant to the self that becomes integrated into identity. The resulting change in identity then alters the individual's subsequent vigilance regarding future age-related changes in other areas of functioning and the behaviors relevant to the threshold just crossed.

A measure developed to assess the multiple threshold is the Self-Perception Scale (SPS) in which the individual is asked to rate on a 4-point scale the extent to which each particular change has affected "the way I feel about myself." In a pilot investigation to evaluate the usefulness of the SPS in detecting multiple thresholds, a sample of 217 healthy adults ranging from 18 to over 65 years of age were tested. The preliminary data from this study indicate that there are different thresholds that individuals use in evaluating the relevance of an age-related change to themselves. Responses to items with the highest percentage of responses are shown in Table 5.1. As can be seen from this table, the thresholds varied for the three age groups according to area of functioning. The chi-square statistics reported in this table represent the age differences within each category of change; a significant chi-square means that the age groups differed on whether a change was considered one of difficulty or not. As can be seen from this table, changes in appearance, including gray hair and wrinkles, were a problem for larger percentages of people ranging from the late 20s through middle age than of those who were over 60 years old. Problems related to mobility began to be reported in the younger ages, but were more prevalent among the older adults, particularly with regard to balance.

Clearly, then, there are varying thresholds for age-related changes across areas; furthermore, scores on the SPS were found to be related to IES assimilation and accommodation scale scores. It was predicted that individuals who use assimilation as a general approach to identity-related

Table 5.1 Percent Within Each Age Group Reporting Problems on the SPS

Age group	Physical Activities	Wrinkles	Gray Hair	Joint Pain	Balance	Hearing Loss
			Area of Functioning on SPS			
18 to 25 (n = 67)	26.87	11.94	5.97	17.91	7.46	4.48
26 to 59 (n = 85)	25.89	27.06	21.18	32.94	7.06	5.58
60 and over (n = 65)	30.77	13.85	7.69	41.54	18.46	16.92
Chi square (all df = 3)	.47	9.87**	8.91**	6.06*	6.99*	7.84*

*p<.05, **p<.01

issues would be less sensitive to age thresholds compared to those who use accommodation and are therefore more sensitive to feedback from events and experiences relevant to aging. Furthermore, by comparing IES-General with IES-Specific Aging scales, the difference between identity processes as general styles of approaching life events could be compared with identity processes relevant to age-specific themes. As shown in Table 5.2, among adults over 60, those who used assimilation both in general and with regard to age changes were less likely to report problems in physical or psychological functioning on the SPS. However, among younger adults, assimilation with regard to aging but not in general was related to the tendency not to report problems in functioning. A large effect was observed on the accommodation-aging scale among those over 60 years. Individuals more likely to report problems on the SPS were also more likely to use accommodation with regard to the aging process.

RELATION OF IDENTITY TO CONTROL PROCESSES AND COPING

Data emerging from the analyses reported above regarding the multiple threshold and its relationship to identity are providing some preliminary support, at least at a descriptive level, for these theoretical concepts.

Table 5.2 Correlations of SPS Total With Identity Scales

	Age Group		
	18 to 25	26 to 59	60 plus
Scale	(*n* = 66)	(*n* = 77)	(*n* = 63)
Assimilation–general	.20	.00	–.26*
Assimilation–aging	.12	–.23*	–.27*
Accommodation–general	.12	.20	.09
Accommodation–aging	.20	.17	.64**

*p <.05 **p<.01

However, to be consistent with current research directions as well as to elaborate further on the behavioral correlates of assimilation and accommodation, it is necessary to take into account related concepts that pertain to the ways that individuals conceive of and address their own personal aging. One of these concepts is locus of control which, with regard to the aging process, refers to the individual's intrinsic theories of aging, and whether aging can be controlled (an internal orientation) or whether there is nothing that can be done to alter the inevitable course of age-related decline (external orientation). A similar concept is also described in terms of primary and secondary control (Heckhausen & Schulz, 1995).

An internal or primary control orientation with regard to aging is regarded as highly adaptive in relation to abilities that can be modified through the UIOLI principle. For example, the view that memory is a "muscle" that can be exercised contributes to more positive memory functioning among older adults (Cavanaugh & Green, 1990). Conversely, the belief that memory deficits are inevitable and uncontrollable leads to a self-fulfilling prophecy in which negative memory beliefs lead to lowered levels of effort and hence performance (Elliott & Lachman, 1989). Over time, such beliefs can generalize across situations that reinforce feelings of helplessness and ultimately contribute to further deterioration over time (Lachman, 1990).

A second related concept is that of coping with stress. This concept can be extremely useful for understanding the individual's approach to the aging process, if aging is considered a "stressor" that serves to mobilize coping strategies. Two major categories of coping mechanisms have been identified in the stress literature: emotion-focused and problem-focused coping (Lazarus & Folkman, 1984). In emotion-focused coping, the individual attempts to change the way he or she thinks about or appraises a stressful situation rather than changing the situation itself. Problem-focused coping involves attempts to reduce stress by changing the stressful situation.

Although locus of control can be distinguished at a conceptual level from coping, in practical terms, the two concepts often serve as codeterminants of adaptational outcomes for the individual. For example, in one large investigation of coping and locus of control, it was found that individuals who believed that they can control their own aging were more likely to use problem-focused coping, and those who believed that they were not in control of their aging were more likely to use emotion-focused coping (Krause, 1986). It has also been found that older adults with an internal locus of control are less likely to engage in the emotion-focused coping strategies of escape-avoidance, self-blame, and hostile reaction (Blanchard-Fields & Irion, 1988).

In the present framework, the decision was made to focus on coping rather than on control. There is considerable overlap in the two constructs, but the concept of control has particular difficulties. There are methodological problems involved in assessing locus of control in the elderly (Lachman, 1986), and there is evidence that control beliefs are poor predictors of relevant behavior, such as adherence to exercise (Williams & Lord, 1995). Conceptually, coping strategies are closer to behavior than are control beliefs, which may serve as an implicit backdrop but not as direct predictors of behavior. Furthermore, greater specificity exists in the measurement of coping, due to the development of instruments that are tailored to particular age-related stressful situations, rather than to general beliefs in the causes of the aging process.

Relation Between Coping and Adaptation

There is a wealth of literature from which to draw in identifying the costs and benefits of emotion- and problem-focused coping as applied to changes associated with the aging process. As a general statement, it appears that individuals who use problem-focused coping strategies are more likely to maintain higher activity levels (Preston & Mansfield, 1984; Speake, 1987) and therefore maximize their physical functioning. These individuals view aging as a challenge to which they apply the coping strategies found to be effective in other life domains (Die, Seelbach, & Sherman, 1987). They are better able to meet their perceived physical needs and tailor their expectations and behavior to fit the changes in their physical identity (Hennessy, 1989). Active involvement in sports or exercise, for some elders, not only promotes physical functioning but can serve as an important coping mechanism (O'Brien & Conger, 1991). Coping style also seems to be related to reactions to a variety of physical health problems (Clark, Becker, Janz, & Lorig, 1991). For example, improved levels of coping and the use of social supports (in part, a problem-focused coping measure), were found to be predictive of hospital readmissions for a sample of elderly cardiac patients (Berkman, Millar, Holmes, & Bonander, 1991). Training in problem-focused coping methods proved helpful in facilitating pain management and reducing anxiety among older individuals with chronic knee pain (Fry & Wong, 1991). Similarly, the use of problem-focused coping was found in one study of people recovering from hip fracture to enable individuals to take advantage of rehabilitative methods that assisted in their recovery. As a consequence of more adaptive coping strategies, these hip fracture patients were less likely to experience depressive symptoms that would further have lowered their perceived functional recovery (Roberto, 1992). Along similar lines, older individuals who can be encouraged to overcome anxiety over their physique and participate in exercise can show beneficial effects in body composition as well as reductions in their concerns over appearance (McAuley, Bane, Rudolph, & Lox, 1995).

As the cases of rehabilitation and exercise illustrate, the relationship between coping and health can be seen as cyclical. Individuals who successfully use coping strategies to manage stress may actually experience improved physical functioning. In one investigation, individuals reporting high levels of stress were found to have lower ratios of critical immune system markers (McNaughton, Smith, Patterson, & Grant, 1990). Active efforts to reduce stress through seeking social support or physical exercise can have physiological advantages in terms of improved immune system functioning (Fiatarone et al., 1989; Thomas, Goodwin, & Goodwin, 1985) which in turn lowers vulnerability to other physical diseases.

In contrast to the positive effects of problem-focused coping is evidence of the deleterious effects of emotion-focused coping on psychological and physical health outcomes. Individuals who use avoidance as a coping strategy are also likely to report higher levels of physical and psychological symptoms, depression, and psychosocial difficulties (Aldwin & Revenson, 1987; Billings & Moos, 1981; Bombardier, D'Amico, & Jordan, 1990; Felton, Revenson, & Hinrichsen, 1984) even continuing for months after the stressful situation has subsided (Smith, Patterson, & Grant, 1990). However, emotion-focused coping can have positive adaptive value if the situation is completely out of one's control, or if excessive rumination is harmful to improvement. As long as the individual follows prescribed treatment, the outcome may still be positive. As Lazarus (1981) points out, when faced with an uncontrollable stressor, direct confrontation is not always necessary for successful coping. In fact, in some cases denial may actually be adaptive (Pearlin & Schooler, 1978). The use of denial as a coping mechanism becomes maladaptive, however, if it prevents the individual from taking action that is beneficial to recovery. In diseases or other health problems that require vigilant attention to bodily signs, such as cancer, kidney failure, or diabetes, coping by denial can lead to the development of life-threatening conditions.

Interaction of Identity and Coping

Although the identity and coping models provide insight into the ways that individuals adapt to the aging process, neither model alone may be sufficient to account for individual variations in behavioral and emotional reactions to the changes in physical functioning and health associated with aging. In existing research on coping, the amount of variance accounted for leaves considerable room for the input of variables related to identity and the self. As a way of gaining a more comprehensive prediction of variations in response to challenges to physical identity associated with the aging process, it is possible to combine the dimension of problem- vs. emotion-focused coping with the dimension of identity assimilation and accommodation. Such an approach produces a fourfold matrix to account for adaptation to the physical aging process. Specific behavioral and adaptive predictions can be made for individuals within each of the four cells of this matrix. For the purpose of the present discussion, it is assumed that individuals can be classified on the basis of the predominant identity processes they use in relation to age-related experiences (Whitbourne, 1987) and that they can be classified in terms of predominant coping style. However, it is unlikely that "pure" forms exist, and it is more reasonable to assume that these dimensions are continuous within individuals.

Moving through this hypothetical matrix, specific behavioral predictions can be made for each of the four pure types. Individuals who use identity assimilation and emotion-focused coping are likely to deny the relevance of aging to their identities and, at the same time, engage in few behaviors intended to offset or compensate for aging changes (Felton & Revenson, 1987). Adverse consequences are more likely to occur for aging individuals who take an assimilative approach to age- or disease-related bodily changes and use emotion-focused coping. They may find it more comfortable not to think about the diagnosis or problem and instead go on with life as usual, not changing their identities in response to the knowledge that they are suffering a major change in health or functioning or even have a potentially terminal illness. Consequently, they will not take active efforts to protect and promote their body's ability to fight the condition or disease. They may manage to avoid confronting their problems by severely restricting their lifestyles (Aldwin, 1991), and in the process exacerbate processes of decline in functions that would otherwise respond to the UIOLI principle. On the other hand, these individuals may be protected from the "depressive realism" that can reduce the strivings of accommodative persons who confront and recognize their limitations (Hooker, 1992). They may use ego-enhancing strategies of making optimistic attributions (Heckhausen & Baltes, 1991) to compare themselves favorably with others and maintain a self that is invulnerable to the effects of aging (Baltes & Baltes, 1990).

Individuals who use identity assimilation and problem-focused coping would be predicted to become actively involved in behavioral controls that could serve a preventative or compensatory function with regard to aging. However, they would not integrate into their identities the knowledge that their body has changed in fundamental ways or faces severe health threats. Thus, at the behavioral level, the individual is engaging in appropriate health maintenance and rehabilitative strategies, and is able to take advantage of these strategies in terms of improvements in physical health. However, the individual has chosen not to give particular thought or emphasis to the implications for identity of the problem or disorder. Such a group would correspond to the "foreclosed" categorization of Marcia's identity status (Marcia, 1966) framework for adolescents, in which the individual arrives at a set of identity commitments without engaging in a process of exploration or "identity crisis." Indeed, this style of approaching psychosocial issues related to ego integrity was observed in a study of community elders (Walaskay, Whitbourne, & Nehrke, 1983–84), in which a group of "foreclosed" older persons were identified. These elders had not struggled with existential questions regarding their mortality, but had nevertheless gone ahead and made funeral arrangements, planning the event as if it were a social occasion. Behaviorally, these individuals appeared to have achieved ego integrity, or resolution of their feelings about death, but had not processed these feelings at a deeper psychological level.

Identity accommodation may occur in conjunction with either problem- or emotion-focused coping. Individuals who tend to use accommodation to the point that they overreact to a diagnosis or physical disorder may suffer the same adverse consequences as those who deny through assimilation the significance of physical changes or illness. Such individuals believe that what they do in reaction to these changes or diseases will make no difference, and through the emotion-focused strategies of distancing, denial, or avoidance, fail to take the necessary steps to maximize their functioning (Lachman et al., 1995; Lohr, Essex, & Klein, 1988; Roberto, 1992; Woodward & Wallston, 1987). Their emotions are likely to be highly dysphoric (Rapkin & Fischer, 1992), and they feel a loss of the ability to control or predict the future course of their physical development or changes in health condition (Baum & Boxley, 1983).

Individuals who use accommodation but also take steps to confront changes in physical status or health through problem-focused coping may be likely to take extremely active steps to help reduce their symptoms or the progress of the disease. It is probable that such individuals feel that they are able to control the events in their lives, leading them to be less likely to use palliative coping strategies in favor of ones that address the situation (Blanchard-Fields & Irion, 1989). These individuals would react to disease or physical changes by harnessing their available resources, and they would actively seek further medical treatment as well as less proven alternate treatments. They might be preoccupied with their bodies, but at the same time they would use every opportunity to talk to others and get help, using coping strategies such as confrontation, seeking social support, planful problem solving, and positive reappraisal. If they have a particular disease, they may "become" the disease, which then becomes a major focus of their lives. The risk of this type of coping in combination with identity accommodation is that although the individual adjusts well to the physical identity stressor by taking active steps, he or she may ruminate excessively about the disease.

Research that is currently underway using an expanded Identity and Experiences Scale which includes a scale assessing balance in conjunction with the Ways of Coping scale to measure coping strategies. This research will test the combined identity-coping model, using health-related behaviors as the dependent variable. It is predicted that healthy adaptation within this model involves the balance between assimilation and accommodation in terms of the impact of age changes or disease on identity (Baltes & Staudinger, 1993; Ryff, 1989, 1991). Flexibility of coping style would further promote positive adaptation. Thus, the individuals within the "middle" of the matrix would be assumed to show the most favorable outcomes with regard to the physical aging process. When problems arise, such individuals can focus on the physical identity stressor and are open to seeking help from others, but they avoid being preoccupied with the illness when necessary in order to focus on other concerns, such as family or work involvements. This ability to adapt to the challenges of aging reflects what Clark and Anderson (1967) described three decades ago as characteristic of "successful" aging and, more recently, has been identified as a protective factor against depression in later adulthood (Brandtstadter & Rothermund, 1994).

In this discussion of identity and coping, it is important to emphasize that the individual's use of these processes is not fixed across the span of the aging years. Individuals may use a variety of coping strategies that complement or offset their identity styles. Furthermore, assuming that there is a relationship between identity processes and coping, and given the emphasis in the coping literature on the variable nature of coping processes (Folkman & Lazarus, 1980; Folkman, Lazarus, Gruen, & DeLongis, 1986) it may be more reasonable to propose that the identity processes are used within the same individual on different occasions, or even within the same individual on the same occasion (Brandtstadter & Renner, 1990). As is true for coping strategies, individuals may use one, then another, of the identity processes in their attempts to adapt to changes in the body's appearance, functioning, and health.

ROLE OF CULTURAL STEREOTYPES

A final consideration in this discussion is the interaction of identity and age-related changes in physical and cognitive functioning with the role of cultural stereotypes and myths about the aging process. Age-related norms and expectations within Western society emphasize the uncontrollable losses that accumulate in the later adult years (Heckhausen & Baltes, 1991; Krueger & Heckhausen, 1993). The degree to which individuals ascribe to negative stereotypes about the aging process can have a detrimental impact on the motivation to cope actively with age-related changes (Ryff, 1991). To the extent that individuals come to hold these beliefs, they will be more likely to adopt the passive approaches involved in emotion-focused coping strategies. Further reinforcing this passivity are interactions with younger adults in which the older person is treated in a patronizing, infantilizing manner. Such treatment can lower the individual's feelings of personal control and self-efficacy (Whitbourne & Wills, 1993).

In this regard, it is also important to consider identity in relation to the "isms" of racism, sexism, and ageism. The individual's racial or ethnic identity and gender may be seen as influencing health behaviors to the extent that what is considered appropriate for one's age, sex, and cultural group may determine whether or not the individual maintains a sufficiently high activity level. For example, elderly women of Asian origin are unlikely to see themselves as active or athletic, given their culture's expectations that women are traditionally feminine and dependent. Culture can also influence the individual's diet in that different cultures emphasize different types of food and food preparation measures. In Asian culture, low-fat foods and a diet high in vegetables are a plus in helping older individuals avoid diseases related to high intake of cholesterol and low intake of natural fiber. Other cultures emphasize less healthy foods, such as the matzo balls, cream cheese, fatty cold cuts and sour cream of ethnic Jewish food. Many traditional ethnic foods, ranging from Mexican to French to Southern Italian, also involve reliance on cheeses or other rich dairy products, fatty meats, eggs, and chocolate. To the extent that the individual has been raised on these foods, and continues to eat and prepare them, dietary problems may be expected to ensue in later adulthood.

Health-seeking behaviors may also be influenced by the individual's gender, socialization, and cultural or ethnic background. Those men who believe in a traditionally stoic approach to physical or psychological problems will resist seeking help, as it may seem to be a sign of weakness. In various ethnic cultures, the need for professional help, in particular, may be regarded as non-normative, and rather than use the services of a mental health clinician, the individual feels it is more appropriate to rely on the family for support. Beyond the level of attitudes is the individual's ability to pay for health services. With changes in Medicare and Medicaid looming on the horizon, it becomes even more likely that individuals with limited economic resources will be unable to pay for help, even when the need is acknowledged.

Moving beyond the sphere of health are stressors within the environment whose presence influences the course of psychological development in later adulthood. Again, these stressors may be seen as linked to class, race, and ethnicity. First and foremost, poverty forces the older person to live in urban areas, such as ghettos or public housing. Living within these environments poses a direct threat to the individual's physical well-being, as such environments create the risk of victimization. Not only are there subjective effects in terms of the older individual becoming limited in what he or she can do to compensate for age-related changes, then, but the real effects of the environment can create severe challenges to adjustment in old age.

CONCLUDING OBSERVATIONS

In this chapter, I have attempted to outline a broad model with varying components to describe, explain, and predict interactions between individual identity processes and age-related physical and psychological changes. The identity model provides a rich descriptive metaphor for understanding the individual's internal and external adaptations to the aging process. Furthermore, with the development of the Identity and Experiences Scale, it will be possible to investigate individual differences in primary identity style of mode of relating to the aging process and the implications of these differences for health and preventative behaviors. The identity model also serves a unique function within the personality and social psychology domains in that it provides an elaborated mechanism for describing how individuals affect and are affected by their experiences relevant to the aging process. With its appropriation of concepts from Piagetian theory, the model also provides a developmental perspective with specified predictions for the interaction between the self and experiences in adulthood. Further research on the identity model will involve continued refinement of the IES and study of its relation to theoretically relevant constructs. In this work, it will be possible to unlock some of the secrets of successful aging shown by elders who creatively approach the construction and reconstruction of their identities throughout life.

REFERENCES

Aldwin, C. M. (1991). Does age affect the stress and coping process? Implications of age differences in perceived control. *Journal of Gerontology: Psychological Sciences, 46*, P174–180.

Aldwin, C. M., & Revenson, T. A. (1987). Does coping help? A reexamination of the relation between coping and mental health. *Journal of Personality and Social Psychology, 53*, 337–348.

Baltes, P. B., & Baltes, M. M. (1990). Psychological perspectives on successful aging: A model of selective optimization with compensation. In P. B. Baltes & M. M. Baltes (Eds.), *Successful aging: Perspectives from the behavioral sciences* (pp. 1–34). New York: Cambridge University Press.

Baltes, P. B., & Staudinger, U. M. (1993). The search for a psychology of wisdom. *Current Directions in Psychological Science, 2,* 75–80.

Baum, S. K., & Boxley, R. L. (1983). Age identification in the elderly. *Gerontologist, 23,* 532–537.

Beck, A. T., Rush, A. J., Shaw, B. F., & Emery, G. (1975). *Cognitive therapy of depression.* New York: Guilford.

Berkman, B., Millar, S., Holmes, W., & Bonander, E. (1991). Predicting elderly cardiac patients at risk for readmission. *Social Work in Health Care, 16*(1), 21–38.

Billings, A. G., & Moos, R. H. (1981). The role of coping responses in attenuating the stress of life events. *Journal of Behavioral Medicine, 4,* 139–157.

Blanchard-Fields, F., & Irion, J. (1989). Coping strategies from the perspective of two developmental markers: Age and social reasoning. *Journal of Genetic Psychology, 149,* 141–151.

Blanchard-Fields, F., & Irion, J. C. (1988). The relation between locus of control and coping in two contexts: Age as a moderator variable. *Psychology and Aging, 3,* 197–203.

Bocknek, G., & Perna, F. (1994). Studies in self-representation beyond childhood. In J. M. Masling & R. F. Bornstein (Eds.), *Empirical perspectives on object relations theory* (pp. 29–58). Washington, DC: American Psychological Association.

Bombardier, C., D'Amico, C., & Jordan, J. (1990). The relationship of appraisal and coping to chronic illness adjustment. *Behavior Research and Therapy, 28,* 297–304.

Brandtstadter, J., & Renner, G. (1990). Tenacious goal pursuit and flexible goal adjustment: Explication and age-related analysis of assimilative and accommodative strategies in coping. *Psychology and Aging, 5,* 58–67.

Brandtstadter, J., & Rothermund, K. (1994). Self-percepts of control in middle and later adulthood: Buffering losses by rescaling goals. *Psychology and Aging, 9,* 265–273.

Carstensen, L. L., & Turk-Charles, S. (1994). The salience of emotion across the adult life span. *Psychology and Aging, 9,* 259–264.

Cavanaugh, J. C., & Green, E. E. (1990). I believe, therefore I can: Self-efficacy beliefs in memory aging. In E. A. Lovelace (Ed.), *Aging and cognition: Mental processes, self-awareness, and interventions* (pp. 189–230). Amsterdam: North Holland.

Clark, M., & Anderson, B. (1967). *Culture and aging: An anthropological study of older Americans.* Springfield, IL: Charles C. Thomas.

Clark, N. M., Becker, M. H., Janz, N. K., & Lorig, K. (1991). Self-management of chronic disease by older adults: A review and questions for research. *Journal of Aging and Health, 3,* 3–27.

Die, A. H., Seelbach, W. C., & Sherman, G. D. (1987). Achievement motivation, achieving styles, and morale in the elderly. *Psychology and Aging, 2,* 407–408.

Dittman-Kohli, F. (1990). Possibilities and constraints for the construction of meaning in old age. *Ageing and Society, 10,* 279–294.

Dowd, J. J. (1990). Ever since Durkheim: The socialization of human development. *Human Development, 33,* 138–159.

Elliott, E., & Lachman, M. E. (1989). Enhancing memory by modifying control beliefs, attributions, and performance goals in the elderly. In P. S. Fry (Ed.), *Psychology of helplessness and control and attributions of helplessness and control in the aged* (pp. 339–367). Amsterdam: North Holland.

Erikson, E. H. (1963). *Childhood and society* (2nd ed.). New York: Norton.

Erikson, E. H., Erikson, J., & Kivnick, H. Q. (1986). *Vital involvement in old age.* New York: Norton.

Felton, B. J., & Revenson, T. A. (1987). Age differences in coping with chronic illness. *Psychology and Aging, 2,* 164–170.

Felton, B., Revenson, T., & Hinrichsen, G. (1984). Stress and coping in the explanation of psychological adjustment among chronically ill adults. *Social Science and Medicine, 18,* 889–898.

Fiatarone, M. A., Morley, J. E., Bloom, E. T., Benton, D., Solomon, G. F., & Makinodan, T. (1989). The effect of exercise on natural killer cell activity in young and old subjects. *Journal of Gerontology: Medical Sciences, 44,* M37–45.

Folkman, S., Bernstein, L., & Lazarus, R. S. (1987). Stress processes and the misuse of drugs in older adults. *Psychology and Aging, 2*(4), 366–374.

Folkman, S., & Lazarus, R. S. (1980). An analysis of coping in a middle-aged community sample. *Journal of Health and Social Behavior, 21,* 219–239.

Folkman, S., Lazarus, R. S., Gruen, R., & DeLongis, A. (1986). Appraisal, coping, health status, and psychological symptoms. *Journal of Personality and Social Psychology, 50,* 571–579.

Fox, K. R., & Corbin, C. B. (1989). The physical self-perception profile: Development and preliminary validation. *Journal of Sport and Exercise Psychology, 11,* 408–430.

Fry, P. S., & Wong, P. T. (1991). Pain management training in the elderly: Matching interventions with subjects' coping styles. *Stress Medicine, 7*(2), 93–98.

Grover, D. R., & Hertzog, C. (1991). Relationships between intellectual control beliefs and psychometric intelligence in adulthood. *Journal of Gerontology: Psychological Sciences, 46,* P109–115.

Harris, M. B. (1994). Growing old gracefully: Age concealment and gender. *Journal of Gerontology: Psychological Sciences, 49,* P149–158.

Hart, E. A., Leary, M. R., & Rejeski, W. J. (1989). The measurement of social physique anxiety. *Journal of Sport and Exercise Psychology, 11*, 94–104.

Heckhausen, J., & Baltes, P. B. (1991). Perceived controllability of expected psychological change across adulthood and old age. *Journal of Gerontology: Psychological Sciences, 46*, 165–173.

Heckhausen, J., & Schulz, R. (1995). A life-span theory of control. *Psychological Review, 102*, 284–304.

Heidrich, S. M., & Ryff, C. D. (1993a). Physical and mental health in later life: The self-system as mediator. *Psychology and Aging, 8*, 327–338.

Heidrich, S. M., & Ryff, C. D. (1993b). The role of social comparison processes in the psychological adaptation of elderly adults. *Journal of Gerontology: Psychological Sciences, 48*, P127–137.

Hennessy, C. H. (1989). Culture in the use, care, and control of the aging body. *Journal of Aging Studies, 3*, 39–54.

Hooker, K. (1992). Possible selves and perceived health in older adults and college students. *Journal of Gerontology: Psychological Sciences, 47*, P85–95.

Hooker, K., & Kaus, C. R. (1994). Health-related possible selves in young and middle adulthood. *Psychology and Aging, 9*, 126–133.

Kiecolt, K. J. (1994). Stress and the decision to change oneself: A theoretical model. *Social Psychology Quarterly, 57*, 49–63.

Krause, N. (1986). Stress and coping: Reconceptualizing the role of locus of control beliefs. *Journal of Gerontology, 41*, 617–622.

Krueger, J., & Heckhausen, J. (1993). Personality development across the adult life span: Subjective conceptions vs. cross-sectional contrasts. *Journal of Gerontology: Psychological Sciences, 48*, P100–108.

Labouvie-Vief, G., Hakim-Larson, J., & Hobart, C. J. (1987). Age, ego level, and the life-span development of coping and defense processes. *Psychology and Aging, 2*, 286–293.

Lachman, M., Bandura, M., Weaver, S., & Elliott, E. (1995). Assessing memory control beliefs: The Memory Controllability Inventory. *Aging and Cognition, 2*, 67–84.

Lachman, M. E. (1986). Locus of control in aging research. *Psychology and Aging, 1*, 34–40.

Lachman, M. E. (1990). When bad things happen to older people: Age differences in attributional style. *Psychology and Aging, 5*, 607–609.

Lazarus, R. (1981). The stress and coping paradigm. In C. Eisdorfer (Ed.), *Models for clinical psychopathology* (pp. 177–214). New York: Spectrum.

Lazarus, R. S., & Folkman, S. (1984). *Stress, appraisal, and coping.* New York: Springer Publishing Co.

Lohr, M. J., Essex, M. J., & Klein, M. H. (1988). The relationships of coping responses to physical health status and life satisfaction among older women. *Journal of Gerontology: Psychological Sciences, 43*, P54–60.

Marcia, J. E. (1966). Development and validation of ego-identity status. *Journal of Personality and Social Psychology, 3*, 551–558.

Markus, H., & Nurius, P. (1986). Possible selves. *American Psychologist, 41*, 954–969.

McAuley, E., Bane, S. M., Rudolph, D. L., & Lox, C. L. (1995). Physique anxiety and exercise in middle-aged adults. *Journal of Gerontology: Psychological Sciences, 50B*, P229–P235.

McCrae, R. R., & Costa, P. T. (1988). Age, personality, and the spontaneous self-concept. *Journal of Gerontology: Social Sciences, 43*, S177–185.

McCrae, R. R., & Costa, P. T. J. (1990). *Personality in adulthood.* New York: Guilford.

McNaughton, M. E., Smith, L. W., Patterson, T. L., & Grant, I. (1990). Stress, social support, coping resources, and immune status in elderly women. *Journal of Nervous and Mental Disease, 178*, 460–461.

O'Brien, S. J., & Conger, P. R. (1991). No time to look back: Approaching the finish line of life's course. *International Journal of Aging and Human Development, 33*(1), 75–87.

Pearlin, L., & Schooler, C. (1978). The structure of coping. *Journal of Health and Social Behavior, 19*, 2–21.

Piaget, J. (1975/1977). *The development of thought* (A. Rosin, Trans.). Oxford: Basil Blackwell.

Preston, D. B., & Mansfield, P. K. (1984). An exploration of stressful life events, illness, and coping among the rural elderly. *Gerontologist, 24*, 490–494.

Rapkin, B. D., & Fischer, K. (1992). Framing the construct of life satisfaction in terms of older adults' personal goals. *Psychology and Aging, 7*, 138–149.

Roberto, K. (1992). Coping strategies of older women with hip fractures: Resources and outcomes. *Journal of Gerontology: Psychological Sciences, 47*, P21–26.

Ryff, C. D. (1989). In the eye of the beholder: Views of psychological well-being among middle-aged and older adults. *Psychology and Aging, 4*, 195–210.

Ryff, C. D. (1991). Possible selves in adulthood and old age: A tale of shifting horizons. *Psychology and Aging, 6*, 286–295.

Ryff, C. D., Lee, Y. H., Essex, M. J., & Schmutte, P. S. (1994). My children and me: Midlife evaluations of grown children and self. *Psychology and Aging, 9*, 195–205.

Smith, L. W., Patterson, T. L., & Grant, I. (1990). Avoidant coping predicts psychological disturbance in the elderly. *Journal of Nervous and Mental Disease, 178*, 525–530.

Speake, D. L. (1987). Health promotion activities and the well elderly. *Health Values: Achieving High Level Wellness, 11*, 25–30.

Staudinger, U. M., Smith, J., & Baltes, P. B. (1993). Wisdom-related knowledge in a life review task: Age differences and role of professional specialization. *Psychology and Aging, 7*, 271–281.

Thomas, P. D., Goodwin, J. M., & Goodwin, J. W. (1985). Effect of social support on stress-related changes in cholesterol, uric acid level, and immune function in an elderly sample. *American Journal of Psychiatry, 142*, 735–737.

Walaskay, M., Whitbourne, S. K., & Nehrke, M. F. (1983–84). Construction and validation of an ego-integrity status interview. *International Journal of Aging and Human Development, 18*, 61–72.

Whitbourne, S. K. (1986a). *Adult development*. New York: Praeger.

Whitbourne, S. K. (1986b). *The me I know: A study of adult identity*. New York: Springer Verlag.

Whitbourne, S. K. (1987). Personality development in adulthood and old age: Relationships among identity style, health, and well-being. In K. W. Schaie (Ed.), *Annual Review of Gerontology and Geriatrics* (pp. 189–216). New York: Springer Publishing Company.

Whitbourne, S. K. (1989). Comments on Lachman's "Personality and aging at the crossroads: Beyond stability versus change". In K. W. Schaie & C. Schooler (Eds.), *Social structure and aging: Psychological processes* (pp. 191–198). Hillsdale, NJ: Erlbaum.

Whitbourne, S. K. (1996). *The aging individual*. New York: Springer Publishing Company.

Whitbourne, S. K., & Connolly, L. A. (1998). Theories and models of mid-life development. In S. B. Willis & J. Reid (Eds.), *Middle aging: Development in the third quarter of life* (pp. 25–45). San Diego CA: Academic Press.

Whitbourne, S. K., & Wills, K.-J. (1993). Psychological issues in institutional care of the aged. In S. B. Goldsmith (Ed.), *Long-term care administration handbook* (pp. 19–32). Gaithersburg, MD: Aspen.

Williams, P., & Lord, S. R. (1995). Predictors of adherence to a structured exercise program for older women. *Psychology and Aging, 10*, 617–624.

Woodward, N. J., & Wallston, B. S. (1987). Age and health care beliefs: Self-efficacy as a mediator of low desire for control. *Psychology and Aging, 2*, 3–8.

CHAPTER 6

Self-Development in Adulthood and Aging: The Role of Critical Life Events

Manfred Diehl

INTRODUCTION

Life-span developmental psychology proposes that human development occurs from conception to death and that it involves the intricate interweaving of biological, sociocultural, and psychological processes (Baltes, 1987; Baltes, Reese, & Lipsitt, 1980; Dannefer & Perlmutter, 1990; Erikson, 1959; Thomae, 1979). This perspective has opened researchers' views of developmental processes in middle and later adulthood and has influenced the inquiry into adult development in at least three important ways.

First, after decades of a deficit and decrement orientation toward adult development, most developmentalists have abandoned this orientation and have begun to study the gains and progressions that may occur during the adult years (Baltes, 1987; Brim & Kagan, 1980; Helson & Roberts, 1994; Labouvie-Vief, 1977, 1982; Schaie, 1994; Thomae, 1979). Second, unlike traditional developmentalists whose theories have been strongly influenced

I would like to thank Lise M. Youngblade, Gisela Labouvie-Vief, Carol D. Ryff, and Victor Marshall for their thoughtful comments on previous versions of this chapter. Of course, none of them bears any responsibility for any shortcomings that may remain.

by biological conceptions of growth and maturation (Harris, 1957; Wohlwill, 1973), adult developmentalists have redirected their focus of inquiry from biological to psychological and sociocultural determinants of human development (Baltes, 1987; Brandtstädter, 1984; Dannefer & Perlmutter, 1990), and to the dynamic interplay of biological, psychological, and sociocultural factors (Baltes, Lindenberger, & Staudinger, 1998; Riegel, 1973). Third, in contrast to more traditional theories of development, life-span developmental theory conceptualizes individuals as "*producers of their own development*" (Brandtstädter, 1984; Labouvie-Vief, 1981; Lerner, 1984; Lerner & Busch-Rossnagel, 1981; Riegel, 1975, 1976a). Although some sociologists argue that individuals with different positions in the social structure have greater or lesser affordances to produce their own development (see Dowd, 1990), this view of the role of the individual in development is important with regard to adult development, because adults are seen as being actively involved in the creation of opportunity structures (Marshall, 1995) for their own development. This creation of opportunity structures may occur either in a proactive mode, with the objective of optimizing development, or in a reactive mode, responding to situations that pose a risk or threat to the individual's development and well-being (Labouvie-Vief, 1981; Riegel, 1975).

Thus, at the heart of the life-span approach to human development is the emphasis on the dynamic interrelatedness of the developing individual and the changing sociocultural context (Bronfenbrenner, 1979; Lerner, 1984). The individual is a priori seen as being influenced by the changing sociocultural context, yet at the same time contributes actively to the changing of this context (Brandtstädter, 1984; Labouvie-Vief, 1981; Lerner, 1984; Lerner & Busch-Rossnagel, 1981; Riegel, 1975, 1976a; Ryff, 1987). Acceptance of these propositions of life-span developmental psychology implies that developmental processes during middle and later adulthood cannot be discussed without reference to the micro- and macro-structures of the sociocultural context in which they occur (Dannefer, 1984; Marshall, 1995).

This chapter focuses on critical life events and their role in linking adults' development to micro- and macro-structures of the surrounding sociocultural context. Although life events have been recognized by several theorists as major determinants of life-span development (see Baltes et al., 1980; Brim & Ryff, 1980; Filipp, 1981; Hultsch & Plemons, 1979), I will argue that developmentalists, so far, have looked at life events and their impact on individual development in a rather global way. In contrast, I will argue for a more focused approach with regard to two specific issues.

First, I will argue that scholars of adult development should abandon their somewhat simplistic assumption that life events per se are a developmental force, but should focus on specific types of critical life events. In particular, I will argue that there are two types of critical life events that are of relevance for adults' self-development. These types include events whose occurrence is either self-determined (i.e., high controllability) or beyond a person's control (i.e., low controllability).

Second, I will advocate that researchers should make a greater effort to examine how these types of critical life events are linked to the micro- and macro-structures of individuals' sociocultural context. Specifically, I will try to show that critical life events are frequently tied to a persons' social roles or to their position within a given social structure and, thus, are a means for examining the linkage between individual development and the larger sociocultural context (Marshall, 1995; Ryff, 1987). Both arguments are presented here separately merely for analytical reasons. In reality, the likelihood of the occurrence of self-determined and externally controlled life events varies greatly depending on the socioeconomic status and the social position of the individual (McLeod & Kessler, 1990; Pearlin, Menaghan, Lieberman, & Mullan, 1981). Thus, whether a life event is self-determined or not and what kind of material and social resources an individual has available for coping with a particular life event becomes a more complex question when social structure and sociocultural context are brought to the fore (Dannefer, 1984; Dowd, 1990; Ryff, 1987).

LIFE-SPAN DEVELOPMENT AND CRITICAL LIFE EVENTS

A Triarchic Model of Developmental Influences

Within the theoretical framework of life-span developmental psychology, non-normative or critical life events are considered one of three major forces that influence development across the life span (Baltes et al., 1980; Baltes et al., 1998). As Figure 6.1 shows, besides normative age-graded (i.e., biological and environmental determinants with a strong relation with chronological age) and normative history-graded influences (i.e., biological and environmental determinants associated with historical time and contexts) which are, in a given culture, common to most individuals' developmental history, non-normative or critical life events are seen as the

Figure 6.1

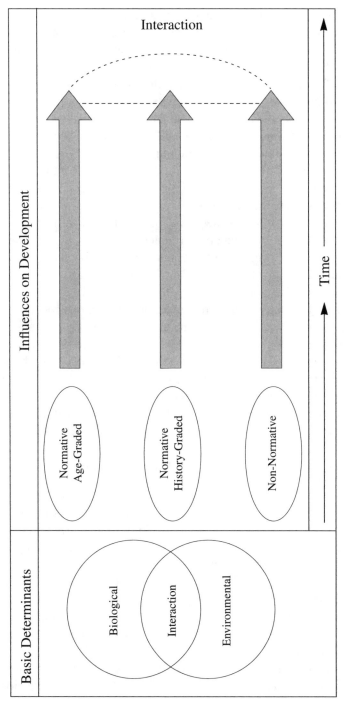

Representation of the operation of three major influence systems on life-span development: normative age-graded, normative history-graded, and non-normative life events. These influence systems interact and differ in their combinatorial profile for different individuals and for different behaviors.

From "Life-Span Developmental Psychology," by P. B. Baltes, H. W. Reese, and L. P. Lipsitt, 1980, Annual Review of Psychology, 31, p. 75. Copyright 1980 by Annual Reviews Inc. Reprinted with permission.

third major force in shaping individuals' development across the life span. Non-normative or critical life events are those kinds of events that "do not occur in any normative age-graded or history-graded manner for most individuals" (Baltes et al., 1980, p. 76). Thus, the attribute of "non-normativeness" refers to the lack of interindividual homogeneity in the occurrence and patterning of the events, whereas the attribute "critical" refers to the impact that the events have on individuals' development.

As Baltes et al. (1998) have noted, critical life events may become especially powerful developmental forces in adulthood and old age because they have great potential for creating conditions of high uncontrollability and unpredictability, thereby challenging a person's adaptation and resilience. This is even the case when unexpected and unplanned life events are positive in nature. Furthermore, Baltes et al. (1980) proposed that since evolutionary-based genetic influences on human development decline with age, non-normative life events are likely to become more salient contributors to development and developmental variation during adulthood than during any other segment of the life span.

This proposition is consistent with two major observations concerning human development. First, development in adulthood and old age seems to be more multidirectional than in childhood and adolescence (Baltes et al., 1980; Baltes et al., 1998). Second, several longitudinal studies (Eichorn, Clausen, Haan, Honzik, & Mussen, 1981; Lehr & Thomae, 1987; Schaie, 1996) have shown that intra- and interindividual variability tends to increase with age. Both of these observations hint at the role of individual life experiences and non-normative influences in shaping individual development.

A Dialectical View of Adult Development

Incorporating critical life events as a developmental force in adulthood and old age is also consistent with a contextualistic-dialectical model of adult development (Lerner, 1984; Riegel, 1975, 1976a). In the early and mid-seventies, Riegel (1975, 1976a, 1976b) criticized the existing paradigms in developmental psychology as being too static and equilibrium-oriented. As an alternative, he brought forward two major propositions. First, he suggested that developmental psychologists direct their attention to individuals' behavior in real world settings. Second, he suggested that developmentalists focus on contradictions and discontinuities as sources of continued development.

With his first proposition, Riegel rejected most developmentalists' preference for studying human behavior in controlled settings and in isolation from the existing social and ecological conditions (see also Bronfenbrenner, 1979). Instead, he advocated that they direct their efforts "toward the concrete actions of the individual in a concrete social world" (Riegel, 1976a, p. 690). With his second proposition, Riegel (1976a, 1976b) challenged developmentalists' preference for stable traits and states of equilibrium, which he saw deeply rooted in Western thinking and strongly influenced by Piaget's (1950, 1952) theory of cognitive development. In particular, Riegel (1975, 1976b) criticized Piaget's theory of cognitive development as insufficient to account for changes during adulthood and aging, because Piaget emphasized the removal of conceptual contradictions and the attainment of a state of equilibrium as individuals' essential developmental task. Instead, Riegel (1975) argued that unlike children and adolescents, adults "need to achieve a new apprehension and an effective use of contradictions in operations and thoughts. Contradictions should no longer be regarded as deficiencies that have to be straightened out by formal thinking but, in a confirmative manner, as the very basis of all activities" (p. 101).

Thus, Riegel (1975, 1976b) suggested that developmentalists focus on states of disequilibrium and discontinuity as constructive confrontations that may serve as impetus for further development rather than disruptions and deficiencies. More formally, Riegel (1976a, 1976b) argued that developmental progressions are initiated by asynchronies among four major dimensions of development: (1) inner-biological, (2) individual-psychological, (3) cultural-sociological, and (4) outer-physical. Whenever two or more of these dimensions are out of step, a state of disequilibrium exists and presents the individual with a "constructive confrontation," a "critical choice point," or an "existential challenge," creating the potential for further development.

Critical life events clearly meet Riegel's requirement of a developmental asynchrony since one of their defining characteristics is that they disrupt or challenge an individual's established person-environment fit (Filipp, 1981). For example, a crisis along the inner-biological dimension, such as a severe illness or incapacitation, is rarely synchronized with the individual-psychological and/or the social-cultural dimension and very often challenges the psychological (i.e., subjective well-being) and social adaptation (i.e., social support system) of the person(s) involved. As a matter of fact, the resultant discrepancies between the inner-biological, the individual-psychological, and the social-cultural dimension will not only reflect differences in biological and psychological resiliency, but the interaction of biological and psychological factors with choice options that are determined by an individual's position within the social structure (e.g., social class membership, ethnicity, socioeconomic status). Similarly, changes in a person's interpersonal or social life, such as a divorce or a change in employment, are likely to require synchronizing efforts along the individual-psychological (i.e., coping with feelings of failure or guilt, coping with new demands) or outer-physical dimension (i.e., relocating to a new place of living). Regardless of the dimensions between which the asynchronies exist, Riegel postulates that individuals will engage in attempts to synchronize the developmental dimensions either through direct actions or through cognitive coping strategies, thus using the disequilibrium as an impetus for change and development.

Although Riegel's dialectical model of human development has been of great heuristic value (Lerner & Busch-Rossnagel, 1981), a cautionary remark also seems to be in order. From a sociological view, Riegel's notion of disequilibria as "constructive confrontations" and "critical choice points" seems to imply that each and every individual within a given sociocultural context has an equal opportunity for positive growth and development. Such a notion, however, appears to be overly optimistic, because it is well documented that there are great differences in individuals' choice options and coping repertoires depending on their position within the social order (Kessler, 1979; Wheaton, 1990). Thus, whether a disequilibrium will be an opportunity for growth and development or a serious threat to a person's well-being depends to some extent on the choice options that are associated with that person's position within the social structure.

Individuals as Proactive Producers and Reactive Responders in Developmental Processes

In contrast to traditional theories of development, life-span developmental theory has also changed researchers' perspective about the role that the individual plays in his or her own development. In particular, life-span developmentalists conceptualize individuals as active, intentional, and planful agents who are influenced by the sociocultural contexts in which they live but who are also involved in shaping these sociocultural contexts (Ford, 1987). Thus, individuals are viewed as "producers of their own development" (Brandtstädter, 1984; Ford, 1987; Labouvie-Vief, 1981; Lerner, 1984; Lerner & Busch-Rossnagel, 1981).

In essence, conceptualizing individuals as producers of their own development means that, within the confines of the opportunity structures defined by their position within a society's social order, individuals "try to actively control their development in functional aspects—such as bodily conditions, sensory functioning, social and cognitive competencies—that, in turn, are important boundary conditions of personal action potentials at a respective age level or developmental stage" (Brandtstädter, 1984, p. 15). Individuals are likely to exert control over their own development either in a proactive or a reactive manner (Ford, 1987). Proactive control of development is exerted when individuals engage in actions with the objective of optimizing their development and associated outcomes. In contrast, individuals are likely to engage in reactive control, either in response to a critical event, or in response to a realized discrepancy between the actual and the socially and/or personally desirable developmental status. In both instances, individuals are likely to engage in planful, self-directed behavior with the objective to optimize developmental processes (Brandtstädter, 1984; Ford, 1987; Labouvie-Vief, 1981).

Despite the emphasis on individuals' active role in their own development, most of the developmental life-event research to date has looked at individuals' reactions to life events rather than at their proactive involvement. Several life-span theorists (Danish, Smyer, & Nowak, 1980; Filipp, 1981), however, have pointed out that a great number of life events are under the decisional control of the individual, thus determining their occurrence, timing, and duration, and providing the person with an opportunity for anticipatory coping and self-directed change.

Critique

Although the theoretical propositions outlined above have resulted in a paradigmatic shift in developmental psychology and have motivated researchers to study development during adulthood and old age, they also have some shortcomings. These shortcomings have important implications for empirical research in general, and for research regarding the developmental impact of critical life events in particular.

In terms of the influences of non-normative life events on adults' development, the major shortcoming of life-span developmental theory (Baltes et al., 1980; Baltes et al., 1998; Lerner, 1984; Riegel, 1975) is that the theoretical propositions lack specificity with regard to the role of the individual, the role of the sociocultural context, and the interrelationships between the two. Concerning the role of the individual, limited knowledge is available about the cognitive-emotional factors that may become critical in the generation of, as well as the response to, critical life events. For example, what are the self-related processes (e.g., favorable or unfavorable self-appraisals, perceived competencies, self-efficacy beliefs, sense of self-esteem) that need to be present to motivate a person to initiate and follow through with changes in his or her life? Or, how are interindividual differences, such as differences in personality, coping styles, or intellectual functioning related to the frequency, types and developmental outcomes of critical life events?

Concerning the role of the micro- and macro-aspects of the sociocultural context that are of relevance in the context of critical life events, only a few attempts (Elder, 1974; Featherman, Hogan, & Sørensen, 1984; Hogan, 1981; McLeod & Kessler, 1990) have been made to link a person's position within the given social structure to his or her susceptibility to and lifetime experience of critical life events. Moreover, little systematic information exists with regard to the extent in which individuals' socialization experiences (e.g., family background, course of education, professional status) and social roles are related to the frequency, types, and developmental outcomes of critical life events. This is a rather disappointing state of affairs, given that several studies have revealed considerable and far-reaching social class differences in the frequency of critical life events (McLeod & Kessler, 1990) as well as in the personal, material, and social resources that individuals have available for coping with these events (e.g., Krause & Borawski-Clark, 1995; Lin, 1982; Thoits, 1995). For example, Lin (1982) has documented that individuals with higher educational attainment tend to be embedded in social networks that are comprised of persons with similar educational background, suggesting the availability of a rich source of knowledge, experience, and problem-solving skills. In contrast, individuals with lower socioeconomic status often lack adequate material (Thoits, 1995) and social coping resources and are, therefore, at a higher risk for experiencing negative physical as well as mental health outcomes as a consequence of stressful life events (see Kessler & Cleary, 1980; Seeman et al., 1993; Seeman & Lewis, 1995).

Thus, in order to advance theory and research on the developmental influence of critical life events, both the role of the individual and the role of the sociocultural context need to be elaborated in more detail. Moreover, the major challenge for developmentally oriented life event researchers is to relate individuals' actions to micro- and macro-aspects of the sociocultural context. In order to do that, a conceptual model is needed that focuses on person as well as context characteristics of critical life events.

CRITICAL LIFE EVENTS AND SELF-DEVELOPMENT: LINKING MICRO- AND MACRO-LEVELS

A Comprehensive Model of the Developmental Effects of Critical Life Events

As developmental life-event researchers (Danish et al., 1980; Filipp, 1981; Hultsch & Plemons, 1979) have noted, critical life events need to be seen as processes rather than as time-limited and localized occurrences. Such a process orientation requires that investigators examine the antecedent and concurrent conditions as well as the short- and long-term consequences of critical life events. Thus, any comprehensive model of the effects of critical life events on individuals' development needs to incorporate not only the relations between the individual and their sociocultural context but also the temporal unfolding of the event. Such a comprehensive model has been outlined by Filipp (1981). As Figure 6.2 shows, Filipp's model conceptualizes critical life events as "naturally occurring developmental interventions" which (1) unfold over time, (2) have high emotional salience, (3) challenge a person's established person-environment fit, and (4) lead to coping behavior with the objective of re-establishing the person-environment fit.

As can be seen in Figure 6.2, Filipp's (1981) model includes as antecedents the person's previous experience and success with critical life events and forms of anticipatory socialization. In tandem with the person characteristics, the context characteristics of the individual's concurrent life situation, and the event characteristics of the critical life event, these antecedents determine a person's coping efforts in response to the critical life event. The person's coping efforts, in turn, are seen as having effects on his or her living conditions, resulting in a reorganization of the fit between person and environment. Under favorable circumstances, this reorganized person-environment fit will result in greater congruence between the needs of the individual and the demands of the environment and, hence, result in enhanced adaption and subjective well-being. Under less favorable circumstances, the newly established person-environment fit will be less than optimal, and may result in a state of incongruence or maladaptation with potentially negative physical or psychological outcomes.

Linking the Individual and the Social Structure

A particular strength of Filipp's (1981) model is that it incorporates reciprocal relationships between individual and sociocultural context as

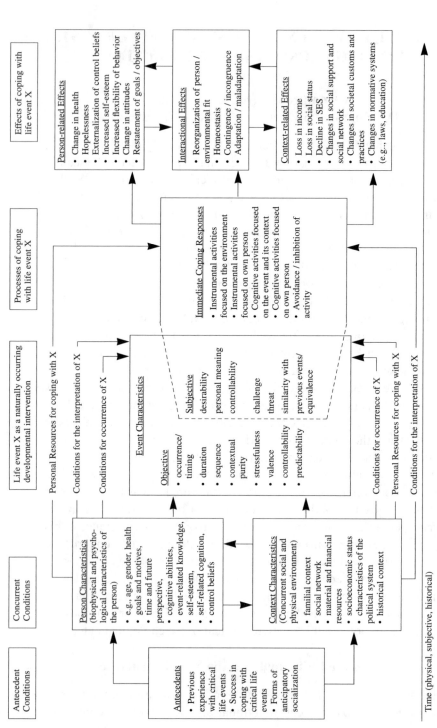

Figure 6.2 A general model for the analysis of critical life events.

From "A General Model for the Analysis of Critical Life Events," by S. H. Filipp 1995. In S.-H. Filipp (Ed.), *Critical Life Events* (3rd ed.) (p. 10). Weinheim, Germany: Psychologie Verlags Union. Copyright 1996 by Psychologie Verlags Union. Adapted with permission.

determinants of an individual's anticipatory and/or actual coping behavior. In this sense, it is the only model in life-event research that has incorporated the calls of theorists such as Dannefer (1984), Elder (1973), Ryff (1987), and Stewart and Healy (1989) who have argued that theories of personality development need to explicate the linkages between individuals' experiences and the sociocultural context in which these individuals are embedded. Thus, incorporation of this model in research on adult development and aging provides a unique framework which can be productively used by life-span psychologists and life-course sociologists alike. For life-span psychologists, adoption of this model represents a challenge not only to statistically control for context and social-structural variables, but to actively conceptualize and investigate the substantive role and the effects of context and social-structural influences in their work. In a similar vein, life-course sociologists are challenged to not neglect person variables over context and social structural influences.

Person Characteristics

In terms of the person characteristics, Filipp's (1981) model focuses on biological, social, and psychological characteristics of the individual. Biological characteristics entail a person's chronological age, sex, race, health condition, and general physiological/neurological functioning. Social characteristics include an individual's social roles, group memberships, social activities, and attainments. Psychological characteristics include a person's cognitive abilities and knowledge, attitudes, values, goals and motives, time and future perspective, self-esteem, and other self-related cognitions such as control beliefs and beliefs of self-efficacy. Thus, the term "person characteristics" refers to all aspects of individuals' bio-psycho-social condition, including their self-related cognitions, which appear to be of particular importance in the context of critical life events.

It is important to note that these person characteristics do not exist and operate in isolation from each other or in isolation from contextual and social-structural influences. Rather, they should be seen as reciprocally influencing each other and as being influenced by context and social-structural variables to produce change and development in individuals' lives. For example, research on the relation between social class and self-esteem (Demo & Savin-Williams, 1983; Rosenberg & Pearlin, 1978) has shown a differential pattern of association depending on the age of the studied individuals. These findings suggest that self-esteem is differently affected by social class variables such as education, occupation, or income at different periods of the life span. In turn, self-esteem is likely to play a different role as a person variable in individuals' response to a critical life event. That is, the same critical life event is likely to be met with different coping resources and is likely to result in different outcomes depending on the age, the social class, and the psychological condition of the person who experiences it.

Context Characteristics

The context characteristics included in Filipp's (1981) model are related to an individual's sociocultural, historical, and physical environment. As such, context characteristics entail as macro-structures (see Bronfenbrenner, 1979) all concurrent historical, economic and social conditions and events that directly or indirectly influence a person's status and well-being. For example, the political and economic status and structures of a nation, and governmental policies that shape the educational, health care, or welfare systems can be seen as context characteristics that affect different individuals and their coping with critical life events in different ways.

At the level of meso-structures, social class membership and socioeconomic status (SES) are relevant and determine persons' access to material and social resources (Kessler & Cleary, 1980; McLeod & Kessler, 1990). For example, it is well documented that individuals with a lower SES report a higher frequency of critical life events (e.g., unemployment, loss of health insurance, and job-related accidents) than individuals with a higher SES (McLeod & Kessler, 1990). At the same time, these individuals are the most disadvantaged with regard to their material/financial as well as their personal and social coping resources (Hurrelmann, 1988; Kessler & Cleary, 1980; McLeod & Kessler, 1990; Pearlin & Schooler, 1978).

At the level of micro-structures, such as school and family, aspects of conflict or cohesion, communication patterns, and availability of social support are important determinants of individuals' coping reactions to critical life events (Antonucci, 1985; Cohen & Syme, 1985; Wellmann & Hall, 1986). For example, in the early stages of critical life events, the social support made available by or actually received from family, friends, or coworkers seems to be one of the strongest predictors of successful coping (Cohen & Wills, 1985).

In summary, the context characteristics specified in Filipp's (1981) model include those features of the sociocultural, historical, and physical environment that directly or indirectly influence either the occurrence of, or a person's reactions to, critical life events. Context characteristics can therefore be seen as conditions that either facilitate or hinder a person's coping efforts.

Event Characteristics

The model also incorporates characteristics that are inherent in the critical event itself. Specifically, Filipp (1981) distinguishes between objective and subjective event characteristics. Objective event characteristics are those aspects of an event that are verifiable in an objective manner and, hence, have a similar effect on all individuals who experience this event. Examples of objective event characteristics are the time of occurrence, duration, the cohort specificity/age relatedness, or the contextual purity of an event (see Brim & Ryff, 1980; Reese & Smyer, 1983).

Subjective event characteristics, on the other hand, are all those aspects of an event for which no objective criteria of verification exist. Subjective event characteristics are based on individuals' cognitive appraisals (Lazarus & Folkman, 1984) or cognitive representations (Thomae, 1979) and include aspects such as the event's desirability and controllability, the degree of threat or challenge triggered by the event, or subjective estimations with regard to one's coping success and self-efficacy (Ruch, 1977; Sarason, Johnson, & Siegel, 1978).

From a developmental perspective, two important features of subjective event characteristics need to be highlighted. First, several theories of coping (Lazarus & Folkman, 1984; Thomae, 1979, 1983) conceptualize individuals' subjective cognitive appraisals of a critical life event as the major determinants of their subsequent coping behavior. As a matter of fact, the great interindividual variability that is seen in individuals' coping reactions may have its primary source in the very nature of their cognitive appraisals. Second, although the actual empirical support for this argument is currently scarce, subjective event appraisals are believed to be influenced to a great extent by the experiences with and the outcomes of previous critical life events. Thus, it is assumed that an individual who has successfully coped with a critical life event in the past will be more likely to perceive future critical life events as a reasonable challenge than a person who has not been successful in his or her coping efforts.

Coping Behavior and Event Outcomes

As Figure 6.2 shows, the combined influences of the antecedent and concurrent conditions (i.e., person, context, and event characteristics) are thought to determine a person's actual coping behavior in the context of a critical life event. Coping behaviors can be overt, problem-oriented, and emotion-oriented actions as well as covert, cognitive strategies that help an individual to negotiate the challenges associated with a critical life event (Lazarus & Folkman, 1984). In turn, the coping behavior will determine the person- and context-related effects of the event, as well as the changed person-environment fit.

Person-related effects of the event may include changes in an individual's health, changes in beliefs of control and self-efficacy, or the redefinition of goals and aspirations. Context-related effects may include changes in a person's socioeconomic and social status (e.g., loss in income, move into a less prestigious job) as well as changes in the social network and the associated support relationships. Similarly, a context-related effect may include that individuals who experience a particular critical life event (e.g., loss of job through downsizing or plant closure) join together through collective action and organize their coping efforts in a systematic way so that they become more effective in their response. In general, it is assumed that if individuals' coping efforts are successful, the person-environment fit will be re-established at a more advanced level of adaptation (i.e., growth or gain), whereas unsuccessful coping efforts will result in a person-environment fit at a lower level of adaptation (i.e., loss or decline).

THE ROLE OF CRITICAL LIFE EVENTS IN ADULT SELF-DEVELOPMENT

The Self in Adult Development and Aging

Over the last decade, there has been an increasing interest in the study of the self across the life span, including self-development in adulthood and aging (Brandtstädter & Greve, 1994; Breytspraak, 1984; Cross & Markus, 1991; Labouvie-Vief, Chiodo, Goguen, Diehl, & Orwoll, 1995; Lipka & Brinthaupt, 1992; Ryff, 1991). Although investigators in this field have drawn on a variety of theoretical frameworks and have used different research methods, their endeavors are based on the shared conviction that the adult self is a multidimensional and dynamic concept (Markus & Wurf, 1987; Noam, Powers, Kilkenny, & Beedy, 1990). Such a view is consistent with cognitive-developmental (e.g., Kegan, 1982; Kohlberg, 1969; Labouvie-Vief, 1992) and action-theoretical (Brandtstädter, 1984; Brandtstädter & Greve, 1994), as well as social psychological approaches to adult development and aging (Breytspraak, 1984; Heidrich & Ryff, 1993; Ryff, 1991).

Moreover, this perspective of the aging self as a dynamic structure is also consistent with sociological perspectives on the self which emphasize more social features of self-making and self-maintenance (Demo, 1992; Rosenberg & Pearlin, 1978; Ryff, 1987), and with the psychological view that adults are actively involved in the production of their own development (Brandtstädter, 1984; Labouvie-Vief, 1981; Lerner & Busch-Rossnagel, 1981). All of these approaches share the basic assumption that individuals' self-understanding and self-concept play a crucial role in how they negotiate personal continuity and change in adulthood and later life (Breytspraak, 1984).

Brandstädter and Greve (1994) have suggested that three major attributes of individuals' self-concepts are relevant in the study of the aging self: (1) continuity and permanence; (2) discriminative relevance; and (3) biographical meaningfulness. In a narrow sense, continuity and permanence refer to those attributes of a person's self-concept that are sufficiently stable and permanent to support his or her sense of self-continuity over time. In a broader sense, self-continuity is also related to an individual's ability to connect self-descriptive attributes with personal life experiences and events in order to construct a coherent and meaningful life story (Brandtstädter & Greve, 1994; Cohler, 1982; McAdams, 1993). In contrast, discriminative relevance refers to those aspects of a person's self-concept that distinguish him or her from others and make him or her the unique individual that he or she is. Finally, the aspect of biographical meaningfulness refers to those aspects of an individual's self-concept that are considered by the individual as important to his or her biography and life plan.

Brandstädter and Greve (1994) also argue that the biological, psychological, and social changes intrinsic to the aging process represent considerable challenges for individuals' self-concepts and sense of self-continuity. As recent research with young, middle-aged, and older adults has shown (Aldwin, 1992; Brandtstädter & Renner, 1990; Diehl, Coyle, & Labouvie-Vief, 1996; Vaillant, 1993), a great number of individuals respond to these challenges by developing resourceful and flexible strategies that prevent damage to their self-concept and permit the maintenance of high self-esteem (see also Heckhausen & Schulz, 1995; Staudinger, Marsiske, & Baltes, 1995). In particular, Brandstädter and Greve (1994) suggest that the preservation and stabilization of a positive self-concept and high self-esteem in adulthood and aging involve the following three interdependent processes: (1) Assimilative activities, (2) accommodative changes and readjustments, and (3) immunizing mechanisms.

As purposeful agents, individuals regulate and modify their behavior and development in correspondence with the views that they hold about themselves and the world (Brandtstädter, 1984). Assimilative activities are based on self-observation and self-evaluation and are related to the goals, expectancies, and self-related beliefs that constitute the structure of self (Bandura, 1989; Markus & Wurf, 1987). Assimilative activities may be instrumental behaviors (e.g., practice of a particular skill), compensatory behaviors (e.g., behavior change to adjust to a functional loss), or self-confirmatory actions (e.g., activities of symbolic self-expression). To the extent that assimilative efforts are futile or too costly, individuals revert to accommodative changes and readjustments. Such accommodative changes and readjustments may involve (1) the disengagement from blocked goals; (2) the adjustment of goals and aspirations to more realistic standards; or (3) self-enhancing social comparisons (Brandtstädter & Renner, 1990). If both assimilative and accommodative activities fail, individuals may engage in immunizing mechanisms (i.e., defensive strategies) to protect the integrity of the self by mitigating the impact of self-discrepant evidence.

Although Brandtstädter and Greve's (1994) model provides a valuable theoretical framework for empirical studies on the aging self, it has, however, one major limitation. In particular, in its current version, this model focuses primarily on the psychological strategies and mechanisms that the aging self employs to adjust to age-related changes and losses, whereas social-structural aspects that may be related to the maintenance of a positive self-concept in later life are surprisingly absent. However, if life-span developmentalists are serious about the notion that the aging self is a product of both micro- and macro-processes, then a more detailed elaboration of the role and life-long effects of social-structural variables (e.g., social class membership, socioeconomic status, occupational career) and their reciprocal interaction with person variables is very much needed (Dannefer, 1984; Dowd, 1990). From a social-structural point of view, one may challenge Brandstädter and Greve's (1994) model by asking whether the use of assimilative, accommodative, or immunizing activities varies systematically with individuals' socioeconomic status or social class membership. For example, one could ask whether individuals with a high SES are, because of their lifelong experiences that have resulted in a greater skill repertoire, higher self-esteem, and more positive self-efficacy beliefs (see Kohn & Schooler, 1969, 1978; Rosenberg & Pearlin, 1978), more likely to use instrumental and self-confirmatory actions compared to persons with low SES. Similarly, one could ask whether accommodative strategies, such as disengagement from blocked goals, shifting one's standards downward, or simply abandoning a goal, are the strategies employed more by individuals with low SES—again reflecting these individuals' experiences throughout their life course. Sociologists such as Dannefer (1987) or Dowd (1990) clearly would argue that the incorporation and linkage of social-structural variables with person variables will greatly enrich the analysis of the aging self, and will lead to a more comprehensive description of micro- and macro-processes in human development across the life span.

It should also be noted that the processes described by Brandtstädter and Greve (1994) bear great similarity to the model of identity processes described by Whitbourne (1985, 1986) and the model of self-related change outlined by Kiecolt (1994). Moreover, Brandtstädter and Greve's model also shows some affinity to phenomenological and narrative approaches to adult development and aging as they have been outlined by Cohler (1982), McAdams (1985, 1993), and Ryff (1986).

The Adult Self and Critical Life Events

Based on Brandtstädter and Greve's (1994) theoretical elaborations, it is reasonable to assume that assimilative, accommodative, or immunizing processes are most likely activated by life events that affect central features of a person's self-structure and, hence, threaten the consistency and internal continuity of the person's self-concept (Atchley, 1989). In particular, two kinds of critical life events appear to be relevant in this context: (1) events that are unanticipated and beyond a person's control (i.e., low controllability), and (2) events that are entirely self-determined (i.e., high controllability) and may produce, to some extent, clashes between the individual's psychological needs and societal norms. Although these two specific types of events differ greatly with regard to the decisional control exercised by the individual, in both instances individuals are faced with situations that have, at least temporarily, highly uncertain outcomes and therefore challenge their coping resources and sense of identity (Kiecolt, 1994; Ryan, 1993). Thus, these two specific types of critical life events are most likely to create situations that Riegel (1976a) referred to as "existential challenge" (p. 693).

Uncontrollable Life Events and the Adult Self

At first glance, the proposition that uncontrollable life events may stimulate self-development in adulthood and aging appears to be quite counterintuitive, because traditional life-event research has provided a great deal of evidence that the experience of uncontrollable events is associated with negative psychological consequences (Cohen, 1988; Glass & Singer, 1972; Seligman, 1975). However, some investigators have pointed out that the relationship between lack of controllability and negative psychological outcomes is not a direct and straightforward one (see Thoits, 1983). Rather, the effect of lack of controllability has been shown (1) to be mediated by individual difference variables such as individuals' locus-of-control beliefs and (2) to differ depending on the life domain and the outcome measures examined (Thoits, 1983). Furthermore, to the extent that individuals' locus-of-control and self-efficacy beliefs differ depending on their social class membership, social class will serve as another mediator with regard to the lack of controllability (Kessler & Cleary, 1980; McLeod & Kessler; 1990; Pearlin & Schooler, 1978). Thus, although controllability is an important event dimension, most of the available life-event research may have examined the psychological effects of uncontrollable life events in a truncated and biased fashion.

It was not until recently that theorists (e.g., Kiecolt, 1994) started to look at events with low controllability as a potential impetus for change and development. Kiecolt (1994) proposed a model specifying some of the conditions under which life events with low controllability may become the impetus for change and development. Based on an extensive literature review, Kiecolt (1994) suggested that a critical life event needs to be identity-relevant and needs to threaten a person's beliefs of competence, self-efficacy, self-esteem, and/or sense of authenticity in order to become a stimulus for change. If a critical life event "causes" these perceptions and the individual appraises his or her personal and social coping resources as sufficient (i.e., the individual believes that self-change is possible and the benefits of change will outweigh the costs), then the critical life event may become the stimulus for coping responses that may result in growth and development.

It needs to be noted that the coping strategies used by the individual do not necessarily have to be overt strategies, but can also include strategies of cognitive reevaluation, social comparison, or impulse control—processes that in control theory are referred to as "secondary control" (Heckhausen & Schulz, 1995; Rothbaum, Weisz, & Snyder, 1992). These latter coping strategies have great importance with regard to affect control and emotion regulation and have been shown to be quite adaptive for middle-aged and older adults (Diehl et al., 1996; Folkman, Lazarus, Pimley,

& Novacek, 1987; Heidrich & Ryff, 1993; Labouvie-Vief, Hakim-Larson, & Hobart, 1987).

Thus, the view that critical life events with low controllability can become the impetus for growth and development in adulthood and aging is consistent with a recently proposed life-span theory of control (Heckhausen & Schulz, 1995), with empirical research on personal control over development (Brandtstädter, 1984), and with several social psychological theories concerning the role of self and self-esteem in the negotiation of existential threat (Solomon, Greenberg, & Pyszczynski, 1991; Steele, 1988). All of these theories have in common that individuals are seen as being highly motivated to protect their self-esteem through efforts of cognitive, behavioral, and affective control (Breytspraak, 1984; Deci & Ryan, 1985, 1991; Heckhausen & Schulz, 1995) and to transform threats to the integrity of their self into experiences of mastery and autonomy (Ryan, 1991, 1993).

Self-Determined Life Events and the Adult Self

Several life-span developmentalists (Brandstädter, 1984; Danish et al., 1980; Filipp, 1981) have noted that a good number of life events in adulthood are under the decisional control of the individual and that the occurrence of such events can be seen as acts of self-determination. Thus, it seems to be warranted for developmentalists to redirect their focus from the depiction of persons as merely reacting entities, toward the intentional and planful actions that individuals engage in to create or contribute to the occurrence of critical life events. Such an endeavor also includes the examination of the developmental antecedents and consequences of self-determined life events (Deci & Ryan, 1985, 1991; Ryan, 1991, 1993).

The proposition that the occurrence of certain kinds of critical life events in adulthood can be conceptualized as an act of self-determination is based on a view of human motivation and action (Bandura, 1997; Brandtstädter, 1984; White, 1959) which conceptualizes human behavior as being motivated not only by physiological deficits and/or environmental pressures but by a system of intrinsic motivations toward self-efficacy, competence, and autonomy (Bandura, 1997; Deci & Ryan, 1985; White, 1959). An essential component of this basic system of intrinsic motivations consists of individuals' actions as they are related to self-regulation, self-enhancement, and self-realization. These actions very often serve the primary purpose of self-esteem maintenance and/or self-enhancement. Specifically, self-esteem maintenance and self-enhancement become important motives in situations where persons' self-esteem is threatened or challenged (Baumeister, 1993), or where their self-development is jeopardized by adverse conditions and the possibility of stagnation and decline (Brandstädter & Greve, 1994; Breytspraak, 1984; Solomon et al., 1991). Thus, I propose that adults are likely to contribute to the occurrence of critical life events, as a form of self-determination or self-regulation, when the threats of the current situation to the person's self-concept and self-esteem outweigh the benefits of that situation (Deci & Ryan, 1995; Kiecolt, 1994).

To illustrate, for a person whose self-concept is to a great extent defined by openness, honesty and affection, the lack of these characteristics in a marital relationship may motivate the person to pursue actions in two different directions. First, the person may strive, for example through marital counseling, to engage the marital partner in endeavors to improve their communication and to increase the presence of openness, honesty, and affection in their relationship. However, if these endeavors fail, then the person may decide to end the marriage and may ask for a divorce. Although such a decision is very likely to result in a critical life event (Chiriboga & Catron, 1991) for both marital partners, to the spouse who requested the divorce it may psychologically be the most appropriate solution if he or she wants to protect the integrity of his/her self-development and maintain a sense of self-esteem.

In summary, it is argued that because of the intrinsic human motivations for competence (White, 1959), self-efficacy (Bandura, 1997), control (Heckhausen & Schulz, 1995), and self-determination (Deci & Ryan, 1985, 1995; Rogers, 1963), adults should be seen as potential creators of critical life events. Moreover, it is suggested that adults are most likely to engage in actions that lead to the occurrence of critical life events if they perceive the consistency and continuity of their self-concept threatened if they do not act, and if other behavioral alternatives have not been successful in protecting their self-concept and self-esteem.

EMPIRICAL EVIDENCE

Although there is a solid theoretical foundation for the conceptualization of uncontrollable and self-determined life events as influences on adults' self-development, to date, the empirical support for these conceptual assumptions is still limited. Nevertheless, the empirical evidence that exists is promising and points to the resourcefulness of the aging self.

Uncontrollable Life Events and Adult Self-Development

The proposition that life events with low controllability may have particular relevance for adults' self-development is supported by empirical evidence from three major areas. First, indirect support for this proposition is provided by several studies showing that despite the losses and deficits that accompany the normal aging process, most older adults manage to maintain a high level of self-esteem and subjective well-being and a sense of mastery (see Pearlin & Skaff, 1995). For example, Bengtson, Reedy, and Gordon (1985) and Filipp and Klauer (1986) have reported a considerable degree of stability in adults' self-descriptions during middle and later adulthood even in the face of age-related losses (e.g., health-related changes, loss of loved ones) that are characterized by low controllability (see also Thomae, 1983). Similarly, Brandtstädter and Greve (1994) noted that there is no convincing evidence for a general decline in self-esteem and subjective quality of life in older adults, at least up to terminal phases where serious health problems become a pervasive concern. Finally, the general assumption that the losses and impairments associated with the aging process would be reflected in a higher prevalence of depressive disorders in older adults is not supported by the existing research literature (see Blazer, 1989; Bolla-Wilson & Bleecker, 1989; Newmann, 1989). In contrast, Blazer (1989) came to the conclusion that older adults may be "protected from the development of major clinical depression" (p. 189), hinting at the resourcefulness of the aging self (see also Pearlin & Skaff, 1995).

The resourcefulness of the aging self has also been shown in studies on adults' mechanisms of coping and defense (Aldwin, 1992; Diehl et al., 1996; Folkman et al., 1987; Labouvie-Vief et al., 1987; McCrae, 1989). All of these studies have more or less shown that the high self-esteem and well-being that characterizes older persons seems to be related to coping strategies that are indicative of greater impulse control and cognitive reappraisal. These coping strategies could well be considered accommodative processes that may be indicative of a form of personal growth unique to later life.

The second area of evidence can be found in the literature on loss and crisis (Montada, Filipp, & Lerner, 1992; Thomae & Lehr, 1986) and on coping with illness and death (Filipp, 1992; Silver & Wortman, 1980). Using a phenomenological approach, Diehl (1984) reported findings from intensive semistructured interviews with adult cancer and heart attack patients indicating that a substantial number of patients coped with their situation by giving their illness a meaning that was consistent with their established self-concept. Moreover, searching for a meaning of one's illness did not mean that these patients engaged in any way in reality-distorting defenses or only in passive and emotion-regulating coping. Rather, they showed a repertoire of coping skills that included both active and problem-focused as well as cognitive and emotion-regulating strategies. During different phases of their illness, these adults also engaged in downward social comparisons to maintain their self-esteem and acknowledged that their illness, despite the fact that it had created a situation of adversity for them, had provided them with an opportunity for change and growth (see also Aldwin, Sutton, & Lachman, 1996).

Similar findings have been reported by Taylor (1983). Based on her research with women with breast cancer, Taylor (1983) described a process of adjustment that centered around three themes: a search for meaning in the experience, an attempt to regain mastery over the event, and an effort to restore self-esteem through self-enhancing evaluations. Taylor found, for example, that the search for meaning involved not only women's attempts to understand why the event occurred, but also its meaning with regard to their self-knowledge or self-change.

With regard to self-enhancing evaluations, Taylor (1983) found that some of the most intriguing self-enhancements were generated in terms of "positive illusions" and were frequently related to the women's downward social comparisons. Positive illusions helped study participants to maintain their self-esteem, regardless of the objective condition of their illness, and contributed to their overall adjustment (see also Affleck, Tennen, & Croog, 1987; Taylor & Brown, 1988, 1994). Although these findings are quite intriguing, it needs to be pointed out that Taylor's study sample consisted primarily of White, upper middle-class women. Therefore it remains to be seen whether women with lower levels of education and a less advantaged socioeconomic background would show similar coping behaviors or whether their coping behavior would be, because of socioeconomic pressures, more focused on instrumental actions.

Finally, Filipp (1992) reported findings from a study conducted in West Germany showing the effect of an uncontrollable life event on adults' self-development. In this study, the coping strategies of 332 cancer patients (age 20 to 74) were assessed longitudinally and related to their adjustment. Filipp found that, overall, the cancer patients used flexible cognitive coping strategies that were similar to the assimilative and accommodative activities described by Brandtstädter and Greve (1994). For example, threat minimization was one of these coping strategies and included intrapsychic, emotion-focused responses such as self-instructions toward positive thinking. Moreover, the use of threat minimizing strategies, which was more pronounced in older adults than in younger adults, was negatively related to symptoms of hopelessness and depression (see also Mummendey, 1981).

The third area of evidence can be found in the literature on the effects of uncontrollable sociocultural/historical events, such as the Great Depression or World War II, on individuals' lives. For example, Elder (1974) showed in his research on the "Children of the Great Depression" that although children from economically deprived families were at a greater disadvantage with regard to the completion of their education and subsequent professional development, economic hardship did not produce noteworthy disabilities in adult accomplishments or health. In a follow-up study, Elder (1979) elaborated on some of the experiences that enabled young men from the Berkeley Guidance Study to overcome the effects of economic hardship during their childhood. In particular, he pointed out that Berkeley men who coped well with the developmental tasks of adulthood often took advantage of specific opportunities such as the G.I. Bill. Moreover, developmental gains were often seen when young men and women who had grown up under economically disadvantaged conditions exposed themselves to situations in which they were forced (i.e., in which they had little control) to fulfill a role that gave them a sense of worth and identity. Thus, Elder's research shows the effects of macro-structures, such as social class membership, on individuals' development, but it also shows how the effects of these macro-structures are modified by specific life events and by the actions of the developing individual (see also Elder, Shanahan, & Clipp, 1994).

In summary, there is growing evidence that life events with low controllability may serve as impetus for adults to engage in behavior that focuses on the protection of the continuity and consistency of their self-concept (see also Ryff & Heidrich, 1997). An important objective of adults' endeavors, regardless of whether they involve instrumental and compensatory activities, accommodative changes and readjustments, or immunizing mechanisms, is the maintenance of their self-esteem and their sense of agency and self-determination. Moreover, these activities may contribute to processes that constitute growth and development in adulthood and aging.

Self-Determined Life Events and Adult Self-Development

Earlier, it was proposed that the occurrence of some critical life events in adulthood can be seen as an act of self-determination and autonomy. Several lines of research support this proposition. For example, research on marital separation and divorce (Chiriboga & Catron, 1991) has shown that one of the major reasons that couples separated was because one of them felt trapped in a relationship that had either a negative impact on their self-concept or hindered their further self-development. That the initiation of such a critical life event can be seen as an act of self-determination is also supported by findings that indicate that the initiator usually copes more successfully with the separation and returns to the pursuit of his or her goals and plans earlier and more successfully than the person who simply responded to the separation (Chiriboga & Catron, 1991; Weiss, 1975).

Perhaps the most direct support for the relevance of self-determined critical life events to individuals' self-development has been provided by Mummendey (1981). He asked 100 adults (age 28 to 47) to report the critical life events that had occurred in different life domains (e.g., family, work, education, health etc.) during the past 5 years and to rate these events in terms of their relevance for changes in individuals' self-concepts. Mummendey (1981) found that critical life events that individuals described as self-initiated (e.g., starting a new relationship, exiting a relationship/separation, job change, change in residence, etc.) showed significant associations with positive self-concept changes. These positive self-concept changes included increases in self-acceptance, psychological mindedness, flexibility, and feelings of responsibility.

Thus, although the current empirical support is scarce, there is some reasonable evidence that self-determined critical life events contribute to adults' personal growth and self-development. Taken together, these findings are consistent with a large body of research showing that individuals who have a sense of being in control of their lives also show higher self-esteem, greater life satisfaction, and better mental health (Heckhausen & Schulz, 1995; Menaghan, 1983; Staudinger et al., 1995).

SUMMARY

Drawing on the theoretical framework of life-span developmental psychology, in general, and on the propositions of Riegel (1975, 1976a), in particular, I argued that most scholars of adult development have looked at critical life events in a somewhat narrow and simplistic fashion. Instead, I advocated that attention should be focused on two specific types of critical life events that seem to be of particular importance for adults' self-development: (1) life events that are unanticipated and beyond a person's control (i.e., low controllability) and (2) life events that are self-determined (i.e., high controllability). Uncontrollable life events threaten the continuity and integrity of adults' self-concept and self-esteem, and individuals' coping efforts should therefore have an effect on their self-development. Self-determined critical life events are proposed to be relevant for adults' self-development because they are expected to support and enhance individuals' sense of mastery and autonomy and, therefore, contribute to a positive self-concept. Empirical evidence in support of these propositions was provided and it was shown that life events can be seen as one avenue of linking aspects of the social structure with aspects of individual development. Throughout it was emphasized that life event researchers need to reflect carefully on the role that contextual and social-structural factors may play in the occurrence and change-producing function of critical life events. In sum, then, there appears to be a rich conceptual foundation and sufficient empirical evidence to warrant a greater investment in the study of critical life events and their effects on adults' self- development.

REFERENCES

Affleck, G., Tennen, H., & Croog, S. (1987). Causal attribution, perceived benefits, and morbidity after a heart attack: An 8-year study. *Journal of Consulting and Clinical Psychology, 55*, 29–35.

Aldwin, C. M. (1992). Aging, coping, and efficacy: Theoretical framework for examining coping in a life-span developmental context. In M. L. Wykle, E. Kahana, & J. Kowal (Eds.), *Stress and health among the elderly* (pp. 96–113). New York: Springer Publishing Co.

Aldwin, C. M., Sutton, K. J., & Lachman, M. (1996). The development of coping resources in adulthood. *Journal of Personality, 64*, 837–871.

Antonucci, T. C. (1985). Personal characteristics, social support, and social behavior. In R. H. Binstock & E. Shanas (Eds.), *Handbook of aging and the social sciences* (2nd ed., pp. 94–128). New York: Van Nostrand Reinhold.

Atchley, R. C. (1989). A continuity theory of normal aging. *The Gerontologist, 29*, 183–190.

Baltes, P. B., Lindenberger, U., & Staudinger, U. M. (1998). Life-span theory in developmental psychology. In W. Damon (Series Ed.) & R. M. Lerner (Vol. Ed.), *Handbook of child psychology: Vol. 1. Theoretical models of human development* (5th ed., pp. 1029–1143). New York: Wiley.

Baltes, P. B., Reese, H. W., & Lipsitt, L. P. (1980). Life-span developmental psychology. *Annual Review of Psychology, 31*, 65–110.

Baltes, P. B. (1987). Theoretical propositions of life-span developmental psychology: On the dynamics between growth and decline. *Developmental Psychology, 23*, 611–626.

Bandura, A. (1989). Self-regulation of motivation and action through internal standards and goal systems. In L. A. Pervin (Ed.), *Goal concepts in personality and social psychology* (pp. 19–85). Hillsdale, NJ: Erlbaum.

Bandura, A. (1997). *Self-efficacy: The exercise of control.* New York: Freeman.

Baumeister, R. F. (Ed.). (1993). *Self-esteem: The puzzle of low self-regard.* New York: Plenum.

Bengtson, V. L., Reedy, M. N., & Gordon, C. (1985). Aging and self-conceptions: Personality processes and social contexts. In J. E. Birren & K. W. Schaie (Eds.), *Handbook of the psychology of aging* (2nd ed., pp. 544–593). New York: Van Nostrand Reinhold.

Blazer, D. (1989). Depression in late life: An update. *Annual Review of Gerontology and Geriatrics, 9*, 197–215.

Bolla-Wilson, K., & Bleecker, M. L. (1989). Absence of depression in elderly adults. *Journal of Gerontology: Psychological Sciences, 44*, P53–P55.

Brandtstädter, J. (1984). Personal and social control over development: Some implications of an action perspective in life-span developmental psychology. In P. B. Baltes & O. G. Brim, Jr. (Eds.), *Life-span development and behavior* (Vol. 6, pp. 1–32). New York: Academic Press.

Brandtstädter, J., & Greve, W. (1994). The aging self: Stabilizing and protective processes. *Developmental Review, 14*, 52–80.

Brandtstädter, J., & Renner, G. (1990). Tenacious goal pursuit and flexible goal adjustment: Explication and age-related analysis of assimilative and accommodative strategies of coping. *Psychology and Aging, 5*, 58–67.

Breytspraak, L. M. (1984). *The development of self in later life.* Boston: Little, Brown.

Brim, O. G., Jr., & Kagan, J. (Eds.). (1980). *Constancy and change in human development.* Cambridge, MA: Harvard University Press.

Brim, O. G., Jr., & Ryff, C. D. (1980). On the properties of life events. In P. B. Baltes & O. G. Brim, Jr. (Eds.), *Life-span development and behavior* (Vol. 3, pp. 367–388). New York: Academic Press.

Bronfenbrenner, U. (1979). *The ecology of human development: Experiments by nature and design.* Cambridge, MA: Harvard University Press.

Chiriboga, D. A., & Catron, L. S. (1991). *Divorce: Crisis, challenge or relief?* New York: New York University Press.

Cohen, L. H. (1988). Measurement of life events. In L. H. Cohen (Ed.), *Life events and psychological functioning: Theoretical and methodological issues* (pp. 11–30). Newbury Park, CA: Sage.

Cohen, S., & Syme, S. L. (Eds.). (1985). *Social support and health.* Orlando, FL: Academic Press.

Cohen, S., & Wills, T. A. (1985). Stress, social support, and the buffering hypothesis. *Psychological Bulletin, 98*, 310–357.

Cohler, B. J. (1982). Personal narrative and the life course. In P. B. Baltes & O. G. Brim, Jr. (Eds.), *Life-span development and behavior* (Vol. 4, pp. 204–241). New York: Academic Press.

Cross, S., & Markus, H. (1991). Possible selves across the life span. *Human Development, 34*, 230–255.

Danish, S. J., Smyer, M. A., & Nowak, C. A. (1980). Developmental intervention: Enhancing life-event processes. In P. B. Baltes & O. G. Brim, Jr. (Eds.), *Life-span development and behavior* (Vol. 3, pp. 339–366). New York: Academic Press.

Dannefer, D. (1984). Adult development and social theory: A paradigmatic reappraisal. *American Sociological Review, 49*, 100–116.

Dannefer, D., & Perlmutter, M. (1990). Development as a multidimensional process: Individual and social constituents. *Human Development, 33*, 108–137.

Deci, E. L., & Ryan, R. M. (1985). *Intrinsic motivation and self-determination in human behavior*. New York: Plenum.

Deci, E. L., & Ryan, R. M. (1991). A motivational approach to self: Integration in personality. In R. Dientsbier (Ed.), *Nebraska Symposium on Motivation: Vol. 38. Perspectives on motivation* (pp. 237–288). Lincoln, NE: University of Nebraska Press.

Deci, E. L., & Ryan, R. M. (1995). Human autonomy: The basis for true self-esteem. In M.H. Kernis (Ed.), *Efficacy, agency, and self-esteem* (pp. 31–49). New York: Plenum.

Demo, D. H. (1992). The self-concept over time: Research issues and directions. *Annual Review of Sociology, 18*, 303–326.

Demo, D. H., & Savin-Williams, R. C. (1983). Early adolescent self-esteem as a function of social class: Rosenberg and Pearlin revisited. *American Journal of Sociology, 88*, 763–774.

Diehl, M. (1984). *Die Krebsdiagnose als kritisches Lebensereignis: Formen der Auseinandersetzung mit einer lebensbedrohlichen Erkrankung* [Diagnosis of cancer as a critical life event: Patterns of coping with a life-threatening illness]. Unpublished master's thesis, Friedrich-Wilhelms-Universität, Bonn, Germany.

Diehl, M., Coyle, N., & Labouvie-Vief, G. (1996). Age and sex differences in strategies of coping and defense across the life span. *Psychology and Aging, 11*, 127–139.

Dowd, J. J. (1990). Ever since Durkheim: The socialization of human development. *Human Development, 33*, 138–159.

Eichorn, D. H., Clausen, J. A., Haan, N., Honzik, M. P., & Mussen, P. H. (1981). *Present and past in middle life*. New York: Academic Press.

Elder, G. H., Jr. (1973). On linking social structure and personality. *American Behavioral Scientist, 16*, 785–800.

Elder, G. H., Jr. (1974). *Children of the great depression*. Chicago, IL: University of Chicago Press.

Elder, G. H., Jr. (1979). Historical change in life patterns and personality. In P. B.

Baltes & O. G. Brim, Jr. (Eds.), *Life-span development and behavior* (Vol. 2, pp. 117–159). New York: Academic Press.

Elder, G. H., Jr., Shanahan, M. J., & Clipp, E. C. (1994). When war comes to men's lives: Life-course patterns in family, work, and health. *Psychology and Aging, 9,* 5–16.

Erikson, E. H. (1959). *Identity and the life cycle.* New York: International University Press.

Featherman, D. L., Hogan, D. P., & Sørensen, A. B. (1984). Entry into adulthood: Profiles of young men in the 1950s. In P. B. Baltes & O. G. Brim, Jr. (Eds.), *Life-span development and behavior* (Vol. 6, pp. 159–202). Orlando, FL: Academic Press.

Filipp, S.-H. (1981). Ein allgemeines Modell für die Analyse kritischer Lebensereignisse. In S.-H. Filipp (Hrsg.), *Kritische Lebensereignisse* (pp. 3–52) [A general model for the analysis of critical life events. In S.-H. Filipp (Ed.), *Critical life events* (pp. 3–52)]. München, Germany: Urban & Schwarzenberg.

Filipp, S.-H. (1992). Could it be worse? The diagnosis of cancer as a prototype of traumatic life events. In L. Montada, S.-H. Filipp, & M. J. Lerner (Eds.), *Life crises and experiences of loss in adulthood* (pp. 23–56). Hillsdale, NJ: Erlbaum.

Filipp, S.-H., & Klauer, T. (1986). Conceptions of self over the life-span: Reflections on the dialectics of change. In M. M. Baltes & P. B. Baltes (Eds.), *The psychology of control and aging* (pp. 167–205). Hillsdale, NJ: Erlbaum.

Folkman, S., Lazarus, R. S., Pimley, S., & Novacek, J. (1987). Age differences in stress and coping processes. *Psychology and Aging, 2,* 171–184.

Ford, D. H. (1987). *Humans as self-constructing living systems: A developmental perspective on behavior and personality.* Hillsdale, NJ: Erlbaum.

Glass, D. C., & Singer, J. E. (1972). *Urban stress: Experiments on noise and social stressors.* New York: Academic Press.

Harris, D. B. (Ed.). (1957). *The concept of development: An issue in the study of human behavior.* Minneapolis, MN: University of Minnesota Press.

Heckhausen, J., & Schulz, R. (1995). A life-span theory of control. *Psychological Review, 102,* 284–304.

Heidrich, S. M., & Ryff, C. D. (1993). Physical and mental health in later life: The self-system as mediator. *Psychology and Aging, 8,* 327–338.

Helson, R., & Roberts, B. W. (1994). Ego development and personality change in adulthood. *Journal of Personality and Social Psychology, 66,* 911–920.

Hogan, D. P. (1981). *Transitions and social change: The early lives of American men.* New York: Academic Press.

Hultsch, D. F., & Plemons, J. K. (1979). Life events and life-span development. In P. B. Baltes & O. G. Brim, Jr. (Eds.), *Life-span development and behavior* (Vol. 2, pp. 1–36). New York: Academic Press.

Hurrelmann, K. (1988). *Social structure and personality development.* New York: Cambridge University Press.

Kegan, R. (1982). *The evolving self: Problem and process in human development.* Cambridge, MA: Harvard University Press.

Kessler, R. C. (1979). Stress, social status, and psychological distress. *Journal of Health and Social Behavior, 20*, 100–108.

Kessler, R. C., & Cleary, P. D. (1980). Social class and psychological distress. *American Sociological Review, 45*, 463–478.

Kiecolt, K. J. (1994). Stress and the decision to change oneself: A theoretical model. *Social Psychology Quarterly, 57*, 49–63.

Kohlberg, L. (1969). Stage and sequence: The cognitive-developmental approach to socialization. In D. A. Goslin (Ed.), *Handbook of socialization theory and research* (pp. 347–380). Chicago, IL: Rand McNally.

Kohn, M., & Schooler, C. (1969). Class, occupation, and orientation. *American Sociological Review, 34*, 659–678.

Kohn, M., & Schooler, C. (1978). The reciprocal effects of the substantive complexity of work and intellectual flexibility: A longitudinal assessment. *American Journal of Sociology, 84*, 24–52.

Krause, N., & Borawski-Clark, E. (1995). Social class differences in social support among older adults. *The Gerontologist, 35*, 498–508.

Labouvie-Vief, G. (1977). Adult cognitive development: In search of alternative interpretations. *Merrill Palmer Quarterly, 23*, 227–263.

Labouvie-Vief, G. (1981). Proactive and reactive aspects of constructivism: Growth and aging in life-span perspective. In R. M. Lerner & N. A. Busch-Rossnagel (Eds.), *Individuals as producers of their development: A life-span perspective* (pp. 197–230). New York: Academic Press.

Labouvie-Vief, G. (1982). Growth and aging in life-span perspective. *Human Development, 25*, 65–88.

Labouvie-Vief, G. (1992). A neo-Piagetian perspective on adult cognitive development. In R. J. Sternberg & C. A. Berg (Eds.), *Intellectual development* (pp. 197–228). New York: Cambridge University Press.

Labouvie-Vief, G., Chiodo, L., Goguen, L., Diehl, M., & Orwoll, L. (1995). Representations of self across the life span. *Psychology and Aging, 10*, 404–415.

Labouvie-Vief, G., Hakim-Larson, J., & Hobart, C. J. (1987). Age, ego level, and the life-span development of coping and defense processes. *Psychology and Aging, 2*, 286–293.

Lazarus, R. S., & Folkman, S. (1984). *Stress, coping and appraisal.* New York: Springer Publishing Co.

Lehr, U., & Thomae, H. (Eds.). (1987). *Formen des seelischen Alterns* [Patterns of psychological aging]. Stuttgart, Germany: Enke.

Lerner, R. M. (1984). *On the nature of human plasticity.* New York: Cambridge University Press.

Lerner, R. M., & Busch-Rossnagel, N. A. (Eds.). (1981). *Individuals as producers of their development: A life-span perspective.* New York: Academic Press.

Lin, N. (1982). Social resources and instrumental action. In P. V. Marsden & N. Lin (Eds.), *Social structure and network analysis* (pp. 131–145). Beverly Hills, CA: Sage.

Lipka, R. P., & Brinthaupt, T. M. (Eds.). (1992). *Self-perspectives across the life span*. Albany, NY: State University of New York Press.

Markus, H., & Wurf, E. (1987). The dynamic self-concept: A social-psychological perspective. *Annual Review of Psychology, 38,* 299–337.

Marshall, V. W. (1995). The micro-macro link in the sociology of aging. In C. Hummel & C. J. Lalive D'Epinay (Eds.), *Images of aging in Western societies* (pp. 337–371). Geneva, Switzerland: Centre for Interdisciplinary Gerontology, University of Geneva.

McAdams, D. P. (1985). *Power, intimacy, and the life story: Personological inquiries into identity*. Homewood, IL: Dorsey.

McAdams, D. P. (1993). *Stories we live by: Personal myths and the making of the self*. New York: Morrow.

McCrae, R. R. (1989). Age differences and changes in the use of coping mechanisms. *Journal of Gerontology: Psychological Sciences, 44,* P161–P169.

McLeod, J. D., & Kessler, R. C. (1990). Socioeconomic status differences in vulnerability to undesirable life events. *Journal of Health and Social Behavior, 31,* 162–172.

Menaghan, E. G. (1983). Individual coping efforts: Moderators of the relationship between life stress and mental health outcomes. In H. B. Kaplan (Ed.), *Psychosocial stress: Trends in theory and research* (pp. 157–191). New York: Academic Press.

Montada, L., Filipp, S.-H., & Lerner, M. J. (Eds.). (1992). *Life crises and experiences of loss in adulthood*. Hillsdale, NJ: Erlbaum.

Mummendey, H. D. (1981). Selbstkonzept-Änderungen nach kritischen Lebensereignissen. In. S.-H. Filipp (Hrsg.), *Kritische Lebensereignisse* (pp. 252–269) [Changes in self-concept following critical life events. In S.H. Filipp (Ed.), *Critical life events* (pp. 252–269)]. München, Germany: Urban & Schwarzenberg.

Newmann, J. P. (1989). Aging and depression. *Psychology and Aging, 4,* 150–165.

Noam, G. G., Powers, S. I., Kilkenny, R., & Beedy, J. (1990). The interpersonal self in life-span developmental perspective: Theory, measurement, and longitudinal case analyses. In P. B. Baltes, D. L. Featherman, & R. M. Lerner (Eds.), *Life-span development and behavior* (Vol. 10, pp. 59–104). Hillsdale, NJ: Erlbaum.

Pearlin, L. I., Menaghan, E. G., Lieberman, M. A., & Mullan, J. T. (1981). The stress process. *Journal of Health and Social Behavior, 22,* 337–356.

Pearlin, L. I., & Schooler, C. (1978). The structure of coping. *Journal of Health and Social Behavior, 19,* 2–21.

Pearlin, L. I., & Skaff, M. M. (1995). Stressors and adaptation in late life. In M. Gatz (Ed.), *Emerging issues in mental health and aging* (pp. 97–123). Washington, DC: American Psychological Association.

Piaget, J. (1950). *The psychology of intelligence*. London: Routledge & Kegan Paul.

Piaget, J. (1952). *The origins of intelligence in children*. New York: International Universities Press.

Reese, H. W., & Smyer, M. A. (1983). The dimensionalization of life events. In E. J. Callahan & K. A. McCluskey (Eds.), *Life-span developmental psychology: Nonnormative life events* (pp. 1–33). New York: Academic Press.

Riegel, K. F. (1973). Dialectical operations: The final period of cognitive development. *Human Development, 16*, 346–370.

Riegel, K. F. (1975). Toward a dialectical theory of development. *Human Development, 18*, 50–64.

Riegel, K. F. (1976a). The dialectics of human development. *American Psychologist, 31*, 689–699.

Riegel, K. F. (1976b). From traits and equilibrium toward developmental dialectics. In W. J. Arnold (Ed.), *Nebraska Symposium on Motivation 1975* (pp. 349–407). Lincoln, NE: University of Nebraska Press.

Rogers, C. (1963). The actualizing tendency in relation to motives and to consciousness. In M. R. Jones (Ed.), *Nebraska Symposium on Motivation, 1962* (pp. 1–24). Lincoln, NE: University of Nebraska Press.

Rosenberg, M., & Pearlin, L. I. (1978). Social class and self-esteem among children and adults. *American Journal of Sociology, 84*, 53–77.

Rothbaum, F., Weisz, J. R., & Snyder, S. S. (1982). Changing the world and changing the self: A two-process model of perceived control. *Journal of Personality and Social Psychology, 42*, 5–37.

Ruch, L. O. (1977). A multidimensional analysis of the concept of life change. *Journal of Health and Social Behavior, 18*, 71–83.

Ryan, R. M. (1991). The nature of the self in autonomy and relatedness. In J. Strauss & G. R. Goethals (Eds.), *The self: Interdisciplinary approaches* (pp. 208–238). New York: Springer-Verlag.

Ryan, R. M. (1993). Agency and organization: Intrinsic motivation, autonomy, and the self in psychological development. In J. E. Jacobs (Ed.), *Nebraska Symposium on Motivation: Vol. 40. Developmental perspectives on motivation* (pp. 1–56). Lincoln, NE: University of Nebraska Press.

Ryff, C. D. (1986). The subjective construction of self and society: An agenda for life-span research. In V. W. Marshall (Ed.), *Later life: The social psychology of aging* (pp. 33–74). Beverly Hills, CA: Sage.

Ryff, C. D. (1987). The place of personality and social structure research in social psychology. *Journal of Personality and Social Psychology, 53*, 1192–1202.

Ryff, C. D. (1991). Possible selves in adulthood and old age: A tale of shifting horizons. *Psychology and Aging, 6*, 286–295.

Ryff, C. D., & Heidrich, S. M. (1997). Experience and well-being: Explorations on domains of life and how they matter. *International Journal of Behavioral Development, 20*, 193–206.

Sarason, J. G., Johnson, J. H., & Siegel, J. M. (1978). Assessing the impact of life changes: Development of the Life Experience Survey. *Journal of Consulting and Clinical Psychology, 46*, 932–946.

Schaie, K. W. (1994). The course of adult intellectual development. *American Psychologist, 49*, 304–313.

Schaie, K. W. (1996). *Intellectual development in adulthood: The Seattle Longitudinal Study.* New York: Cambridge University Press.

Seeman, T. E., Berkman, L. F., Kohout, F., LaCroix, A., Glynn, R., & Blazer, D. (1993). Intercommunity variations in the associations between social ties and mortality in the elderly: A comparative analysis of three communities. *Annals of Epidemiology, 3*, 325–335.

Seeman, M., & Lewis, S. (1995). Powerlessness, health, and mortality: A longitudinal study of older men and mature women. *Social Science and Medicine, 41*, 517–525.

Seligman, M. E. P. (1975). *Helplessness: On depression, development, and death.* San Francisco, CA: Freeman.

Silver, R. L., & Wortman, C. B. (1980). Coping with undesirable life events. In J. Garber & M. E. P. Seligman (Eds.), *Human helplessness: Theory and applications* (pp. 279–340). New York: Academic Press.

Solomon, S., Greenberg, J., & Pyszczynski, T. (1991). A terror management theory of social behavior: The psychological functions of self-esteem and cultural worldviews. In M. P. Zanna (Ed.), *Advances in experimental social psychology* (Vol. 24, pp. 93–159). San Diego, CA: Academic Press.

Staudinger, U. M., Marsiske, M., & Baltes, P. B. (1995). Resilience and reserve capacity in later adulthood: Potentials and limits of development across the life span. In D. Cicchetti & D. J. Cohen (Eds.), *Developmental psychopathology: Vol. 2. Risk, disorder, and adaptation* (pp. 801–847). New York: Wiley.

Steele, C. M. (1988). The psychology of self-affirmation: Sustaining the integrity of the self. In L. Berkowitz (Ed.), *Advances in experimental social psychology* (Vol. 21, pp. 261–302). New York: Academic Press.

Stewart, A. J., & Healy, J. M., Jr. (1989). Linking individual development and social changes. *American Psychologist, 44*, 30–42.

Taylor, S. E. (1983). Adjustment to threatening events: A theory of cognitive adaptation. *American Psychologist, 38*, 1161–1173.

Taylor, S. E., & Brown, J. D. (1988). Illusion and well-being: A social psychological perspective on mental health. *Psychological Bulletin, 103*, 193–210.

Taylor, S. E., & Brown, J. D. (1994). Positive illusions and well-being revisited: Separating fact from fiction. *Psychological Bulletin, 116*, 21–27.

Thoits, P. A. (1983). Dimensions of life events that influence psychological distress: An evaluation and synthesis of the literature. In H. B. Kaplan (Ed.), *Psychosocial stress: Trends in theory and research* (pp. 33–103). New York: Academic Press.

Thoits, P. A. (1995). Stress, coping, and social support processes: Where are we? What next? *Journal of Health and Social Behavior, Extra Issue*, 53–79.

Thomae, H. (1979). The concept of development and life-span developmental psychology. In P. B. Baltes & O. G. Brim, Jr. (Eds.), *Life-span development and behavior* (Vol. 2, pp. 281–312). New York: Academic Press.

Thomae, H. (1983). *Alternsstile und Altersschicksale: Ein Beitrag zur Differentiellen Gerontologie* [Styles of aging and fates of aging: A contribution to differential gerontology]. Bern, Switzerland: Huber.

Thomae, H., & Lehr, U. M. (1986). Stages, crises, conflicts, and life-span development. In A. B. Sørensen, F. E. Weinert, & L. R. Sherrod (Eds.), *Human development and the life course: Multidisciplinary perspective* (pp. 429–444). Hillsdale, NJ: Erlbaum.

Vaillant, G. E. (1993). *The wisdom of the ego*. Cambridge, MA: Harvard University Press.

Weiss, R. S. (1975). *Marital separation*. New York: Basic Books.

Wellmann, B., & Hall, A. (1986). Social networks and social support: Implications for later life. In V. W. Marshall (Ed.), *Later life: The social psychology of aging* (pp. 191–231). Beverly Hills, CA: Sage.

Wheaton, B. (1990). Life transitions, role histories, and mental health. *American Sociological Review, 55*, 209–223.

Whitbourne, S. K. (1985). The psychological construction of the life span. In J. E. Birren & K. W. Schaie (Eds.), *Handbook of the psychology of aging* (2nd ed., pp. 594–618). New York: Van Nostrand Reinhold.

Whitbourne, S. K. (1986). *The me I know: A study of adult identity*. New York: Springer Verlag.

White, R. W. (1959). Motivation reconsidered: The concept of competence. *Psychological Review, 66*, 297–333.

Wohlwill, J. F. (1973). *The study of behavioral development*. New York: Academic Press.

PART 2

Socioeconomic Structures and the Self

Practical Consciousness, Social Class, and Self-Concept: A View From Sociology

Jon Hendricks

INTRODUCTION

S elf-concept, practical consciousness, and meaningful experience are familiar constructs in social science that are too often used without sufficient attention to how they interrelate. Sociologists, in particular, have shown a penchant for mechanical models as organizational metaphor. Allowing for certain exceptions, they have focused on macro-level factors and most frequently characterized actors as passive reactors to external stimuli or structural circumstances (Elder & O'Rand, 1995; George, 1990; Gubrium, Holstein & Buckholdt, 1994; Marshall, 1995; Riley, Kahn, & Foner, 1994). Psychologists have been better at parsing individual-level determinants but have not always been attuned to social forces (Bem, 1967, 1972; Epstein, 1973; Hooker & Kaus, 1994; Markus & Ruvolo, 1989; Ryff, 1986, 1991; Sullivan, 1940; Suls, 1982; Whitbourne, 1986). Perhaps a melding of the two perspectives may shed some much-needed light on how self-concept and practical consciousness coalesce with contextual variables to yield meaningful experience.

This discussion is intended primarily for social gerontologists and focuses on the cohesion of practical consciousness, purpose-at-hand, or intentionality, and self-concept as an outgrowth of an actor's social circumstances. It will be asserted that self-concept is adjoined to practical consciousness, an actor's definition of meaningful experience and the social categories to which he/she belongs. As one facet changes, so, too, will others. Self-concept will be characterized as an expression of personal agency as well as an outgrowth of social participation. Closer explication of the constitutive properties of self-concept should prove helpful in analyzing how these issues are affected by age. As will become apparent, each issue is linked to important questions in social gerontology.

Concern with various aspects of personal agency has long been at the heart of social science; it has also been a persistent conundrum (Dallmayr, 1981). Does action reflect reactive response or proactive intent? Resolution of that question has become muddled, characterized by internecine battles rather than insight. Despite considerable effort (Dallmayr, 1981; Denzin, 1989; Ellis & Flaherty, 1992; Giddens, 1984, 1986; Harre, 1986; Kemper, 1981; Thoits, 1989; Weber, 1947), examinations of personal agency within sociology are among those "stalled revolutions"—apparently not enhancing our understanding of the human condition (Hochschild, 1989; Wolfe, 1992). Inquiries into the nature of self-concept are only marginally better off. One hurdle is that constitution of self is elusive, belying easy explanation (Breytspraak, 1984; Dannefer, 1989; Gecas, 1982; Gergen, 1991; Goethals & Strauss, 1991; Gordon & Gergen, 1968; Gubrium & Holstein, 1994; Kohli, 1986a; Rosenberg, 1979; Taylor, 1989; Wiley, 1994). Social gerontology will benefit as the link between macro- and micro-level provisions is clarified and the relationship explored. Besides, as Marshall (1995, p. 363) ardently put it, "The analytical distinction between self and society is inherently false."

This chapter provides a synopsis of relevant constructs, an identification of parallels and suggests ways the dimensions interact. Part I highlights the intersect of self-concept, practical consciousness, and actors' interpretation of experience. The focus is on individual-level factors revolving around reflexivity. Part II illustrates how actors' perceptions are central to social gerontology. Part III brings social resources into the mix, asserting that social capital is crucial to practical consciousness and all facets of self-concept are molded by categorical memberships. As will be apparent, one consequence of categorical memberships, ranging across gender, ethnicity, and age, to social class categories and the like, is an enduring commonality conferred upon actors and the social resources upon which they draw (Bourdieu, 1986). Part IV illustrates contingencies of self-concept as shaped by social capital associated with social class. The organizing rationale behind the presentation is a belief that exploration of self-concept and practical consciousness in a relational framework is over-due. Hopefully, it will provide impetus for refined measures of self, clar-ify ambiguities in empirical/conceptual treatments, help point to the effect of life-course changes, and foster an explication of the relevance of social resources for social psychological dimensions of aging.

SETTING THE STAGE: INTENTIONALITY AND APPREHENSION OF THE WORLD

The self can be said to be the relational nexus to which all interaction and perception is referred. But how does the process work? Trying to figure it out necessitates bringing in Descartes and Hume. Descartes' dictum, *cog-ito ergo sum* is well known—but what does it mean? Descartes was forth-right: "My mind, by which I am what I am, is entirely and truly distinct from my body." Both Descartes and Hume asserted that personal aware-ness is at the heart of interpretation, the organization of experience and formation of self-concept. By exercising self-conscious reflexivity, actors gain awareness of themselves—accretion of experience *per se* is not suf-ficient. Disembodied reason is empty; yet surely actors bring to experience some kind of template for making sense of what they encounter. Descartes and Hume envisioned a primary role for the thinking actor as it is by means of cognitive processing that meaning is created. However, each left sufficient latitude so that followers could interpret cognition as being latent and actors minds, tabula rasa—a blank slate upon which experience writes large. What has been lacking is attention to actors as active agents, as opposed to passive reactors to what comes their way. Couch's (1987) con-tention that every observation is inherently intentional exemplifies the view that purpose is portentous for an actor's knowledge of the world. That is, knowing is an outgrowth of ongoing reflexive processes, not some-thing that springs full-blown from experience alone.

In the post-modernist dialogue running through social science, there is renewed interest in personal agency and the link between perception, inter-action and "objectivity." Post-modernists assert that the objectivity attrib-uted to the noumenal world and the world of perception are flip-sides of the same coin, mutually dependent and reflective of one another (Dallmayr,

1981; Groeben, 1990). Harding (1992) asserted that the concept of objectivity, as the most vaunted form of neutrality, is widely regarded to have been supplanted in social science (Harding, 1992). She cut the Archimedean high ground from a singular scientific method and challenged claims that "empiricism" has a better handle on what is real than other viewpoints. In speaking of how inquiry shapes what is regarded as evidence, Harding was clear, "an excessively restricted notion of research methods, has ensured that only weak standards of objectivity will be required of research projects" (Harding, 1992, p. 577). Her point was that what is "factual" is contingent on both instrumentation and vantagepoint of observers. Definitions of "factuality" involve an observing eye, all the baggage that eye brings to observation, and the constraints implicit in the process of information-gathering and categorization.

INDIVIDUALS AND MEDIATED EXPERIENCE

Mead's (1934) pronouncements on the self are the lodestar. He labeled "self" as the phenomenon that is the recognized outcome of an actor's experience. "Self" is simultaneously subject and object, known through its own reflexively (Wiley, 1994). Insightful as they are, Mead's views are not explicitly phrased in terms of the ebb and flow of real life or real aging. The obvious question is, how are self-concept and life experience joined? How does what an actor is *about* affect what it is they see as the world around them? Then, too, how do actors gain and maintain a sense of themselves as ontological entities and how might it be affected by aging?

Constructing Our Selves

Because questions about self-concept resist easy resolution, greater explication is warranted. That brand of sociological theorizing called social constructionism has something to offer. Social constructionists assert that the social world and meanings attached to it, including actors' self-concept, are socially constituted (Berger & Luckmann, 1966; Harre, 1986). Actors interacting with others in similar circumstances for periods of more than momentary duration create communal interpretative templates via negotiated meanings and mutual definitions of their situation. The very success of their interaction serves as its own reinforcement. The need to understand how experience is structured through social participation is seen as paramount, as participation is the mechanism by which meaning is created. Self-concept can thus be said to be a realization of practical consciousness, shaped through interaction. At the same time, the act of perception is inexorably concept-laden, and responses mediated by actors' purpose and relative locale within their milieu (Armond-Jones, 1986; Averill, 1980).

For social constructionists, practical consciousness is the perspectival lens through which sensory input is mediated, distilled, and assembled into cognition—whether that is termed emotion or rational thought. It is through intentionality, neé, practical consciousness, reflecting an actor's purpose-at-hand, that the "stuff" of experience is rendered into meaningful categories labeled "factual" data. Intentionality is first and foremost pragmatic, it focuses attention and leads to the created life-world that is reflexively known. Perception embodies anticipation as well as sensory input. Whatever a person, thing, or experience means, that meaning is assuredly purposive, part of some sort of schema, socially negotiated and communal. Apart from socially constituted definitions, such phenomena have no discernable ontological status on their own, regardless of their apperception as such. Social constructionists also assert that knowledge is necessarily contingent and consensual, a result of the creative process that *is* personal agency (Berger & Luckmann, 1966; Dallmayr, 1981; Giddens, 1986; Harre, 1986).

An important implication is that actors can be conceived of as conceptually active authors of their life-world. An interesting parallel between an actor's life-world and scholarly inquiry emerges when attention is focused on the extent to which the purpose and intent of inquiry give rise to the categories later utilized to validate the processes by which knowledge was formulated (Hacking, 1992; Turner, 1994). Real life and science are comparable insofar as the creation of that which is called knowledge is grounded in the intent of the knower. In either instance, how we know what we know becomes self-authenticating (Hacking, 1992). In gerontology, social constructionism is unevenly represented, but in no place is it more clearly applied or useful than in recent examinations of how reckoning the life-course colors the way it is lived (Gubrium et al., 1994).

Groeben (1990) added a valuable codicil by his comment that the significance of theories of intentionality lies in their appraisal of the cohesion between self-concept, experience and action—constitutive elements of conscious behavior. They are the mechanisms through which meaning is attached, thereby yielding a concept-laden life-world. There is a tacit aspect to Groeben's avowal insofar as intentionality is at the heart of many facets of perception; it is the bridge between self, agency, and meaning-ful experience. There are at least two challenges to unraveling what inten-tionality implies. To begin with, no action is a freestanding interpretative act, detached from other interpretations. It is through intentional action that actors develop portfolios of meaning and their self-concept. Then, too, action is the "object," the behavioral event, upon which social science explanation focuses (Groeben, 1990). In other words, the second-order constructs of scholarly analyses derive from first-order constructs formu-lated by actors in the course of their own activity, and the two must be consonant.

Attempts to grapple with the intentional character of perception are hardly new. Even though sociology has been slow to take up the quest, Gestalt psychology, and later variations discussed under the rubric of field theory, was built on the premise that meaningful experience is an organic whole, comprised of integrated thematic constituents that cannot be deduced apart from consideration of the complete experience. As the twentieth century was dawning, Wertheimer, Koffka, and other psycho-logical scholars in Germany, James, Pierce, Dewey, and a few contempo-raries in the United States, were asserting that the interpretation of experience is intrinsically propositional (Murphy & Longino, 1990). Dewey's particular twist was to suggest that it is through that most per-sonal of human reactions, emotion, that experience is imbued with mean-ing. If the prospect of emotionally laden comprehension rankles, it would not do injustice to Dewey if emotions were thought of as tantamount to a state of mind. This is not to imply emotions are the same as rationality, only to suggest that emotions are analogous to a state of mind insofar as they color interpretation. In the same vein, practical consciousness is self-stabilizing to the extent that it shapes subsequent interpretation by pro-viding a template through which meaning is sorted and experience assimilated (Gergin & Semin, 1990; Giddens, 1986; Hacking, 1992). As Whitbourne and Primus (1996) noted, one's self-concept is akin to a pred-icate; it is the schema by which the life-world is organized. Actors attach meaning to experience via self-referential filtering processes. One effect of this reading of practical consciousness is that the division between sub-jective perception and what is casually termed objective reality becomes equivocal due to the character of practical consciousness (Groeben, 1990; Schutz, 1973). The components of this model of personal meaning are shown in Figure 7.1. As should be apparent and as will be discussed below, it is a bilateral process.

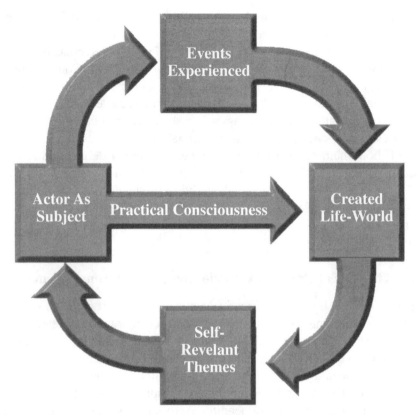

Figure 7.1 Practical consciousness and the creation of self and meaning.

Self-Concept and the Origins of Meaning

If self-concept is a lens through which experience is filtered, it is important to understand how an actor's sense of self is acquired, maintained, or altered. Following a storied history involving considerable passivity ascribed to actors, sociological analysis took a seminal turn with Rosenberg's (1979) landmark explication. In addition to his acumen, Rosenberg posed a dilemma by identifying self-concept as "the totality of the individual's thoughts and feelings having reference to himself as an object" (1979, p. 7). Years earlier, the psychologist Harry Stack Sullivan (1940, p. 21) had spoken of the self as what one takes oneself to be. Epstein (1973) advanced a similar definition by alluding to self-concept as the theory individuals have about themselves as an object. In Felson's (1992) precis, self-concept is said to be all the ways actors describe themselves. In social gerontology, George (1987) assayed self-identity as the global picture individuals have of themselves. What should be apparent is that social scientists refer to a bundle of interrelated concepts when speaking of self-concept (Breytspraak & George, 1982). Consequently, analysts have labored to distinguish cognitive and affective dimensions of selfhood (Breytspraak, 1984). Self-concept has been defined in terms of cognitive operations, yet as a passive consequence of social involvement. Self-esteem has been cast as the emotional or affective "valence" actors hold about themselves. In their present guise, neither delineation is adequate, and each misses the predicate logic that self-concept implies. Foucault (1988) offered a valuable addition by suggesting that definition and redefinition of self is a corollary of actors producing objects, new knowledge, relationships, modes of behavior, or conduct to optimize a sense of well-being.

The Role of Practical Consciousness and Personal Agency

The axiom that human beings are agenetic has been part of social science from the beginning. There is agreement that actors organize, select, attend to, or otherwise act upon their environment (Gergin & Semin, 1990; Kohli, 1988). In a substantial way, self-concept provides the mental architecture by which meaning is wrought from the welter of experience. Lyotard (1984) asserted that self-concept is a condition of knowledge, a cornerstone of the construction of meaning. Actors produce their self-concept concurrently to engaging the world. As actors deal with occurrences, they continuously monitor, select for self-relevance, and formulate meaning— that is what human development is (Brandtstadter, 1990; Markus & Cross, 1990; Whitbourne & Primus, 1996) The process is the mechanism by which the life-world is created. Some scholars characterize its operation as "interpretative practice," with the results simultaneously creating and corroborating the "logic" of ways of knowing. Others refer to intentionality or practical consciousness; the outcome is the same. Once in existence, the constructed life-world functions as a primary reality. It yields precedents and principles, undergirds world-views, facilitates ensuing interpretation, and connotes the operation of pragmatic rules implicit in an actor's purpose-at-hand (Gubrium & Holstein, 1994; Turner, 1994).

Rosenberg (1979) incorporated the melding of self-concept and created life-worlds into his characterization by asserting that sense of self is contingent on ability to think reflexively about oneself and one's world. Reflexivity is the key and because of it, actors conceive of themselves as a consequence of experience. Though self-concept is envisaged as being epiphenomenal, it is also deemed to have ontological status. One corollary is that an actor's self-concept evolves as his or her abilities or circumstances change (Lawton & Nahemow, 1973). If ability to affect one's situation is altered, self-concept will embody that fact. Based on a review of sixty-two studies, Bengtson, Reedy, and Gordon (1985) concluded: (a) self-concept is stable over time, (b) levels of most dimensions of self-concept remain stable over time, and (c) levels of some dimensions do change over time, yet (d) those that change do so not for developmental reasons but in response to changes in social milieu.

Referring again to Figure 7.1, it depicts the interaction of experience, self-concept, and the distillation of meaning. It originates from a contention that perception is concept-laden, reflecting the practical canons of the perceiving actor. The workings implied are dynamic and predicated on an assumption that actors' practical consciousness colors what they deduce and distill from experience. As intentional beings, actors create self-referential life-worlds out of the phenomena of experience as filtered by practical consciousness. In so doing, they employ what amounts to a predicate logic, wherein purpose-at-hand and self-referential precedents, drawn from previous experience, function as scrims though which succeeding experiences are refined, labeled and categorized.

Accordingly, an actor's practical consciousness, their purpose-at-hand, engenders the mental map by which experience is contoured, interpreted, and given narrative unity. None of this is to say that all things going on around actors are attended to as salient, as not all are consonant with practical purpose. Barring an intrusive breech, practical consciousness, or focused intentionality, determines what is heeded and how it is categorized. Once in existence, this created life-world is presumed to be assumptive, self-evident, and permeated by unquestioned truths. Prominent features of the created life-world are then utilized to forge self-relevant constructs that are reiteratively self-validating, accorded ontological status, taken-for-granted, incorporated back into self-concept and used as cynosures for sequent interpretation. Gubrium (1988) grappled with the entire process and referred to it as a form of practical ethnography. It is as though actors act as ethnographers, utilizing constructs to foster a recursive order in emergent interpretation with each step being referenced to the others.

As self-concept is corroborated, it reinforces self-relevant leitmotifs, affirming the premise while simultaneously standing as precedent. Thus, self-concept is mediator and generative consequence of recursive patterns (Giddens, 1986). That is, experience is rendered meaningful through the sorting schemata of self-referential information processing. Meaning is thus created by virtue of the fact that actors are most sensitive to "self-relevant stimuli" (Markus & Kitayama, 1991, p. 230). Self-concept personifies intentionality in ways analogous to the ways other definitions of a situation incorporate orienting assumptions and self-relevant patterns. As will be discussed, these individual-level pattern-generating mechanisms are bracketed by meanings inherent in social milieus.

INDIVIDUAL INTERPRETATION IN
AGING RESEARCH

The literature of social gerontology has tended to sidestep explication of the role of interpretation in the configuration of experience. Be that as it may, actors' assessments of their circumstances are inseparable from the first-order explanatory constructs they formulate. No better examples of the interaction of individual and macro-level factors can be found than in the exploration of meaning attendant to caregiving, assessments of health status, or plain old "lived experience."

George (1990, p. 193) observed that actors' interpretative frameworks are the cornerstones of many constructs in social gerontology. But she cautioned that the origins of those meaning structures are too frequently glossed over. Though many researchers build on individualized interpretative schema, a concentration on instrumentation and analytic technique overshadows their constitutive components. Illustrating her point, George delineated how the perception of social integration signifies actors' interpretative frameworks and is intertwined with diverse evidence of social support, integration, and morale (Liang, Dvorkin, Kahana, & Mazian, 1980; Liang, Kahana, & Doherty, 1980). Of course, the same principle applies to perception of financial well-being, caregiver burden, health, and other everyday issues.

In many respects, the social-psychological paradigm is an attempt to grasp how the meaning individuals render shapes attitudes and behaviors (George, 1990). She reminded researchers that there is no shortage of social-psychological measures of actors' perceptions and experiences. Extrapolating from a synopsis by Maddox and Campbell (1985), George concluded that actors' perceptual schema are definitive for such constructs as anxiety, morale, life-satisfaction, well-being, and burden. For example, social-psychological measures of happiness ask for personal estimations of emotional states and treat responses as ordinal (if not interval) scales of the valence individuals attach to experience. Regardless of scalar debates, estimates of happiness attempt to encapsulate personal readings and imbue them with objective properties by dint of consensual psychometric properties and estimation procedures without sufficient concern being given to how meaning is constituted.

Despite the frequency with which social gerontologists utilize exactly this process, the structuring of perception has received little attention (Gubrium, 1986; Gubrium & Buckholdt, 1977; 1994; Kaufman, 1986). To clarify the process: Those who study changes in the person over the life-course would be well-advised to attend to the constitution of interpretative knowledge. If social gerontologists are to understand how meaning is constructed, researchers must enhance their appreciation of how actors interpret events, thereby infusing their lives, experiences, and social interaction with thematized content. In other words, the pragmatic focus of an actor's practical consciousness, delimited by their purpose-at-hand, is central to the way interpretative frameworks are created and the life-world organized.

Interpretative Meaning: Illustrations From Daily Life

As caregiving burden has received considerable attention, it is an appropriate concept to demonstrate how interpretative frameworks work. Hartung (1993) and Lawton (1993) engaged in a revealing colloquy about the role of interpretative meaning and perception of the hardships associated with caregiving. Responding to an earlier comment by Lawton, Hartung (1993, p. S33) described a "counter intuitive relationship between race and (caregiving) burden, with Black Americans experiencing lower perceived burden and less depression." Her contention was that the perception of burden is greater among more affluent Black caregivers than among their less-affluent counterparts, whereas that relationship is reversed among White caregivers. She also noted that similar relationships are often reported for other variables. If the prospect of interaction effects is taken into account, the incongruity grows even more pronounced. Why the difference?

Hartung enumerated a series of caveats, the proverbial bottom line being that attempts to explain the relationship between income and perceived burden require observant elaboration of an actors' reading of their own situation. Conjectures about burden must be couched in terms of actors' sense of "relative deprivation" as it is played out in diminished income, savings thresholds, and their significance for various income and racial categories. Put less elegantly: Gerontologists risk misinterpretation by relying on income, treated as an interval scale, and attributing explanatory power to the differences. Hartung postulated that crossing back over a "savings threshold" to become nouveau poor precipitates a greater sense of burden among Black caregivers than never being able to save in the first place, or not being close to the threshold. It is the recrossing of the threshold that prompts the sense of burden, not the expense of caregiving relative to financial status. Though it is possible to quarrel or qualify, Hartung's point has merit. Lawton responded that her insights "significantly advance our ability to conceptualize a surprisingly neglected area, the subjective experience of the continuum that runs from wealth to poverty" (Lawton, 1993, p. S34). Who is to say how much of a given variable is enough? Actors know what something means to them, so responses must be interpreted *in situ* as their judgements structure their expectations and ultimately the way they feel (Whitbourne, 1985).

Another illustration from the health care field might be illuminating. Markides, Lee, Ray, and Black (1993) offered a glimpse of the unintentional reification of interpretative practice. In examining how diagnoses were made and coded in the Hispanic Health and Nutrition Examination Survey (H-HANES), they offered cautionary counsel. Though explorations of subjective assessments of health are well established, the focus has been on patients' perception of their own health, with physicians' diagnoses juxtaposed as the comparative "gold standard". It has been assumed that patients are more "subjective". Certainly they are not trained observers, but, as Markides and colleagues advise, the latter does not preclude personalized interpretation from informing diagnoses. It is their contention that physicians' personal experience and practical consciousness affect what they perceive—same as for any actor. They asserted that physicians' normative expectations are factored into their diagnoses. Markides and colleagues aver that physicians perceive what they expect to see, given the experiences they have had and their "beliefs" about categories of patients. An interesting prospect, to be sure, one fraught with research potential and one that goes to the dialectical bond between "objective" and "subjective" information.

Consider, too, the potential import of another aspect of health-physical capacity. Individual capacities are ineluctably connected to the ways actors assimilate information from their environment and, therefore, the way they think of themselves. Regardless of potential opportunities, actors must have the wherewithal, the sensory capacity, and the personal resources, to act effectively, to engage their environment, and exercise their options. There is no gainsaying the fact that an array of personal and social resources are incorporated into practical consciousness. Barred by health or impaired functioning from engaging the unfolding of events, impaired actors find it arduous to sustain meaningful participation. An option is simply not an option if an actor is unable to take action, to exercise choice, or to perceive subtle changes in the ebb and flow of events. None of this is to say there is not considerable latitude, only to assert that certain sensory, physical, and psychological thresholds exist and cannot be ignored when analyzing self-concept.

Taken together, age and health have profound implications for self-concept. In the process of investigating identity in middle and latter life, Logan, Ward, and Spitze (1992), maintained that perceptions of personal age, one facet of self-concept, stem from a compounding of age and health status—both rooted in socially constructed categorizations. There is consensus that health status is inherent in self-concept and definitions of meaning (Grove, Ortega, & Style, 1989; Heidrich & Ryff, 1993; Hooker & Kaus, 1994). There is reasonable unanimity that actors who feel sicker, or are seen as sicker by others, are perceived to be older than their chronological peers and feel themselves to be older (Logan et al., 1992). As deteriorating health impinges on sense of self, there is a rebalancing of the relative prominence of different components of self-concept. Cain (1964) referred to "age-status asynchronization" to suggest asynchronies that may characterize actors who find themselves emersed in a complex set of roles that may be internally inconsistent, incongruent, are buffeted by displacing ill-health, or are otherwise out of synchrony with other arenas of their lives.

One last illustration will ring familiar. The notion of lived experience provides another demonstration of the importance of interpretative frameworks. In everyday discourse actors routinely make reference to the concept. "Not being a ——, how can you understand . . . ," "You cannot really know what it is like to have to retire until you. . . ," or "Until you have been in my shoes how can you possibly. . . ." The point of such rejoinders is that meaning is difficult to fathom apart from first-hand contact with the context in which it is created. As Ellis and Flaherty (1992) argued, the whole intent of "subjective research" is to enable investigators to better apprehend the world as actors perceive it from the vantage point of their structural location within a given milieu.

SELF AND SOCIAL CLASS: AN ECOLOGICAL PERSPECTIVE

There is another dimension of the creation of self-concept that needs to be considered: self-concepts are not created *ex cathedra*. In a seminal commentary, Clausen observed, "Human life is the product of many forces— genetic, physiological, ecological, social and cultural" (1972, p. 462). The implication for self-concept is that how actors think of themselves is comprised of individualized interpretative frameworks bracketed by social circumstances. In this section, attention is on the influence of social resources in shaping self-concept. Except for a few noteworthy exceptions (Clausen, 1972, 1986; Dannefer & Perlmutter, 1990; Elder & O'Rand, 1995; Gergen, 1977; George, 1990, 1992; Kohli, 1986b; Markus & Cross, 1990; Marshall, 1986; Riegel, 1973; Ryff, 1986; Smelser & Smelser, 1970; Stryker, 1981), the gerontological literature has treated self-concept primarily as a personal project. The effects of social resources such as socioeconomic roles have not been widely recognized as germane (Markus & Cross, 1990). Fortunately, a change is afoot, and more relational perspectives are refocusing attention on the reciprocal fusion of social resources and social psychological characteristics (Bourdieu, 1986; Ritzer & Gindoff, 1994; Elder, & O'Rand, 1995).

The foregoing discussion about personalized interpretative templates underlying the organization of self-concept should not be seen as a claim that self-concept is a singular expression of an actor's volitional mind-set. On the contrary, though the process of meaning construction takes place as part of individual reflexivity, self-concept also reflects the recursive sweep of social roles that provide social capital. It is grounded in and defined by means of interaction and the cumulative effect of the "crescive bond" that create "institutionally formulated scripts" that function as primers leading to shared biographical perspectives among those occupying a communal life space (Gubrium et al., 1994; Hagestad & Marshall, 1980; Schutz, 1973). Membership in many types of collectivities resonates with meaning and furnishes an ecological backdrop as well as an interpretative auspice through the emotional presence of shared group life (Gergen & Semin, 1990; Taylor, 1989). In short, participation provides archetypal representations that supply the characteristic lens actors use for interpretation (Bourdieu, 1989). Each coalition confers meaning in the minds of its members, meanings that result in a "natural attitude" that supports personal interpretation while connoting and maintaining structural differentiation (Bourdieu, 1989; Schutz, 1973). That attitude construes the world as being "just so," and not any other way. Regardless of subtype, affinity groups shape experience insofar as they provide the social resources that are the origin of sociocentric world-views adhering in the minds of individuals (Hendricks, 1995).

One's action space, wherein actors are agenetic in the creation of meaning through person-environment transactions, reflects divers forces beyond individual volition in an intersubjective world of communal meanings (Brandtstadter, 1990; Schooler, 1989). It means that actors do not create life-worlds entirely of their own choosing, but do so within the penumbra of social and personal resources (Bourdieu, 1989; Brandtstadter, 1990). It also means developmental processes, including how actors conceive of themselves, are configured by the referential power of social resources. Variations in social class presage variation in mediated life scripts and augur divergence in knowledge, personality, and subjective attributes or outcomes connoting differential self-concepts (Kohn & Slomczynski, 1990; Rosenberg, 1981; Ryff, 1987; Schooler, 1989;). This is what the ecology of human development implies—that the life-course is relational and contextualized (Bronfenbrenner, 1979).

Self-concept, then, stands as the ultimate amalgam, melding micro- and macro-level factors as filtered through practical consciousness (Ritzer & Gindoff, 1994). Whereas relativity is presumed, it is neither absolute nor solipsistic; actors act in concert and through tacit agreement. In so doing, they are abetted by underlying representations, resonant definitions of what is real and appropriate, a sense of "objective" reality that is "subjectively appropriated in the process of socialization" and affirmed through practice (Carugati, 1990, p. 130). For all intents and purposes, socially relevant categorical membership "sets limitations upon what can be produced and by whom. . . . Any social structure will limit and restrain the production of future alternative[s]" (Wardell & Benson, 1978, p. 5).

Brandtstadter captured the symmetry between social resources and personalized intent in his remark, "As these contextualized conditions undergo change, so do the modal patterns and constraints for individual development" (Brandtstadter, 1990, p. 84). These social resources are extra-individual, "deep structures", which do not always receive deliberative attention but are key to self-concept. What such an assertion portends for self-concept is that ecological niche and social location help fashion the relational processes involved in how actors see themselves (Hendricks, 1992; Kohli & Meyer, 1986).

Riley and colleagues (Riley, Johnson, & Foner, 1972; Riley et al., 1994) have focused on the role social structure plays in assessments of individual life course change and intercohort variation. It may be that changes in structural arrangements are the bedrock of individual and collective characteristics, as structural circumstances are vital to the way actors apprehend the world (Dannefer, 1987, 1988a, 1988b; Dannefer & Perlmutter, 1990). Accordingly, it would be newsworthy if research did not find generational or maturational differences. Giddens (1979) labeled the bond between actors and social milieu structuration—the spawning of generative and emergent outcomes tacitly shaped by the conventions of interaction. Through the syntax of actors' motives, and the referential power of social resources, the essence of the group is actualized via individual behavior. Giddens (1991) considered the salience of social resources to be inextricably fused with key features of personal awareness. No matter how elusive, it would be egregious to assert that actors acquire personal identity unfettered by social bonds (Dannefer, 1984; Dowd, 1990).

Concentrating the Focus

There is a bilateral bond between actor and social resources. Though a host of social and communal factors need explication, my efforts will focus on social class as a constitutive property of self-concept. The rationale is that social class provides the social capital that is incorporated into the "webs of significance" in which actors dwell (Geertz, 1973, p.5). In a review, George (1990) asserted that much research treats structural factors, including social class, as independent variables, social-psychological states as dependent outcomes, and social processes as mediating the two (George, 1990; House, 1977). However, there is an even more organic bond. It is not so much an interface of external or internal factors as an instantiation—a bringing into existence, a potentiation of that which had previously been latent. As actors emerge from structural circumstances by way of social roles, occupational pursuits, or other types of involvement that promote integration, they simultaneously realize a reflexive self-concept (Bourdieu, 1986; George, 1990).

In an interlocutory analysis of self-concept, social class is essential to the negotiated interpretations incorporated into sense of self (Giddens, 1986; George, 1990; Markus & Cross, 1990). Actors are enveloped by social circumstances the way fish are immersed in water—they cannot otherwise exist. Actors are socialized to why the world is as it is through language, tacit conventions, social prescriptions, and so on. These ideas are incorporated into group identity and help fashion the formative experiences incorporated into consciousness (Carugati, 1990). Insofar as social classes are differentiated, actors will hold diverse views predicated on proximity to a given range of social conditions. In reference to psychological functioning as a consequence of social class, Kohn and Slomczynski (1990) contended, "People's social class positions and their place in the stratification order affect their psychological functioning mainly by their decisive influence on proximate conditions of life. It is these proximate conditions of life that influence personality" (p. 3).

Social Class and Social Relativity

Though the gravitational pull of social class is intangible, its leverage is manifested in individual interpretations. The norms implicit in class membership are inculcated in individuals. Far from being simply a mosaic of occupational, educational, and financial resources, social class wields considerable sway over all aspects of an actor's situation, including what they discern as meaningful or how they age. The import of social class is that it connotes the social conditions of knowledge that manifest themselves in the behavior/action of real people. Giddens (1986) was of the opinion that the interaction of people and their memberships is reciprocally defined, dynamic, and lifelong.

As Weber (1921, 1968) pointed out, the challenge is to develop explanatory models that do not disconnect actor from the distinctions intrinsic to status groupings or structural circumstance. As he and others have noted, normative expectations, regularities, and consistencies characterizing groups of actors are illustrative of the transcendent and emergent mediation between social class and self (House & Mortimer, 1990; Settersten and Hagestad, 1996; Smelser & Smelser, 1970). Without getting bogged down in tangents about formation or endurance, suffice it to say there is consensus that social class is the origin of ideas, knowledge, routine, and agency. In probing why social class may be more portentous for self-concept at some points in life than others, Rosenberg and Pearlin (1978) specified four distinctive models, each of which accedes a prominent role to social class as a medium for expression of self-concept. In a cross-cultural exploration of the role of social resources in the United States and Poland, Kohn and Slomczynski asserted that "A more advantaged position in the class structure, and a higher position in the social-stratification order, result in valuing self-direction more highly, in greater intellectual flexibility and in a more self-directed orientation" (1990, p. 106).

From the Outside in: Stratification and Interpretation

Social stratification is rooted in the socially acclaimed merit of relative contributions, modes of production, and the political/ideological trappings corroborating the rationale. Characteristics that distinguish social classes stem from market-based differentiation that signals how "precious" a society regards a commodity or attribute to be. In short, we assess human capital the way we tally any recognized asset. Sociologists refer to an aggregated measure of social class comprised of occupation, education, and income levels—three prominent features of human capital. Yet, social class is more holistic than is implied by a composite indicator, it assures communal lifestyles. Without diverting into a disquisition on why class matters, or its operationalization, suffice it to say, social class blends together ascribed and achieved characteristics that provide recognized social resources.[1]

The relevance of social class is that it provides social resources affecting noneconomic arenas such as health, access to opportunity, and the experience of aging. At the same time, the accoutrements of social class sustain differentiated life-styles, world-views, or normative expectations that are leavened into self-concept. Social class is also relational, defined in terms of relative standing compared to other social classes, coloring the way actors interact with and label one another. It would not be overstating the case to suggest that far from being solely an ordering of social positions, social class plays out in an actor's world-view, responses to phenomena, sense of self, and how others perceive them. Degradation in any of the constitutive elements on which social class or life styles are built will bring about a reappraisal of actors insofar as social resources are integral to their persona and their ability to negotiate with others or their environment.

Personal interpretation and social class fuse together to frame what actors perceive—what they know to be the case. The same process pertains to self-concept; sense of self is comprised of a commingling of individual intentionality and social capital; it is the synthesis of all taken-for-granted assumptions about the world. In part, surety issues from consensus—to say something is "so," in a social sense, is to acknowledge tacit agreement

---

1. Although social class underlies differences in the apportionment of opportunities and the distribution of societal rewards, the basis for assignment to any particular social class is not seen solely as a consequence of human capital. In recent years, an element of political economy has been added as commentators have asserted that social class membership is not merely the result of status attainment, but reflects an allocation of opportunities based on group characteristics. Regardless of the basis for assignment, position in the hierarchy is a major influence over access to any number of important resources relevant to self-definition. The relevance of social class raises many questions, among them is how the accoutrements of lifestyle affect social psychological factors and the way selves are shaped.

among participants that it is indeed thus. The "legitimated grammar of individualism" that is so much a part of modern life does not gainsay that contention in the least (Giddens, 1991; Huber, 1988).

In his landmark exposition of the composition of the self, Rosenberg (1979) outlined four operative processes. He spoke of attribution, whereby judgements are made about entire personalities based on observation of a finite range of behaviors. He also alluded to other aspects that may be even more germane. In going about their routines, actors adhere to or violate normative expectations for people in their approximate circumstances. Through reflected appraisals perceived in the responses of others, actors monitor how well they match expectations (Felson, 1992; Rosenberg, 1979;). Kuypers and Bengtson (1973) built their social breakdown model of unsuccessful aging on reflected appraisals and their work helped set the stage for a relational analysis of self-concept as formed by micro- and macro-level factors. Breytspraak (1984) and Karp (1988) also considered reflected appraisals in light of the increasing frequency of negative "aging messages" encountered by middle-aged actors. Regardless of the loading, self-concept will encompass perceived feedback filtered through self-referential constructions of meaning (Gergen & Semin, 1990; Heidrich & Ryff, 1993).

Normative expectations influence actors via social comparisons with others thought to be in comparable circumstances. Attributes such as age, education, gender, health, and other salient characteristics are used to select others for comparison (Felson, 1992, p. 1745; Rosenberg, 1979). Such referential role models remain part of an actor's frame of reference as they age, especially for those prone to "self-in-relation-to-other" comparisons (Heidrich & Ryff, 1993; Hendricks, 1992; Markus & Kitayama, 1991). Wood (1989) identified three purposes served by social comparisons: self-evaluation, self-improvement and self-enhancement. Comparing oneself to others may have a salutary effect for those who see themselves as doing well compared to their peers and a negative effect on those who see themselves doing less well (Heidrich & Ryff, 1993; Hendricks, 1992; Ryff & Essex, 1992). However derived, social comparisons are significant for purposes of self-appraisal and differentiation (Breytspraak, 1984; Markus & Cross, 1990).

Normative expectations are always part of actors' biographies. Ryff (1991) examined how actors conceive of themselves and concluded they may carry around a set of self-referential expectations brought into play as they appraise their status. Actors often have anticipated scripts, future life histories, and trajectories in mind. Their projected scripts are both proleptic and dynamic, exerting sway on current thinking though future states are not yet realized (Hendricks & Peters, 1986; Markus & Ruvolo, 1989; Seltzer & Troll, 1986). These anticipated selves function like incentives, paving the way for future recourse, providing license while simultaneously furnishing interpretative beacons (Ryff, 1991). To the extent expectations incorporate an actor's perception of events relative to their present status, these self-appraisals are incorporated into self-concept. Felson asserted that "specific self-appraisals of ability affect performance" (1992, p. 1747). Ryff framed the issue in terms of actors holding personal standards based on self-assessments of improvement, maintenance, or declining abilities and competencies (Ryff, 1991). It may even be that with advancing age, self-comparisons exert a greater influence over self-concept that social comparisons (Giddens, 1991; Suls & Mullen, 1982). Likely there is fluidity in self and social comparisons affecting how actors construe themselves because of age or situational changes (Bengtson et al., 1985; Kohli & Meyer, 1986). In making self-assessments, actors monitor their physical and psychological capacity vis-à-vis anticipations of what they thought they would be like (Whitbourne, 1985: Whitbourne & Primus, 1996). It may be that some personality types rely more extensively on interdependent relationships, while others rest on independence self-definitions (Markus & Kitayama, 1991).

As a concomitant of social class, actors encounter differential privilege and reward that help establish identifiable lifestyles and other social resources that seem to exist independently. Social class not only entails a distribution of valued commodities; it also embodies routinized patterns of interaction along with accompanying linguistic, normative, and moral practices. At the same time, social class connotes distribution of values; norms and world-views to which actors are socialized (Rosenberg, 1981; Ryff, 1987). As Weber (1921, 1968) asserted, from social class categories flow variations in human experience that are powerful, indelible, and amazingly subtle, yet ubiquitous.

Because of the consanguinity of groups, social conventions are produced and reproduced via the associative social relationships of daily practice (Weber, 1921, 1968). The resulting norms, mores, and symbolic representations are reflexively acquired by actors and contribute the sense of ipsative stability carried across transitions and from one context to another (Elder & O'Rand, 1995). Because perceptions grounded in social class possess what amounts to an ontological status, they provide a sense of stability, providing a palpably "assumptive world"—taken as undeniably real, as "second nature" and without further ado.

Heterogeneity and Social Relativity

Age-grading typifies the kind of social relativity that characterizes expectations inherent in social locale. So, too, do timing norms for life-course transitions (Settersten & Hagestad, 1996). Most transitions are predicated on nomological patterns sorted according to the beliefs and values of localized subcultures. Bronfenbrenner (1979) referred to the "ecology of human development" to underscore how proximate conditions structure the experience of aging. A variety of situational factors, ranging from physical conditions to social class and occupational roles, racial, ethnic, and gender-based experiences impose substance and form to age-graded transitions that differentiate actors. Settersten and Hagestad (1996) noted that despite ample ambiguity, timing norms are slightly more pronounced for American men than women. Acknowledging generalized patterns, Hogan and Astone (1986) pointed out, "This means that the pace of biological, psychological, and social development may vary between individuals, and there need be no uniformity in the ordering in which development stages on the different dimensions occur" (p. 111).

Rowe and Kahn (1987, 1997, 1998) champion an even more expansive proposition. They maintain that the elemental biological and physiological substrates upon which much of our conceptualization about human development and aging are based are not immutable in the face of social diversity. They distinguish between usual and successful aging, grounding each in social contingencies, asserting that even basic biogenetic functions are expressed through behavioral consequences given form by social resources. In successful aging, social and environmental factors play a neutral or positive role. Optimal social conditions yield optimal physical outcomes. Social class, abetted by public policies, produces discernable lifestyles capable of modifying normative changes that otherwise accompany chronological age. That is, age-related processes are realized within parameters set by socially determined statuses and spheres of activity. Without belaboring their argument, Rowe and Kahn postulate that successful aging is a benefit accruing from advantageous social circumstances (Rowe & Kahn, 1998). One illustration will make the point: Personal and social resources affect nutritional status, thereby affecting such things as the timing of onset and duration of menses, incontrovertibly part of self-concept among women.

A lifetime's experience of social class may explain the heterogeneity found in surveys of elderly persons. Though variances are often seen as anomalies, else attributed to unspecified disparities in life experience, such indicia may represent the reverberations of social class categories in shaping attitudes and behavior. It would be shortsighted to attribute variations to individual personalities or dismiss them as aberrations without further inquiry (Dannefer, 1984; House, 1981; Smelser & Smelser, 1970). Commenting on the lack of focus on the relevance of disparities that may result from social class, Dannefer (1988a, 1996) noted how ironic it is that "the idea that social structure and social processes play a regulative or constitutive role in the production of aged diversity is less familiar although no less promising" than psychological or physiological explanations (p. 11).

What is needed to decipher the relativity of personal attributes and assorted manifestations of difference found among older persons is recognition that social class and social capital have an undeniable reach over actors (Bourdieu, 1986; Dannefer, 1988b, 1996; Fry & Keith, 1982; George, 1990; Kohli, 1986a; Riley et al., 1994). Those social processes implicit in daily practice that are characteristic of disparate status groupings or categorical memberships may account for a significant portion of the heterogeneity found among older persons, including self-concept (Dannefer, 1988a, 1996; Kohli & Meyer, 1986). Social experience shaped by access to opportunity, normative roles, transitions, timetables, and age-role incongruities need to be investigated to see if they are implicated in shaping self-relevant perceptions of meaning.

SOCIAL CONTINGENCIES AND SELF-CONCEPT

The dearth of explanations for "old-age heterogeneity" may stem from a conflating of factors associated with social capital or with human capital. For example, going to work full time reflects a combination of personal and class-based resources while serving as prologue to the sequencing of adult life (O'Rand, 1990). The initial transition is the origin of subsequent duration dependent consequences and serial transitions (Spilerman, 1977). The timing of the passage is indexed to formative experiences anchored in social class in a consistent but inverse relationship (Elder & O'Rand, 1995; O'Rand, 1990; Settersten & Hagestad, 1996; Spilerman, 1977).

Contingent Transitions and Social Class

Those young people unable to affect voluntary entry, who find themselves full-time members of the labor force while their age peers are continuing their education, also find themselves catapulted into adult preoccupations.

They experience an unfolding of sequelae that may be quite disparate when compared to those who delayed entering the labor force (Elder & O'Rand, 1995). Those who delay entry experience an extended adolescence, a compression of work or childbearing years, and the period they spend as grandparents. Those who leave school experience a prolonged work life, earlier marriage, differential retirement, and grandparenthood (O'Rand, 1990; Settersten & Hagestad, 1996). Working or going to school are portentous for self-concepts when the transition occurs and over the ensuing years. Those who have the resources to continue their education, defer full-time labor force participation, and other rites of passage likely to shape their self-concepts will have a different sense of aging than is the case for those who lacked comparable resources (Elder & O'Rand, 1995; O'Rand, 1990; Spilerman, 1977).

Work itself also augurs an effect on self-concept. It is widely held that the nature of work provides a "crucial explanatory link between positions in the class and stratification structure and psychological functioning" (Kohn & Slomczynski, 1990, p. 5). Jobs that permit autonomy or creativity and provide emoluments such as retirement annuities will foster a distinctive old age, not to mention a sense of futurity, compared to jobs that are closely supervised, routinized, or permit neither economic security nor personal growth. A succession of entry-level positions or recurrent or protracted unemployment is unlikely to provide comparable fodder for inclusion in self-concepts, as they lead to disordered or disrupted transitions in other arenas of life (Cain, 1964; Rindfuss, Swicegood, & Rosenfeld, 1987). By contrast, stable jobs permitting self-direction, advancement, pension coverage, or options for self-creation will have different effects on actors in terms of sense of futurity, the perception of and timing of retirement, and overall self-concept (O'Rand, 1990).

Another illustration is apropos. In a discussion of the effects of automation on aging workers, I suggested that the advent of computer technology might lead to both a flattening and a bifurcation of traditional occupational categories and status differentials (Hendricks, 1983). The presumption was that hi-tech innovation could bring a leveling of substantive complexity, autonomy, self-pacing, or even physical mobility across a broad range of occupations. The prospect of task routinization and a decline in opportunities for self-direction in upper- and middle-level white-collar positions will have as great an impact as it had in blue-collar pursuits. In short, technology may restructure the way jobs are done and workers will have less latitude in their performance. It is reasonable to assert that a larger proportion of tomorrow's labor force will have blue collar-like job experiences by virtue of the fact that fewer of them will have control over the "doing" of their jobs—occupational titles notwithstanding. At the same time, it is likely that educational requirements and relative wage levels or benefit packages will eventually reflect shifts wrought by alterations in worker autonomy. According to Kohn and Slomczynski (1990), "Occupational self-direction plays a pivotal role in explaining the effects of social structure on personality and the effects of personality on position in the social structure" (p. 235).

If predictions are accurate, many of the accoutrements of occupational status and job performance may be flattened across much of the labor force. Consequently, there may be fewer hierarchical status rankings among tomorrow's workers. Surely there will be a segment that continues to have careers characterized by autonomy, definitional power over job structuring, substantive complexity, and intellectual exploration. Another segment, something on the order of 80%, will have a different experience[2]. Still another segment will find itself on the periphery, moving in and out of jobs at irregular intervals, experiencing disjunctive career paths or unstable employment. In the face of technological innovation, retooling may be tantamount to detooling as the rationale for worker autonomy shifts. In the face of such prospects, what happens to notions of occupation advancement, mobility, life course trajectories, passages, or, for that matter, self-concept? On the latter point: if career ladders are no longer the norm, if jobs do not allow ideational flexibility or self-direction, what are the implications for workers' self-concepts? Normative time tables and the nature of transitions themselves help forge sense of self (Elder & O'Rand, 1995; Featherstone & Hepworth, 1989; Hogan & Astone, 1986; Marini, 1984a, 1984b)

Figure 7.2 is intended to depict self-concept as emerging from personal resources and an array of social resources associated with social class. While it is difficult to picture the dynamic quality of the interaction among the constituents, the figure represents sense of self as an ecological construct emerging from an interplay of contextualized social factors. As is

---

2. Society is currently seeing one aspect of this flattening in terms of revenues flowing into the coffers of the Social Security trust fund by virtue of sector-related employment patterns. Similarly, the vast and growing service sector of the economy is evidencing dramatic cutbacks in the type and level of its retirement plans.

More relevant for this volume is the way changes in the structure of work are altering the subjective meaning of the work experience across all levels and types of employment. For example, an analogous redefinition may also be observed among pharmacists, among physicians employed by HMOs, or executives and white-collar workers in companies that are downsizing.

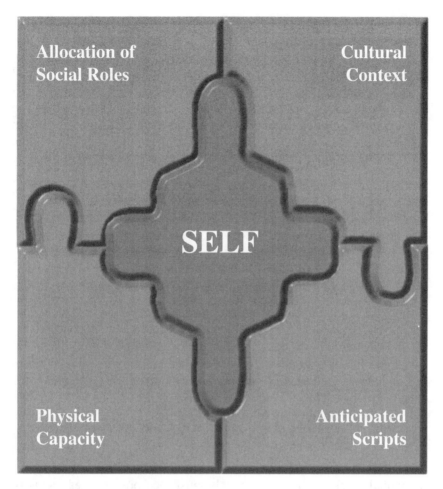

Figure 7.2 Self as contingent outcome.

evident, sense of self may be seen as akin to a figure-ground relationship. The relevance of each element derives from its juxtaposition to other elements and none can be apprehended apart from their mutuality.

In the scenario presented, self-concept emerges as a structural consequence of contextualized resources. What the figure does not adequately convey is that the factors shown in no way exhaust the influence of structural processes, or that each has a relativity affected by social capital associated with social class, ethnicity, gender, and macro-level features that facilitate or constrain access to opportunity. With the pertinence of each dimension mediated by personal agendas, the only way to assess their impact is to attend to the ways mediation occurs (Kohli, 1988; Marshall, 1995; Ryff, 1986; Sorensen, 1986).

Keeping the reciprocity of personal agency and social resources in mind, a relational analysis of self-concept would focus on how societal forces channel and individual intentionality defines meaningful experience. Marshall was prescient in discerning the constant tension between stability issuing from structural factors and instability flowing from human intentionality (Marshall, 1995, 1996). Recognizing much the same thing, Ryff (1986) commented on the relativity of knowledge and the difficulty of generalizing about sources of self-concepts. As she and others caution, if social gerontology is to unravel the dynamic interaction between the two dimensions, analyses must consider agency and structure simultaneously.

CONCLUSION

Although there is renewed interest in the linkage between practical consciousness, sense of self and meaningful experience, a more conceptually grounded explication is due. This discussion is intended preliminary for social gerontologists in that the goal has been to suggest ways in which self-concept is a contingent process and one that varies by age. Actors undertake personal interpretations based on their purpose-at-hand, but their judgements are not entirely of their own volition; factors related to social capital are always relevant. Self-concept reflects a coterie of roles, awareness of age norms, age-appropriate behavior, social norms, anticipated timetables, interaction patterns, and shifting personal priorities. At the individual level, explanatory models must incorporate assessments of experience, the internalization of age-norms derived from social class categories, cognizance of age-appropriate behavior, health, and physical capacity. At the macro level, explanations must recognize that actors' perceptions are cradled in the values, anticipated timetables, and structural constraints implicit in formal and informal relationships (Cutler, 1982; Hendricks, 1987, 1994).

By conceiving of sense of self as a transformative, mediational filter through which meaning is created, the bond between self-concept, intentionality, and self-referential meaning may be better understood. Being more attentive to the role self-concept plays in assembling experience into meaningful categories should have practical utility for understanding life-course changes and issues of identity in later life. Having a better handle on the process will lessen the gulf between scientific explanation and the first-order precepts of the constructed life-world. Incorporating practical consciousness and the ordinary theorizing of actors into scientific perspectives on how meaning is created and how self-concept evolves will bring a closer alignment to what happens in real life (Gubrium & Wallace, 1990; Ryff, 1986).

Dannefer (1989) has been among those calling for a broadening of theoretical models in the sociology of aging. In his view, "A theory of aging must systematically consider the implications for aging of different modes of action, consciousness and selfhood and their relationship to different social forms" (p. 4). This discussion has asserted that it is through the self-referential focus of practical consciousness that the created life-world is constituted and it is through practical consciousness that an actor's self-concept takes shape. In many respects, self-concept is first and foremost a theoretical statement created by actors and only secondarily utilized by social scientists (Epstein, 1973). Without overworking the analogy, an actor's theory of self is not unlike any other conceptual model; its postulates are corroborated through their application.

Self-concept exemplifies the synthetic quality; the seemingly objective "thing" that emerges as experience is distilled into self-relevant meaningful relationships. But experience never takes place in a vacuum; it is not insulated from the effects of macro-level memberships or strictures. Accordingly, self-concepts are conditional, allocentric, and bound to situational impositions. Breytspraak highlighted the social origins of sense of self when she referred to it as emerging from "the point of articulation between the individual and society" (Breytspraak, 1984, p. 31). Actors weave webs of significance that relate one to another, with sense of self as an organizational nexus (Giddens, 1991). Markus and Cross (1990) referred to "working-self concepts" to connote how situational identities replicate principal forms of involvement at any point in time.

Social resources play an integral role among the factors thought to influence composition of self-concept. Accordingly, such social factors as social class, gender, race or ethnicity, subculture, or structural location, to name but a few, are instrumental in determining resources and thereby the broad outlines of the arena within which self-concept is formulated. Certainly each has been implicated in explanatory frameworks in previous research, and each is tied to institutionalized pathways to opportunity (Featherman, 1986; George, 1990; O'Rand, 1990;). Without oversimplifying it, differential self-concepts accrue from differences in social capital that mediate social experience and the reflexive sense actors have of themselves (Featherman & Lerner, 1985; Featherstone & Hepworth, 1989). Dowd's synopsis is apt: "Developmental opportunities and, therefore, development itself varies in direct correspondence with social class or economic and social well-being" (1990, p. 150).

If inquiry is to make sense of changes in self-concepts, a relational approach is needed, one that attends to the social construction of self and its integrative/mediational role (Kohli & Meyer, 1986). It means that the distinction between actor, as autonomous being, and positionality, or communal circumstance, must be breached. There are not many lone wolves out there, nor do many people grow old without ties to referential others or normative expectations. Lastly, it means accounts of self must incorporate the ways in which access to opportunity, resources, and role involvements vary across the broad spectrum of variables that constitute social capital.

Although these cautionary remarks are not sufficient in themselves to bring about a reconstruction of the paradigm, they may initially blur and in the long run contribute to a more evocative conceptualization. A recentering is in order in the social and behavioral sciences, not to mention in social gerontology. The reality of self-concept and aging processes broadly considered is that they are based on interpersonal, fiduciary, and social-psychological resources anchored in social class, occupation, racial and ethnic subcultures, as well as gender, health and other factors beyond the control or even the purview of individual actors.

REFERENCES

Armond-Jones, C. (1986). The thesis of constructionism. In R. Harre (Ed.), *The social construction of emotions* (pp. 32–56). Oxford: Basil Blackwell.

Averill, J. (1980). A constructionist view of emotions. In P. Plutchik & H. Kellerman (Eds.), *Emotion theory, research, and experience* (pp. 305–339). New York: Academic Press.

Bem, D. (1967). Self-perception: An alternative interpretation of cognitive dissonance phenomena. *Psychological Review, 74*, 183–200.

Bem, D. (1972). Self-perception theory. In L. Berkowitz (Ed.), *Advances in experimental social psychology* (pp. 1–62). New York: Academic Press.

Bengtson, V., Reedy, M., & Gordon, C. (1985). Aging and self-conceptions: Personality processes and social contexts. In J. Birren & K. W. Schaie (Eds.), *Handbook of the psychology of aging* (2nd ed., pp. 544–593). New York: Van Nostrand-Reinhold.

Berger, P., & Luckmann, T. (1966). *The social construction of reality*. Garden City, NY: Anchor.

Bourdieu, P. (1986). The forms of capital. In J. Richardson (Ed.), *Handbook of theory and research for the sociology of education* (pp. 241–258). Westport, CT: Greenwood Press.

Bourdieu, P. (1989). Social space and symbolic power. *Sociological Theory, 7,* 14–25.

Brandtstadter, J. (1990). Development as a personal and cultural construction. In G. Semin & K. Gergin (Eds.), *Everyday understanding: Social and scientific implications* (pp. 83–107). Newbury Park, CA: Sage.

Breytspraak, L. & George, L. (1982). Self-concept and self esteem. In D. Mangen & W. Peterson (Eds.), *Research instruments in social gerontology: Vol. 1. Clinical and social psychology* (pp. 241–302). Minneapolis: University of Minnesota Press.

Breytspraak, L. (1984). *The development of self in later life.* Boston: Little, Brown.

Bronfenbrenner, U. (1979). *The ecology of human development.* Cambridge: Harvard University Press.

Cain, L. (1964). Life course and social structure. In R. Farris (Ed.), *Handbook of modern sociology* (pp. 272–309). Chicago: Rand McNally & Company.

Carugati, F. (1990). Everyday ideas, theoretical models and social representations: The case of intelligence and its development. In G. Semin & K. Gergen (Eds.), *Everyday understanding: Social and scientific implications* (pp. 130–150). Newbury Park, CA: Sage.

Clausen, J. (1972). The life course of individuals. In M. Riley, M. Johnson & A. Foner (Eds.), *Aging and society: Vol. 3. A sociology of age stratification* (pp. 457–514). New York: Russell Sage Foundation.

Clausen, J. (1986). *The life course: A sociological perspective.* Englewood Cliffs, NJ: Prentice-Hall.

Couch, C. (1987). Objectivity: A crutch and club for bureaucrats/subjectivity: A haven for lost souls. *Sociological Quarterly, 28,* 105–118.

Cutler, N. (1982). Subjective age identification. In D. Mangen & W Peterson (Eds.), *Research instruments in social gerontology: Vol. 1. Clinical and social psychology* (pp. 437–461). Minneapolis: University of Minnesota Press.

Dallmayr, F. (1981). *Twilight of subjectivity.* Amherst, MA: University of Massachusetts Press.

Dannefer, D. (1984). Adult development and social theory: A paradigmatic reappraisal. *American Sociological Review, 49,* 100–116.

Dannefer, D. (1987). Aging as intracohort differentiation: Accentuation, the Matthew effect, and the life course. *Sociological Forum, 2,* 211–236.

Dannefer, D. (1988a). Differential gerontology and the stratified life course: Conceptual and methodological issues. In G. Maddox & M. P. Lawton (Eds.), *Annual Review of Gerontology* (Vol. 8, pp. 128–150). New York: Springer Publishing Company.

Dannefer, D. (1988b). What's in a name? An account of the neglect of variability in the study of aging. In J. Birren & V. Bengtson (Eds.), *Emergent theories in aging* (pp. 128–150). New York: Springer Publishing Company.

Dannefer, D. (1989). Human action and its place in theories of aging. *Journal of Aging Studies, 3,* 1–20.

Dannefer, D. (1996). The social organization of diversity, and the normative organization of age. *The Gerontologist, 36,* 174–177.

Dannefer, D., & Perlmutter, M. (1990). Development as a multidimensional process: Individual and social constituents. *Human Development, 33,* 108–137.

Denzin, N. (1989). *Interpretative interactionism.* Newbury Park, CA: Sage.

Dowd, J. (1990). Ever since Durkheim: The socialization of human development. *Human Development, 33,* 138–159.

Elder, G., & O'Rand, A. (1995). Adult lives in a changing society. In K. Cook, G. Fine, & J. House (Eds.), *Sociological perspectives on social psychology* (pp. 452–475). Needham Heights, MA: Allyn and Bacon.

Ellis, C., & Flaherty, M. (Eds.). (1992). *Investigating subjectivity: Research on lived experience.* Newbury Park, CA: Sage.

Epstein, S. (1973). The self-concept revisited: Or a theory of a theory. *American Psychologist, 28,* 404–416.

Featherman, D. (1986). Biography, society and history: Individual development as a population process. In A. Sorensen, F. Weinert, & L. Sherrod (Eds.), *Human development and the life course: Multidisciplinary perspectives* (pp. 99–152). Hillsdale, NJ: Erlbaum.

Featherman, D., & Lerner, R. (1985). Ontogenesis and sociogenesis: Problematics for theory and research about development and socialization across the lifespan. *American Sociological Review, 50,* 659–676.

Featherstone, M., & Hepworth, M. (1989). Ageing and old age: Reflections on the postmodern life course. In B. Bytheway, T. Keil, P. Allatt, & A. Bryman (Eds.), *Becoming and being old: Sociological approaches to later life* (pp. 143–157). London and Newbury Park, CA: Sage.

Felson, R. (1992). Self-Concept. In E. Borgatta & M. Borgatta (Eds.), *Encyclopedia of sociology* (pp. 1743–1749). New York: MacMillan.

Foucault, M. (1988). Technologies of the self. In L. Martin, H. Gutman, & P. Hutton (Eds.), *Technologies of the self: A seminar with Michel Foucault* (pp. 16–49). Amherst: University of Massachusetts Press.

Fry, C., & Keith, J. (1982). The life course as a cultural unit. In M. Riley, R. Abeles, & M. Teitelbaum (Eds.), *Aging from birth to death,* (Vol. 2, pp. 51–70). Boulder, CO: Westview Press.

Gecas, V. (1982). The self-concept. *Annual Review of Sociology, 8,* 1–33.

Geertz, C. (1973). *The interpretation of cultures.* New York: Basic Books.

George, L. (1980). *Role transitions in later life: A social stress perspective.* Monterey, CA: Brooks/Cole.

George, L. (1987). Self-esteem in later life. In G. Maddox (Ed.), *Encyclopedia of aging* (pp. 593). New York: Springer Publishing Company.

George, L. (1990). Social structure, social processes, and social-psychological states. In R. Binstock & L. George (Eds.), *Handbook of aging and the social sciences* (3rd ed., pp. 186–204). New York: Van Nostrand Reinhold.

George, L. (1992). Economic status and subjective well-being: A review of the literature and an agenda for future research. In N. Cutler, D. Gregg, & M. P. Lawton. (Eds.), *Aging, money, and life-satisfaction* (pp. 69–99). New York: Springer Publishing Company.

Gergen, K. (1977). Stability, change and chance in human development. In N. Datan & H. Reese (Eds.), *Life-span development psychology* (pp. 135–158). New York: Academic Press.

Gergen, K. (1991). *The saturated self.* New York: Basic Books.

Gergen, K., & Semin, G. (1990). Everyday understanding in science and daily life. In G. Semin & K. Gergen (Eds.), *Everyday understanding: Social and scientific implications* (pp. 1–18). Newbury Park, CA: Sage.

Giddens, A. (1979). *Central problems in social theory.* London: MacMillan.

Giddens, A. (1984). *The construction of society.* Berkeley: University of California Press.

Giddens, A. (1986). Action, subjectivity, and the constitution of meaning. *Social Research, 53*: 529–545.

Giddens, A. (1991). *Modernity and self-identity: Self and society in late modern age.* Stanford, CA: Stanford University Press.

Goethals, G., & Strauss, J. (Eds.). (1991). *Multidisciplinary perspectives on the self.* New York: Springer Verlag.

Gordon, C., & Gergen, K. (Eds.) (1968). *The self in social interaction.* New York: Wiley.

Groeben, N. (1990). Subjective theories and the explanation of human action. In G. Semin & K. Gergen (Eds.), *Everyday understanding: Social and scientific implications* (pp. 19–44). Newbury Park, CA: Sage.

Grove, W., Ortega, S. & Style, C. (1989). The maturational and role perspectives on aging and self through the adult years: An empirical evaluation. *American Journal of Sociology, 94*, 1117–45.

Gubrium, J. (1986). The social preservation of mind: The Alzheimer's disease experience. *Symbolic Interaction, 9*, 37–51.

Gubrium, J. (1988). *Analyzing field reality.* Newbury Park, CA: Sage

Gubrium, J., & Buckholdt, D. (1977). *Toward maturity: The social processing of human development.* San Francisco: Jossey-Bass.

Gubrium, J., & Holstein, J. (1994). Grounding the postmodern self. *The Sociological Quarterly, 35*, 685–703.

Gubrium, J., Holstein, J., & Buckholdt, D. (1994). *Constructing the life course.* Dix Hills, NY: General Hall.

Gubrium, J., & Wallace, B. (1990). Who theorizes age? *Ageing and Society, 10*, 131–149.

Hacking, I. (1992). "Style" for historians and philosophers. *Studies in History and Philosophy of Science, 23*, 1–20.

Hagestad, G., & Marshall, V. (1980). Discontinuity versus flexibility: The need for a social psychological approach to men's and women's adult roles. Paper presented to 32nd Annual Meeting of the Gerontological Society of America, San Diego, November, 1980.

Harding, S. (1992). After the neutrality ideal: Science, politics, and "strong objectivity." *Social Research, 59,* 567–587.

Harre, R. (1986). An outline of the social constructionist viewpoint. In R. Harre (Ed.), *The social construction of emotions* (pp. 2–14). Oxford: Basil Blackwell.

Hartung, R. (1993). On Black burden and becoming *nouveau poor. Journal of Gerontology: Social Science, 48,* S33–S34.

Heidrich, S., & Ryff, C. (1993). The role of social comparisons processes in the psychological adaptation of elderly adults. *Journals of Gerontology: Social Science, 48,* 127–136.

Hendricks, J. (1983). Impact of technological change on middle-aged and older workers: Parallels drawn from a structural perspective. In P. Robinson, J. Livingston, & J. Birren (Eds.), *Aging and technological advances* (pp. 113–124). New York: Plenum.

Hendricks, J. (1987). Age identification. In G. Maddox (Ed.), *Encyclopedia of aging* (p. 15). New York: Springer Publishing Company.

Hendricks, J. (1992). Learning to act old: Heroes, villains or old fools. *Journal of Aging Studies, 6,* 1–11.

Hendricks, J. (1994). Social class and adult development. In R. Kastenbaum (Ed.), *Encyclopedia of aging and human development* (pp. 467–472). Phoenix, AZ: Oryx.

Hendricks, J. (1995). The social construction of ageism. In L. Bond, S. Cutler, & A. Grams (Eds.), *Promoting successful and productive aging* (pp. 51–68). Thousand Oaks, CA: Sage.

Hendricks, J., & Peters, C. (1986). The times of our lives: An integrative framework. *American Behavioral Scientist, 29,* 662–676.

Hochschild, A. (1989). *The second shift.* New York: Viking.

Hogan, D., & Astone, N. (1986). The transition to adulthood. In R. Turner (Ed.), *Annual Review of Sociology: Vol. 12* (pp. 109–130). Palo Alto: Annual Reviews.

Hooker, K., & Kaus, C. (1994). Health-related possible selves in young and middle adulthood. *Psychology and Aging, 9,* 126–133.

House, J. (1977). The three faces of social psychology. *Sociometry, 40,* 161–177.

House, J. (1981). Social structure and personality. In M. Rosenberg & R. Turner (Eds.), *Social psychology: Sociological perspectives* (pp. 525–561). New York: Basic.

House, J., & Mortimer, J. (1990). Social structure and the individual: Emerging theories and new directions. *Social Psychology Quarterly, 53,* 71–80.

Huber, B. (1988). Social structures and human lives: Variations on a theme. In M. Riley, B. J. Huber, & B. Hess (Eds.), *Social structures and human lives* (pp. 346–363). Newbury Park, CA: Sage.

Karp, D. (1988). A decade of reminders: Changing age consciousness between fifty and sixty years old. *The Gerontologist, 28,* 727–738.

Kaufman, S. (1986). *The aging self.* Madison, WI: University of Wisconsin Press.

Kemper, T. (1981). Social constructionist and positivist approaches to the sociology of emotions. *American Journal of Sociology, 87,* 336–362.

Kohli, M. (1986a). Social organization and subjective construction of the life course. In A. Sorensen, F. Weinert, & L. Sherrod (Eds.), *Human development and the life course: Multidisciplinary perspectives* (pp. 271–292). Hillsdale, NJ: Erlbaum.

Kohli, M. (1986b). The world we forgot: A historical view of the life course. In V. Marshall (Ed.), *Later life: The social psychology of aging* (pp. 271–303). Beverly Hills: Sage.

Kohli, M., & Meyer, J. (1986). Social structure and the social construction of the life stages. *Human Development, 29*, 145–156.

Kohli, M. (1988). Ageing as a challenge for sociological theory. *Ageing and Society, 8*, 367–394.

Kohn, M., & Slomczynski, K. (1990). *Social structure and self-direction.* Oxford: Basil Blackwell.

Kuypers, J., & Bengtson, V. (1973). Social breakdown and competence: A model of normal aging. *Human Development, 25*, 181–201.

Lawton, M. P. (1983). Environment and other determinants of well-being in older people. *The Gerontologist, 23*, 349–357.

Lawton, M. P. (1993). Reply to Hartung. *Journals of Gerontology: Social Science, 48*, S34.

Lawton, M. P., & Nahemow, L. (1973). Ecology and the aging process. In C. Eisdorfer & M. P. Lawton (Eds.), *The psychology of adult development and aging* (pp. 619–674). Washington, DC: American Psychological Association.

Liang, J., Dvorkin, L., Kahana, E., & Mazian, F. (1980). Social integration and morale: A reexamination. *Journal of Gerontology, 35*, 746–757.

Liang, J., Kahana, E., & Doherty, E. (1980). Financial well-being among the aged: A further elaboration. *Journal of Gerontology, 30*, 409–420.

Logan, J., Ward, R., & Spitze, G. (1992). As old as you feel: Age identity in middle and later life. *Social Forces, 71*, 451–467.

Lyotard, J. (1984). *The postmodern condition.* Minneapolis: University of Minnesota Press.

Maddox, G., & Campbell, R. (1985). Scope, concepts, and methods in the study of aging. In R. Binstock & E. Shanas (Eds.), *Handbook of aging and the social sciences* (2nd ed., pp. 3–34). New York: Van Nostrand-Reinhold.

Marini, M. (1984a). Age and sequencing norms in the transition to adulthood. *Social Forces, 63*, 229–244.

Marini, M. (1984b). The order of events in the transition to adulthood. *Sociology of Education, 57*, 63–84.

Markides, K., Lee, D., Ray, L., & Black, S. (1993). Physicians' ratings of health in middle and old age: A cautionary note. *Journals of Gerontology: Social Science, 48*, S24–27.

Markus, H., & Cross, S. (1990). The interpersonal self. In L. Pervin (Ed.), *Handbook of personality: Theory & research* (pp. 576–608). New York: Guilford Press.

Markus, H., & Kitayama, S. (1991). Culture and the self: Implications for cognition, emotion, and motivation. *Psychological Review, 98*, 224–253.

Markus, H., & Ruvolo, A. (1989). Possible selves: Personalized representations of goals. In L. Pervin (Ed.), *Goal concepts in personality and social psychology* (pp. 211–241). Hillsdale, NJ: Erlbaum.

Marshall, V. (1986). Prominent and emerging paradigms in the social psychology of aging. In V. Marshall (Ed.), *Later life: The social psychology of aging* (pp. 9–31). Beverly Hills, CA: Sage.

Marshall, V. (1995). The micro-macro link in the sociology of aging. In C. Hummel & C. J. L. D'Epiny (Eds.), *Images of aging in western societies* (pp. 337–371). Geneva: Center for Interdisciplinary Gerontology, University of Geneva.

Marshall, V. (1996). The state of theory in aging and the social sciences. In R. Binstock & L. George (Eds.), *Handbook of aging and the social sciences* (4th ed., pp. 12–30). San Diego: Academic Press.

Mead, G. (1934). *Mind, self and society*. Chicago: University of Chicago Press.

Murphy, J., & Longino, C. Jr., (1992). What is the justification for a qualitative approach to ageing studies. *Ageing and Society, 12*, 143–156.

O'Rand, A. (1990). Stratification and the life course. In R. Binstock & L. George (Eds.), *Handbook of aging and the social sciences* (3rd ed., pp. 130–148). San Diego: Academic Press.

Passuth, P., & Bengtson, V. (1988). Sociological theories of aging: Current perspectives and future directions. In J. Birren & V. Bengtson (Eds.), *Emergent theories in aging* (pp. 333–355). New York: Springer Publishing Company.

Rachlin, A. (1991). Rehumanizing dialectic: Toward an understanding of the interpenetration of structure and subjectivity. *Current Perspectives in Social Theory, 11*, 255–269.

Riegel, K. (1973). An epitaph for a paradigm. *Human Development, 16*, 1–7.

Riley, M., Johnson, M., & Foner, A. (Eds.) (1972). *Aging and society: Vol. 3. A Sociology of Age Stratification*. New York: Russell Sage Foundation.

Riley, M., Kahn, R., & Foner, A. (Eds.) (1994). *Age and structural lag*. New York: Wiley Interscience.

Rindfuss, R., Swicegood, C., & Rosenfeld, R. (1987). Disorder in the life course: How common and does it matter? *American Sociological Review, 52*, 785–801.

Ritzer, G., & Gindoff, P. (1994). Agency-structure, micro-macro, individualism-holism-relationism: A metatheoretical explanation of theoretical convergence between the United States and Europe. In P. Sztompka. (Ed.), *Agency and structure: Reorienting social theory* (pp. 3–23). Yverdon, Switzerland: Gordon and Breach.

Rosenberg, M. (1979). *Conceiving the self*. New York: Basic Books.

Rosenberg, M. (1981). The self-concept: Social product and social force. In M. Rosenberg & R. Turner (Eds.), *Social psychology: Sociological perspectives* (pp. 593–624). New York: Basic Books.

Rosenberg, M., & Pearlin, L. (1978). Social class and self-esteem among children and adolescents. *American Journal of Sociology, 84*, 53–77.

Rowe, J., & Kahn, R. (1987). Human aging: Usual and successful. *Science, 237*, 143–149.

Rowe, J., & Kahn, R. (1997). Successful aging. *The Gerontologist, 37*, 433–440.

Rowe, J., & Kahn, R. (1998). *Successful aging.* New York: Pantheon.

Ryff, C. (1986). The subjective construction of self and society: An agenda for life-span research. In V. Marshall (Ed.), *Later life: The social psychology of aging* (pp. 33–74). Beverly Hills: Sage.

Ryff, C. (1987). The place of personality and social structure: Research in social psychology. *Journal of Personality and Social Psychology, 53*, 1192–1202.

Ryff, C. (1991). Possible selves in adulthood and old age: A tale of shifting horizons. *Psychology and Aging, 6*, 286–295.

Ryff, C., & Essex, M. (1992). The interpretation of life experience and well-being: The sample case of relocation. *Psychology and Aging, 7*, 504–517.

Schooler, C. (1989). Social structure effects and experimental situations: Mutual lessons of cognitive and social science. In K. W. Schaie & C. Schooler (Eds.), *Social structure and aging: Psychological processes* (pp. 129–153). Hillsdale, NJ: Lawrence Erlbaum.

Schutz, A. (1973). *Collected papers I. The problem of social reality.* The Hague: Martinus Nijhoff.

Seltzer, M., & Troll, L. (1986). Expected life history: A model in nonlinear time. *American Behavioral Scientist, 29*, 746–764.

Settersten, R., & Hagestad, G. (1996). What's the latest? II. Cultural age deadlines for educational and work transitions. *The Gerontologist, 36*, 602–613.

Smelser, N., & Smelser, W. (Eds.). (1970). *Personality and social systems.* New York: Wiley.

Sorensen, A. (1986). Social structure and mechanisms of life-course processes. In A. Sorensen, F. Weinert, & L. Sherrod (Eds.), *Human development and the life course: Multidisciplinary perspectives* (pp. 177–197). Hillsdale, NJ: Erlbaum.

Spilerman, S. (1977). Careers, labor market structure, and socioeconomic achievement. *American Journal of Sociology, 83*, 551–593.

Stryker, S. (1981). Symbolic interactionism: Themes and variations. In M. Rosenberg & R. Turner (Eds.), *Social psychology: Sociological perspectives* (pp. 3–29). New York: Basic Books.

Sullivan, H. (1940). *Conceptions of modern psychiatry.* New York: Norton.

Suls, J. (Ed.) (1982). *Psychological perspectives on the self.* Hillsdale, NJ: Lawrence Erlbaum.

Suls, J., & Mullen, B. (1982). From the cradle to the grave: Comparison and self-evaluation across the life-span. In J. Suls (Ed.), *Psychological perspectives on the self* (Vol. 1, pp. 97–128). Hillsdale, NJ: Lawrence Erlbaum.

Taylor, C. (1989). *Sources of the self: The making of modern identity.* Cambridge: Harvard University Press.

Thoits, P. (1989). The sociology of emotions. *Annual Review of Sociology, 15*, 317–342.

Turner, S. (1994). *The social theory of practices: Tradition, tacit knowledge, and presuppositions*. Chicago: University of Chicago Press.

Wardell, M., & Benson, K. (1978). A dialectical view: Foundation for an alternative sociological method. Paper presented at Midwest Sociological Society, Omaha, Nebraska [quoted in Rachlin].

Weber, M. (1968). *Economy and society*. New York: Bedminster Press. Originally published 1921.

Weber, M. (1947). *The theory of social and economic organization*. New York: Free Press.

Whitbourne, S. (1985). The psychological construction of the life span. In J. Birren & K.W. Schaie (Eds.), *Handbook of the psychology of aging* (2nd ed., pp. 594–618). New York: Van Nostrand Reinhold.

Whitbourne, S. (1986). *The me I know: A study of adult identity*. New York: Springer Verlag.

Whitbourne, S., & Primus, L. (1996). Physical identity in later adulthood. In J. Birren (Ed.), *Encyclopedia of gerontology* (pp. 733–742). San Diego: Academic Press.

Wiley, N. (1994). History of the self: From primates to present. *Sociological Perspectives, 37*, 527–545.

Wolfe, A. (1992). Weak sociology/strong sociologists: Consequences and contradictions of a field in turmoil. *Social Research, 59*, 759–779.

Wood, J. (1989). Theory and research concerning social comparisons of personal attributes. *Psychological Bulletin, 106*, 231–248.

CHAPTER 8

Educational Attainment and Self-Making in Later Life

Melissa M. Franks, A. Regula Herzog, Diane Holmberg, & Hazel R. Markus

Question: How would you describe yourself?
Answers:

I'm an independent old lady.

("Hester", 85-year-old woman, 10th grade education).

I'm strong-minded, and I believe in truth and sanctity.

("Joan", 71-year-old woman, high school degree).

I'm usually cheerful, and I enjoy things that are going on. I enjoy people and family, and I enjoy retirement. I'm easy to get along with. With most people, I enjoy helping them and doing things with them. With other people, I tend to be critical.

("Carlotta", 68-year-old woman, college degree).

These quotes represent three individuals' responses when asked to characterize themselves, or to give insight into their self-concepts. Hester focusses on one key aspect of her self-concept, namely her independence. Similarly, Joan emphasizes her independence of thought, but also goes on to describe some beliefs and values. Of the three, Carlotta gives by far the

Data used in this chapter were from the Self Portraits survey. These data were collected by A. Regula Herzog and Hazel R. Markus with funding provided by the National Institute on Aging grant AG08279. The survey was conducted through the University of Michigan's Survey Research Center.

most diverse picture of herself. She describes her personality, her likes and dislikes, and also gives some insight into the variable nature of her self-concept. Are these descriptions merely diverting, yet essentially uninformative, images? Current views of selfhood suggest not; these views portray the self as a multidimensional and dynamic entity that is actively involved in psychological and social processes (see review by Markus & Wurf, 1987). Each of these three women possesses a different view of self; we would anticipate that they would each, in turn, possess different hopes, dreams, goals, memories, values, and preferred activities. Their views of themselves are thus anticipated to affect many aspects of their lives; yet how did these influential views of themselves arise in the first place?

In current theorizing, the self-system can be described as an ongoing interpretive process influenced not only by the individual's own thoughts, feelings, and desires, but also by cultural imperatives and social expectations (Herzog & Markus, 1999; Markus & Herzog, 1991). This perspective on selfhood posits that individuals continue to define who they are throughout their life, and suggests that an individual's life experiences importantly influence how the self is constructed and maintained or modified. Thus, in understanding why these three women are who they say they are, it is essential to consider where they have been, what experiences they have had in life, and where they fit within the social structure. Consistent with this view of self, this volume explores the influence of social structure in setting the stage for the important life experiences which facilitate or impede the construction of the self into later life.

In this chapter, we focus on one key aspect of our respondents' life experiences which may have altered their life trajectories, setting the stage for very different views of self even decades later: namely, their educational experiences. Clearly, American society is stratified by socioeconomic status, and individuals in our society are advantaged or handicapped by their position in the social hierarchy (Dowd, 1990). Hester, with her 10th-grade education, likely has led a very different life in many respects than college-educated Carlotta, especially given that they grew up in a time when college education was rarer than it is today. It is reasonable to expect that such divergent experiences will importantly influence their views of themselves. Thus, in this chapter, we focus on educational attainment and its relevance to the richness of the self-system in older adulthood.

Certainly the view that those who inhabit very different social worlds will develop very different selves is not new. For example, a great deal of theoretical and empirical work has been done in recent years investigating the influence of culture on the self (e.g., Markus & Kitayama, 1991;

Markus, Mullally, & Kitayama, 1997; Triandis, 1995). Even within a given culture, however, individuals inhabiting different social strata may possess different values, goals, opportunities, and life tasks. In a meritocratic society, education is a prime candidate for such a life- and self-altering stratification variable. Surprisingly, however, very little empirical evidence exists linking education and the self. For example, the recent comprehensive treatment of the self by Gergen (1991) does not address the issue of the effects of education. Even a recent review in the *Annual Review of Psychology* concerning the self in the social context (Banaji & Prentice, 1994) reviews only social interactions but not social-structural factors. The goal of this chapter is to begin to fill this void by exploring the potential contribution of educational attainment to the diversity of the older adult self-system. We first briefly describe the importance of a multifaceted self to successful aging. We next turn to the influence of social context on the development and maintenance of the self, then focus specifically on the contributions of education to the self-system.

THE SELF AND SUCCESSFUL AGING

Examinations of the self from a sociological perspective, conceptualized as salient roles or identities, have detailed the importance of multiple role identities for sustaining well-being in adulthood. Such studies have long indicated that the more roles individuals occupy, the better their mental health (e.g., Coleman & Antonucci, 1983; Linville, 1987; Thoits, 1983). Moreover, the benefit to psychological well-being of multiple role involvements recently was demonstrated in a study of older adults (Adelmann, 1994b). In this study, those older adults occupying a greater number of roles experienced less depression, higher life satisfaction, and greater self-efficacy than did those occupying fewer roles. In general, these studies suggest that multiple role involvements allow individuals greater opportunity for positive self-evaluations in that negative experiences resulting from failure in (or departure from) one valued role can be offset when other equally valued roles are available.

Other research in an aging context also has indicated the importance of self in maintaining psychological well-being. Such work has demonstrated, for example, that older adults benefit most from emotional support specific to stress experienced in domains of self they find most important (Krause & Borawski-Clark, 1994) and that effective use of social comparisons by older women can enhance self-evaluation and thereby enable maintenance of positive mental health, even in the event of poor physical health (Heidrich & Ryff, 1993). In sum, this work illustrates the benefit to well-being of possessing a complex, multifaceted self, as opposed to a simpler, unitary self-concept. A more diverse self offers advantages through the protection of highly valued domains of self and the selection of positive self-aspects for social comparison.

A growing literature on successful aging further establishes an important role of self-processes in adapting to late life. Successful aging has been summarized as the maximization of the benefits associated with aging together with the minimization of the losses (Baltes & Baltes, 1990). Echoing the results of the previously cited literature, research and theory concerning successful aging also finds that the maintenance of a rich and flexible self is an important factor in responding to the challenges of older adulthood (e.g., Baltes & Baltes, 1990; Brandtstadter, Wentura, & Greve, 1993). These approaches each posit that successful aging is achieved through continued adjustment of one's environment as well as one's goals and expectations for functioning to offset the demands of the aging mind and body. It has been argued that the multifaceted dynamic self of recent vintage serves as the manager of such adaptive processes (e.g., Herzog, Franks, Markus, & Holmberg, 1995; Markus & Herzog, 1991), and thus is critical to the maintenance of well-being in older age.

Much of the research on self in an aging context has been focused on the self at present. Past and possible selves too can be argued to be importantly involved in successful adjustment to older adulthood. Past selves may represent autobiographical memories thought to provide the basis for reminiscence and life review. Past selves also enable reflection on past accomplishments and as such, serve as sources of pride and well-being (see review by Markus & Herzog, 1991). Past selves may also serve as a counterpoint to the current self, allowing assessments of progress made in key life domains. Future or possible selves are thought to activate motivation for behaviors that are performed to bring about hoped-for selves or to avoid feared selves (Markus & Nurius, 1986). In a recent study, older adults' endorsements of possible selves in the domain of health were important predictors of current health behaviors (Hooker & Kaus, 1992). Possible selves thus may reflect the selection and revision of goals so central to the thinking on positive aging posited by Carstensen (e.g., Carstensen, 1992) and Brandtstadter (e.g., Brandtstadter et al., 1993). The self of the past and that of the future are current constructions, however, and as such, are strongly influenced by the self of today. What is central in the making of the current self is likely to be recalled (or more noticeably absent) in the self of yesterday, and similarly is likely to be hoped for (or feared) in the self of tomorrow.

Thus, it can reasonably be argued that the structure and function of the self is a key factor in the physical and mental health functioning of older adults. Further, it can be noted that a rich, diverse, flexible self-system provides substantial advantages over a more constrained self-system. Based on these premises, the remainder of this chapter explores the role of educational attainment in the formation and support of a rich, multifaceted self-system throughout the life course. Although health and well-being are not examined empirically here, it is our expectation that a multifaceted self contributes considerably to successful adaptation to the challenges of aging in our society.

THE SELF-SYSTEM

The self most often is conceptualized as a system of knowledge structures in which one's experiences are organized (see review by Markus & Wurf, 1987). These structures have been variously labeled as self-schemas (Markus, 1977), salient identities (Stryker, 1986) or core conceptions (Gergen, 1977). The self-system further is posited to extend beyond the self at present to include the self of the past as well as the anticipated self for the future (both hoped for and feared; cf. Markus & Herzog, 1991; Markus & Nurius, 1986). These temporal aspects of self illustrate both continuity and change in the self-system. The self at present is evaluated against the self of the past and it also sets the course for the self hoped for (or changes the course to avoid the feared self) in the future.

It is not presumed that the representation of the past self is an accurate reflection of who we once were, any more than the anticipated future self is presumed to be a true depiction of who we will become (see review by Markus & Herzog, 1991). Rather, the self of the present is the lens through which the self in the past and the self anticipated for the future are viewed. In this way, the current self plays a selective role in choosing to adopt and elaborate past and possible selves which are consistent with or support current selves and to discard or modify those which are inconsistent with current self-views. It is in this way that the self-system engineers a sense of continuity or change. The posited influence of the current self on that of the past and of the future is consistent with memory research, which has shown that recall of prior ratings of attitudes and personality traits are biased by current perceptions (see review by Ross, 1989).

The process of organizing the various traits, identities, and roles which comprise the self is referred to here as self-making (Herzog & Markus, 1999). Self-making in older age, and at all ages, is conceptualized not as a uniform process, but rather as a very unique and individual process in response to the experience of aging in a social context. Self-making further is believed to be a continual process of integrating into the self-system the knowledge gained from experiences encountered in the social context. As such, the environment in which individuals exist importantly affects the formation and maintenance of self. The absence of novel stimuli in one's environment reduces opportunities for challenges to self-definition and thereby limits the making of the self. Conversely, a social context which affords variety in experience provides opportunities for integrating new information into the self-system and thus, facilitates self-making. It is our hypothesis that educational attainment is an important marker of the experiences and resources available to reinforce and expand the self.

EDUCATION AND SELF

The effect of education on the adult self-system can be thought of in a number of different ways. Substantial evidence for a relationship between education and the formation of attitudes, expectations, and values has been reported. For example, Inkeles and Smith (1974) reported in their groundbreaking work on becoming modern that education was one of the most powerful factors predicting modern attitudes such as openness to change, sense of efficacy, planning and aspirations, use of information and opinions, and awareness of diversity. There is, therefore, good reason to expect that education influences self-construction through the values that it communicates and the experiences that it affords.

What sort of values might the educational system communicate that would aid in the construction of a rich, diverse self? First, education (especially higher education) teaches students that thinking is important—that it is important to answer abstract questions such as "Who am I?", even if such questions have no immediate practical outcomes. Students learn that there may be many correct answers to any given question, and that one should consider a problem from a variety of different angles. Thus, education may indirectly communicate to students that the self is an object worthy of study, and that there are many ways to conceptualize the self.

Education may also give students the tools they need to communicate what they have learned about the self to others. As education progresses, students learn to note similarities and differences, to draw abstractions, and to organize a diverse array of information into coherent units. These skills, once learned, can be applied to any set of complex information, including information about the self. Assessments of the self in social-psychological research generally assume that respondents are able to generate abstractions about the self (e.g., decide the extent to which trait or role descriptors define the self; generate spontaneous verbal descriptions of the self). The tools to note and communicate such abstractions may be especially prevalent in those with higher education. Selves under less scrutiny, such as may be common in less educated individuals, are difficult to verbalize or communicate to others.

In addition to the values and skills it provides, education also provides experiences which may contribute to the formation of a complex self. For example, through teaching of history, geography or literature, students learn about cultures, lifestyles, and career options other than those available in their immediate environment. Awareness of these alternatives provides a rich backdrop against which to develop one's own identity, and, as such, may result in a more extensive and reflective self. In addition to learning about diversity through the curriculum, higher education may provide individuals with the opportunities to experience diversity first-hand. Especially for the older adults considered in this chapter, going away to college might have been the first opportunity for a student to meet individuals from a variety of backgrounds. Seeing how different others around you are from yourself may inspire you to examine exactly what constitutes "yourself".

These suggestions outline just a few of the ways in which the initial experiences of education may encourage one to form a rich, complex view of the self. Education also affords many life experiences following the completion of formal schooling that may continue to influence self-making in later life. In older adulthood, higher levels of educational attainment have been shown to be associated with better cognitive functioning (cf. Pedersen, Reynolds, & Gatz, 1996), reduced functional impairment (e.g., Maddox & Clark, 1992) and better health (e.g., House et al., 1990), as well as with greater feelings of personal control (Mirowsky, 1995). Such research has identified several corollaries of education that may explain the influence of education on physical and mental functioning in older age, and by extension, on self-making in later life.

First, educational attainment is critical to occupational and economic attainment (Sewell & Hauser, 1975). Although itself affected by parental socioeconomic status, the level of formal education affects labor force participation, occupational status, income, and assets. These economic advantages may then facilitate self-making through the enrichment of life experiences and opportunities. This linkage might be termed a materialistic interpretation of the role of education on self-making.

A second, and related, interpretation might be called an intelligence or skills interpretation. Higher education may stimulate cognitive capacity by increasing the demands on neuronal activity (Pedersen et al., 1996). In turn, greater cognitive capacity may then encourage more or more elaborated thoughts about many topics, including the self. For example, more educated adults, with greater training in analytical reasoning, may be better able than are adults with less education to abstract and categorize information relevant to the self and to compare self with others.

Thus, whether it has its effects directly through the ways of thinking it encourages or the behaviors it affords, or whether the effects are more indirect, mediated through occupational status, income, or intelligence, we propose that education has implications for self-making; furthermore, these repercussions for self-making extend beyond the completion of formal schooling in late adolescence or early adulthood. The level of education attained during or before the early adult years is posited to set the stage for the presentation of experiences and opportunities throughout the remainder of one's life. Thus, given the fuller range of opportunities afforded by educational achievement in American society, we hypothesize that more educated older adults will possess a more elaborated representation of self which, according to recent theory and research, is important in successful aging.

Returning to our sample respondents, it may be no accident that Carlotta gives a more elaborated self-description than Joan, who gives a more elaborated description than Hester. Their different experiences years ago in the educational system may have encouraged Carlotta and Joan to begin to form a more complex and elaborated view of self. Since then, they likely have been set on different life trajectories; maintaining, and perhaps exacerbating, initial differences in self-concept. Thus, by older age, we anticipate that those with higher education would have more elaborated and complex selves than those with less education. We now explore this hypothesis, along with potential mediating variables.

EDUCATION AND SELF-MAKING IN OLDER AGE

Sample and Methods

Before addressing the primary objective of this chapter, to examine the influence of educational attainment on self-making in later life, we briefly will describe self-making in older adulthood more generally. After describing the older adult self, we next will examine the influence of education on the self-system. Data from a recent survey of adults in a Midwestern city are used to explore self-making in older adulthood and its relationship to educational attainment. Analyses were conducted using weighted data to adjust for variations in sampling and response rates.

Self Portraits is a recent survey of 1471 adults in a large Midwestern city. This study used a multistage stratified area probability sample of persons aged 30 years and over. The interviews were conducted in 1992 by interviewers from the University of Michigan's Survey Research Center. The total sample reflects a response rate of 74% of those capable of completing the interview. Interviews were conducted in the respondents' homes by trained interviewers and took, on average, 93 minutes to complete. The average respondent in the overall sample was 59 years of age (SD = 15.7; range = 30–93) and had completed 12.4 years of education (SD = 2.9; range = 0–17).

The subset of this sample aged 65 and older (n = 679) is used here to describe the self in older adulthood and to explore the relationship between education and the construction of self. In this subsample of older adults, the average respondent was 73.2 years of age (SD = 6.4; range = 65 –93). The average older adult respondent had completed 11.3 years of education (SD = 3.2; range = 0–17). Approximately 60% of these respondents had a high school education (34%) or beyond (28%). Almost 20% of these older adults had attained only an 8th-grade education or less.

To explore the self-system of adults, respondents in the Self Portraits survey were first allowed the opportunity to describe themselves in their own words. Respondents were asked to describe themselves currently, as they were at any time in the past and as they expect to be in the future. Responses were coded for up to six descriptors of self offered by respondents. The question pertaining to the future was composed of two parts: what respondents hoped to become, and what they were afraid of becoming.

Following the self-generated descriptions, respondents then were asked to rate how well each of a series of words or phrases described them on a 5-point scale (ranging from 1 "extremely well" to 5 "not at all"). After extensive pilot work, 44 potential self-descriptors were included in the survey. The selection of descriptors was designed to maximize coverage of various aspects of social roles, personal attributes and personality, as well as sociodemographic descriptors of the self.

Exploratory factor analysis with varimax rotation was used to determine the underlying factor structure of the descriptors of self at present for the total sample. This analysis resulted in eleven factors including: mental health (e.g., *depressed, content*); upstanding (e.g., *organized, responsible*); social (e.g., *caring, friend*); vocation (e.g., *involved in paid work, hardworking*); accommodating (e.g., *tolerant, realistic*); attractive (e.g., *physically attractive, intelligent*); inventive (e.g., *curious, sense of humor*); avocation (e.g., *involved in hobbies/leisure activities, active*); family roles (e.g., *being a mother/father, being a husband/wife*); social characteristics (*aware of race or ethnic background, aware of being a man or woman*); and autonomy (e.g., *dependent, independent*). The highest-loading (positively valenced) item from each factor was selected to represent the domains of the multidimensional older adult self. The resulting eleven aspects of self included: *content, organized, caring, involved in paid work, tolerant, physically attractive, curious, involved in hobbies or leisure activities, being a mother/father, aware of your race or ethnic background,* and *independent.*

Of the 55 bivariate associations among the 11 aspects of self, two-thirds (63 %) were significantly ($p < .01$) related. These associations ranged from $r = .10$ to $r = .26$ (the mean was $r = .16$), suggesting limited empirical overlap among the eleven self-descriptors. Thus, the multifaceted self is conceptualized as the number of the 11 items rated as self-descriptive (rated as either 1 "extremely" or 2 "very" descriptive). Three measures (one each for current, past, and possible self) were created by summing the number of items endorsed as describing the self. In this way, endorsement of a greater number of these aspects as self-descriptive reflects a more diverse, complex, and multifaceted self-system.

Self-Making in Older Adulthood

The analyses focus primarily on the 11 rated descriptors, with results from the self-generated descriptors reported to provide additional support for the findings and conclusions. In describing the older adult self, we first examined the extent to which the conceptualization of self as multidimensional was demonstrated in the reports of the respondents aged 65 years and older in the Self Portraits study. A multidimensional self indeed was reported by most respondents. At least 95% endorsed more than one item as self-descriptive for each of the temporal components of self. Of the eleven rated descriptors examined, respondents endorsed, on average, 6.5 ($SD = 2.0$; range = 0–11) current aspects of self, 7.2 ($SD = 2.3$; range = 0 –11) past, and 6.1 ($SD = 2.6$; range = 0–11) possible aspects of self.

Turning now to the responses provided when respondents described themselves in their own words, at least three-fourths of respondents generated multiple self-descriptors for each component of self (past, current, and future). For each of the three temporal components, the average number of descriptors generated was about 3. The mean number of self-generated descriptors of the current self was 3.1 ($SD = 1.6$; range = 0 –6); of the past self, the mean number of self-descriptors was 2.8 ($SD = 1.5$; range = 0–6); and of the possible self, the mean was 3.2 ($SD = 1.3$; range = 0–6). The mean number of hoped-for self-aspects generated was 1.8 ($SD = 0.8$; range = 0 –3), and the mean number of feared self-aspects was 1.5 ($SD = 0.7$; range = 0 –3). These findings further support the conceptualization of the older adult self as multidimensional. Unlike Hester, most respondents do not focus on just one salient aspect of the self; instead, most mention and endorse a number of different self-aspects.

Having demonstrated that the older adult self is multifaceted, a finding consistent with theory and research primarily focused on younger adults, we next explored the extent to which the multifaceted nature of self is systematic across the three temporal components. Using both the rated self-descriptors and those generated by respondents, findings suggest that the degree to which the self is multidimensional was found to be consistent across the temporal components of self. In other words, those with a more complex self in the present also describe themselves in a more complex way in the past and in the future. That is, endorsing more rated descriptors of the current self was correlated ($p < .001$) with both the past self ($r = .48$) and with the possible self ($r = .61$). In addition, endorsing more past self-aspects was correlated ($r = .56$) with endorsing more possible aspects. Albeit to a lesser extent, generating more descriptors of the self in the present was associated with mentioning more past descriptors ($r = .30$) and more possible descriptors ($r = .23$). Again, generating more past aspects of self was correlated ($r = .31$) with generating more possible aspects.

Breaking apart the aggregated picture of the rated self painted thus far, Table 8.1 displays the percentage of respondents endorsing each item as either extremely or very descriptive of the self. With a few notable exceptions, (*involved in paid work, physically attractive* and *involved in activities*), each of the descriptors was endorsed by at least one-half of

Table 8.1 Percentage of Respondents Endorsing Each Domain as Self-Descriptive

	Current Self	Past Self	Possible Self
Caring	93%	92%	89%
Parent	86	79	81
Aware of race or ethnic identity	75	68	65
Independent	74	73	68
Content	67	63	63
Organized	57	62	56
Tolerant	57	58	56
Curious	50	55	48
Involved in hobbies or leisure activities	42	44	42
Physically attractive	31	53	30
Involved in paid work	20	72	13

respondents. Looking first at the current self, caring was the most often endorsed descriptor and was rated as self-descriptive by 93% of respondents. *Parent* was the second most frequently endorsed descriptor with 86% of respondents rating it as descriptive.

For the past self, only one descriptor (*involved in activities*) was endorsed by fewer than one-half of the respondents. Consistent with the current self, *caring* and *parent* were the most frequently endorsed past self-descriptors. Notable changes in the rank order of endorsement from the current self include: *involved in paid work*, which was endorsed as descriptive of the past self by 72% of respondents, compared with 20% for the current self; and *physically attractive* and *awareness of race.*

For the possible self, the ranking of frequency of endorsement was very similar to that for current self-descriptors. Again, *caring* and *parent* were the most frequently endorsed descriptors of the self expected in the future. In addition, *involved in paid work* was endorsed as a possible self by only 13% of respondents. The most notable deviations from the endorsements of the current self are *awareness of race* and *independent*. About two-thirds of respondents expect each of these to be descriptive in the future, as compared with approximately three-quarters of respondents endorsing each as currently descriptive.

Education and Self-Making

We now begin to address our hypothesis that greater educational attainment is associated with a more multifaceted self-system. The bivariate relationships between the three temporal components of the rated self and educational attainment showed that a higher level of education was related to a broader current self ($r =.21$; $p <.001$), possible self ($r = .19$; $p < .001$), and past self ($r = .11$; $p < .01$). A similar pattern of findings was detected for the self-generated descriptors with more education being related ($p < .001$) to the production of more descriptors of the self currently ($r = .19$), in the past ($r = .15$), and in the future ($r = .24$).

The bivariate relationship between education and each of the 11 rated self-descriptors (current, past, and possible) are presented in Table 8.2. Education was associated with five of the eleven current and possible self descriptors investigated (*content, tolerant, curious, involved in activities, independent*) and was associated with four of the past descriptors (*work, tolerant, curious, involved in activities*). The aspect of self most strongly

Table 8.2 Bivariate Correlation of Education With 11 Domains of Self

	Current Self	Past Self	Possible Self
Caring	−.06	−.04	−.07
Parent	−.01	.07	−.02
Aware of race or ethnic identity	−.04	.03	.00
Independent	−.16***	−.03	−.12***
Content	−.17***	−.03	−.15***
Organized	−.03	.00	−.02
Tolerant	−.18***	−.15***	−.20***
Curious	−.17***	−.15***	−.17***
Involved in hobbies or leisure activities	−.23***	−.19***	−.27***
Physically attractive	.02	.01	.00
Involved in paid work	−.07	−.07*	−.02

*p < .05. **p < .01. ***p < .001.

related to education was *involvement in activities*, suggesting that in fact education leads to the time, resources, or inclination to engage in a wide variety of activities, perhaps fostering a more complex self. Moreover, three descriptors (*tolerant, curious, and involved in activities*) were associated with greater education across all three temporal components of self, suggesting that education does not just result in temporary differences in self-concept at the time it is being experienced, but instead can color views of self throughout the life course.

Path analysis was then conducted using LISREL VIII (Joreskog & Sorbom, 1993) to further explore the relationship of education to the construction of the self-system. It was hypothesized that greater education would be associated with the making of an expansive current self, and thereby result in a more broadly constructed past self and possible self. These analyses further control for the effects of age and gender, but for ease of presentation, only the effects of education are shown and discussed here.

The estimated path coefficients are presented in Figure 8.1. The model showed an acceptable fit to the data (χ^2 (1) = 117.51; $p < .001$; GFI = .95; NFI =.83). Findings demonstrated a strong total effect of education on all three components of self (current, past, and future). As hypothesized, a direct effect of education on the current self was detected. In addition, a significant indirect effect of education on the past self ($B = .10$; $p < .001$) and on the possible self ($B = .13$; $p < .001$) through the current self was found. As shown, no direct effects of education were detected for the past self or for the possible self. Because the three temporal components of self were significantly associated each with the others, two additional models were tested (but not shown). In both of these models, direct effects of education on the current self remained significant after controlling for the past or for the possible self.

Thus, our overall hypothesis that education would be associated with self-making was supported. Moreover, the detected relationships support our hypothesis that the association of education to the self would flow through the current self to the past self and the possible self. In other words, these findings suggest that educational attainment influences how older adults describe themselves currently and, in turn, the resultant richness of the current representation of self broadens the reconstruction of the self of the past and the projection of the self into the future.

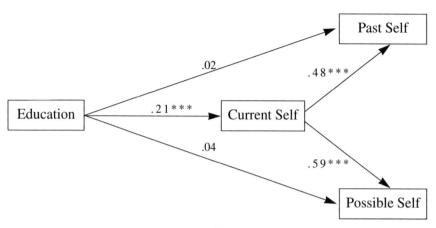

Figure 8.1 Direct effects of education on the self-system.
*p < .05   **p < .01   ***p < .001

Potential Mediators of the Relationship Between
Education and Self-Making

Based on the foregoing analysis suggesting that education exerts its influence on the past and the possible self indirectly through bolstering the current self, and for simplification, the following analyses focused only on self-making at present. Path analysis using LISREL VIII (Joreskog & Sorbom, 1993) was again conducted to test three possible mediators of the association between education and the self: income, intelligence, and occupational prestige. Income and occupation were selected to represent the materialistic interpretation of the effect of education on self-making, and intelligence was chosen to represent the skills interpretation. As with the previous model, the effects of age and gender were controlled in the following analysis, however, only the direct effects of education are depicted in Figure 8.2.

In the Self Portraits survey, income was assessed by one item asking respondents to estimate their annual household income. The median annual household income for this subsample was between $15,000 and $20,000. Occupational prestige was represented through the occupational codes of the 1970 census. For this sample of older adults, only 13% were currently employed, and thus occupational prestige, by and large, was represented by respondents' previous employment. In terms of levels of occupation, 18% of respondents had been employed as laborers, 26% had been

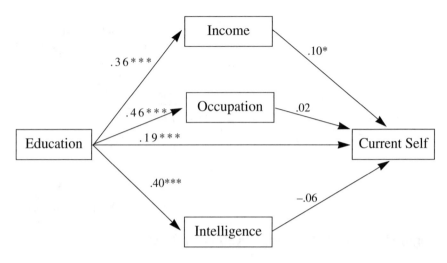

Figure 8.2 Potential mediators of the relationship between education and the current self.
*p < .05   **p < .01   ***p < .001

employed as craftsmen, 29% were employed as clerical or sales personnel, and 21% had held professional or managerial positions. The remainder either had never been employed for pay (4%) or had missing data.

Intelligence was represented by an abbreviated version of the similarities subtest from the WAIS-R (Wechsler, 1981). Respondents were asked to describe the way in which two nouns were similar, and their answers to six pairs of nouns were coded as to whether they represented an abstract (for a score of 2 points), a concrete (1 point), or an incorrect (0 points) similarity. The similarities subtest measures abstract reasoning, and is thought to be, in part, an indicator of crystallized intelligence or a form of cognitive ability. Scores on this measure could range from 0 to 12 with higher scores representing greater cognitive ability. The mean level of intelligence was 5.5 ($SD = 2.8$; range = 0 –12). These three potential intervening mechanisms were significantly correlated with one another. Occupation was associated with both income ($r = .41$) and intelligence ($r = .35$), and income and intelligence were correlated at $r = .28$.

Although the model demonstrated an acceptable fit to the data ($\chi^2(3) = 102.00$; $p < .001$); GFI = .96; NFI = .84), the hypothesized intervening variables offered little toward the explanation of the relationship between education and self-making. A significant direct effect of education on the current self was still detected. Education was a significant predictor of all three potential mediators, but of these three, only income was related to self-making. Moreover, the indirect effect of education on self through the mediators examined in the present model was not significant. The tested mediators added only a small (1.8%) but significant ($p < .01$) amount of variance to the prediction of self beyond that contributed by age, gender, and education. It should be noted that when income was examined alone as a mediator (model not shown), a significant indirect effect of education through income was detected. That is, education was related to higher reported household income, which in turn, was related to more current self-descriptors.

In summary, a significant direct effect of education on self-making still emerged in the model including the hypothesized intervening mechanisms. Some evidence was found to suggest that income mediated the relationship between education and the current self. No evidence was found to indicate mediating effects of either occupational prestige or intelligence on self-making.

DISCUSSION OF FINDINGS

Data from the Self Portraits survey provided evidence that the older adult self, like that of younger adults, is not unidimensional, but rather is varied and multifaceted. Evidence also was found to support the hypothesis that more years of education would augment the making of a multifaceted self-system. Findings further revealed that the effect of education on the older adult self-system was, for the most part, direct and was not mediated by such educational corollaries as income, occupational prestige, or intelligence.

In the present investigation, educational attainment was shown to influence self-description in the later years of life. For these older adults, the attainment of a higher level of education was associated with rating more items as descriptive of self. Moreover, this finding was confirmed in that those older adults with more education also provided more self-generated descriptors than did less educated older adults. This positive association between education and self-representation was detected across the current, past, and possible components of the self-system.

The demonstrated relationship between education and a fuller representation of self is particularly noteworthy in that it may have implications for the well-being of older adults. Theory and research on successful aging (e.g., Baltes & Baltes, 1990) and on multiple roles (e.g., Adelmann, 1994a, 1994b) have posited the importance of an adaptive and resilient self in the maintenance of health and well-being in the later stages of life. Together with the present findings, results of prior research raise the possibility that self-processes may help to explain the physical and psychological health advantage for more highly educated older adults over those less educated. That is, education attained earlier in life may encourage the acquisition of a broad array of self-aspects and open the possibility of further expanding the self in the future. In this way, education bolsters the self-system and processes of the self (e.g., personal control, self-esteem) which, in turn, may be beneficial for sustaining health and well-being throughout life. In future work, we will investigate the relationship of the multidimensionality of the self-system to the health and well-being of older adults. For now, however, we see that those with more education do indeed create more multifaceted selves.

Although education is associated with a more complex self in general, some domains show stronger effects than others. For example, the investigation of education with the domains of self revealed that education was most strongly related to describing oneself as *involved in hobbies and leisure activities*. Previous research focused on leisure activity and aging has demonstrated that education is an important indicator of the amount and types of activities pursued by older adults (see reviews by Lawton, 1985, and Cutler & Hendricks, 1990). More specifically, socioeconomic status indicators including income and educational, and occupational attainment have been shown to increase participation in active and intellectually stimulating leisure activities. Thus, those with more education are particularly likely to engage in the sort of leisure activities which can continue to provide intellectual challenges throughout life. Likewise, they are particularly likely to be curious (interested in learning new things) and tolerant (perhaps respectful of diversity). Moreover, these differences exist in individuals whose formal education was completed 40–60 years ago.

The present findings provided support for the hypothesis that the influence of education on the construction of the past and of the possible self is carried through its relationship to self-making at present. Education did not directly influence the making of the past or possible self, but rather was related to these components of self indirectly through the making of the current self. Adults who continue their education may be set on a course of life different from those who do not pursue further training (see review by Dannefer, 1988). As a result, when more educated older adults are asked to recall the self of the past and project the self into the future, they may be looking backward and forward from a different frame of reference than might less educated older adults.

This is not to say that less educated individuals necessarily possess a simplistic self associated with negative well-being outcomes. First, note that some of the domains of self (e.g., caring, parent, physically attractive) are not significantly related to education; these domains are equally accessible to all. A relatively complex self potentially still could be constructed within these domains.

Second, it should be noted that it is the self as measured by survey instruments which is related to education. More educated individuals appear better able to articulate a self-description in response to an open-ended question, and more readily endorse closed-ended self-descriptors, and thus, according to such measures of the self, they have a more rich and complex self-system. It is possible, however, that less-educated individuals have a rich and complex self-system which is not tapped by such measuring devices. Ways of measuring the self were largely developed in a college student population; more attention must be paid to methodology which may be more appropriate for other populations. It is possible that common self measures have a high-education bias for abstract, verbally articulated answers, which may make it more difficult to hear the voices of less-educated respondents. It should be recognized, however, that more educated respondents in this study revealed a more complex self in both open- and closed-ended responses, covering roles, traits, and activities, in the past, the present, and the future. It remains fair to say that, to the best of our knowledge, using a variety of different questions, more educated respondents have a more rich and diverse self than less-educated respondents.

The process of becoming educated demands new behaviors and activities which may not be emphasized in the lives of those who receive little education. If self-representation is rooted in behavior (Cross & Markus, 1990), then doing becomes being. It is through tackling intellectual challenges that we may develop a view of self as curious; it is through accepting a wide variety of new ideas, beliefs, and people that we may develop a view of self as tolerant. Thus, in addition to the values it transmits or rewards, it is the new behaviors and exposure to diversity, both within the curriculum and in the types of people one meets, that may explain the influence of education on the self. These effects may continue far beyond the end of formal education, as those who have formed the education habit continue to be involved in activities, to learn new things, and to keep in contact with a wide variety of people. For example, education may be related to self-making throughout the lifespan via such social processes as social support from and social comparisons to others in one's social network. Social networks of those with more or less education may be quite different. As such, how we define who we are, who we were, and who we may become may be importantly influenced by others in our social world; whom those others will be may depend on our educational level.

An alternative causal order also may explain the association between education and such aspects of self, however. The educational system may serve as a selection mechanism whereby those individuals who possess a variety of relevant self aspects are successful, and as a result, are encouraged to progress to higher levels of education. In this view, a complex self is less a consequence of educational attainment and more a precursor for progress in the educational system. The true sequence of these causal connections cannot be determined with the current cross-sectional data. It is likely, however, that the cause and effect flows in both directions.

Education may also have more indirect effects on self-making, via its relationship to other important variables such as occuption, income, or intelligence. However, findings from this study suggest that the relationship of education to self-making is not clearly mediated through these other variables. This finding differs from previous work on the influence of education on such outcomes as physical and cognitive functioning. For example, Ross and Wu (1995) demonstrated the relationship of education and physical health to be mediated by work and economic conditions, as well as by psychosocial resources such as control and social support and by performance of healthy (or avoidance of unhealthy) behaviors. Similarly, Pedersen et al. (1996) provided evidence that the effect of education on the cognitive functioning of older adults could, in large part, be explained by general cognitive ability.

The findings of the present investigation were consistent with those of previous work examining the role of education in the association between age and sense of control in older adults, however (Mirowsky, 1995). In addition to education, the research by Mirowsky included other indicators of socioeconomic status: i.e., income, employment, earnings, and marital status. Of these, only income was demonstrated to contribute beyond education, and to a much lesser extent. In explaining this pattern of findings, it was suggested that education may be a more general representation of status in the social hierarchy which precedes and subsumes other status indicators and thus, demonstrates a stronger effect on self-processes.

Although the present findings are consistent with previous research on education and intrapersonal resources (i.e., sense of control), it is possible that the presumed mediators were not measured with enough precision in the current study to facilitate detection of the hypothesized effects. It also is possible that these constructs did not operate as mediators in the present study because most of the respondents were no longer working for pay. It may be that the prestige of one's occupation and level of income do not have the same influence on self after employment has terminated.

Finally, although the expected relationships of education to the self-system were detected, it should be noted that educational attainment was conceptualized simply as the number of years of formal schooling, and did not encompass the content or quality of the educational experience. It is possible that the influence of education on self-making differs depending on the type of training pursued. In future generations, more adults will have had some training beyond high school, and thus the content and quality of the education may be more important influences on the construction of self than simply the number of years in school.

In conclusion, the findings reported here contribute to the growing literature investigating the influence of social structural characteristics on self and personality. The present research demonstrated that more years of formal schooling was associated with a more elaborated self-system (conceptualized as consisting of a greater number of current, past and possible self-aspects) in older age. Thus, it is in fact no accident that Carlotta has a more complex and articulated self-description than Hester; the fact that Carlotta has much more education than Hester seems to have a great deal to do with her more complex self. Further, this educational effect on self was not mediated by such resources as income, occupation, or intelligence, but instead seems to come relatively directly, via the values the educational system transmits or the opportunities for new behaviors and meeting new people it affords.

The purpose of this paper primarily was to describe the influence of education on selfhood in late life. As we anticipated, several aspects of the self appeared to be bolstered by advanced educational attainment. Taken together, the findings from this paper reinforce the position that the social context in which we are embedded importantly affects who we are and who we might become as we grow older. Much work lies ahead, however, in understanding how the self-system is shaped throughout life by placement in the larger structure of a society, as well as the extent to which structural advantages engender self-processes which promote successful aging.

REFERENCES

Adelmann, P. K. (1994a). Multiple roles and physical health among older adults: Gender ethnic comparisons. *Research on Aging, 16*, 142–166.

Adelmann, P. K. (1994b). Multiple roles and psychological well-being in a national sample of older adults. *Journal of Gerontology: Social Sciences, 49*, S277–S285.

Baltes, P. B., & Baltes, M. M. (1990). Psychological perspectives on successful aging: A model of selective optimization with compensation. In P. B. Baltes & M. M. Baltes (Eds.), *Successful aging: Perspectives from the behavioral sciences* (pp. 1–34). New York: Cambridge University Press.

Banaji, M. R., & Prentice, D. A. (1994). The self in social contexts. *Annual Review of Psychology, 45*, 297–332.

Brandtstadter, J., Wentura, D., & Greve, W. (1993). Adaptive resources of the aging self: Outlines of an emergent perspective. *International Journal of Behavioral Development, 16*, 323–349.

Carstensen, L. L. (1992). Social and emotional patterns in adulthood: Support for socioemotional selectivity theory. *Psychology and Aging, 7*, 331–338.

Coleman, L. M., & Antonucci, T. C. (1983). Impact of work on women at midlife. *Developmental Psychology, 19*, 290–294.

Cross, S. E., & Markus, H. R. (1990). The willful self. *Personality and Social Psychology Bulletin, 16*, 726–742.

Cutler, S. J., & Hendricks, J. (1990). *Leisure and time use across the life course.* In R. H. Binstock & L. K. George (Eds.), *Handbook of aging and the social sciences* (3rd ed.) (pp. 169–185). New York: Academic Press.

Dannefer, D. (1988). Differential gerontology and the stratified life course: Conceptual and methodological issues. In G. L. Maddox & M. P. Lawton (Eds.), *Annual Review of Gerontology and Geriatrics* (Vol. 8, pp. 3–36). New York: Springer Publishing Company.

Dowd, J. J. (1990). Ever since Durkheim: The socialization of human development. *Human Development, 33*, 138–159.

Gergen, K. J. (1977). The social construction of self-knowledge. In T. Mischel (Ed.), *The self: Psychological and philosophical issues* (pp. 139–169). Totowa, NJ: Rowman and Littlefield.

Gergen, K. J. (1991). *The saturated self: Dilemmas of identity in contemporary life.* New York: Basic Books.

Heidrich, S. M., & Ryff, C. D. (1993). The role of social comparison processes in the psychological adaptation of elderly adults. *Journal of Gerontology: Psychological Sciences, 48*, P127–P136.

Herzog, A. R., Franks, M. M., Markus, H. R., & Holmberg, D. (1995). Productive activities and agency in older age. In M. Baltes & L. Montada (Eds.), *Produktives leben im alter [Productive activities in later life]* (pp. 323–343). New York: Campus Verlag.

Herzog, A. R., & Markus, H. R. (1999). The self concept in life span and aging research. In V. L. Bengtson & K. W. Schaie (Eds.), *Handbook of theories of aging* (pp. 227–252). New York: Springer Publishing Company.

Hooker, K., & Kaus, C. R. (1992). Possible selves and health behaviors in later life. *Journal of Aging and Health, 4*, 390–411.

House, J. S., Kessler, R. C., Herzog, A. R., Mero, R. P., Kinney, A. M., & Breslow, J. (1990). Age, socioeconomic status, and health. *The Milbank Quarterly, 68*, 383–411.

Inkeles, A., & Smith, D. (1974). *Becoming modern.* Cambridge, MA: Harvard University Press.

Joreskog, K. G., & Sorbom, D. (1993). *LISREL 8.* Chicago: Scientific Software International, Inc.

Krause, N., & Borawski-Clark, E. (1994). Clarifying the functions of social support in later life. *Research on Aging, 16*, 251–279.

Lawton, M. P. (1985). Activities and leisure. In C. Eisdorfer, M. P. Lawton, & G. L. Maddox (Eds.), *Annual Review of Gerontology and Geriatrics* (Vol. 5, pp. 127–164). New York: Springer Publishing Company.

Linville, P. W. (1987). Self-complexity as a cognitive buffer against stress-related illness and depression. *Journal of Personality and Social Psychology, 4*, 663–676.

Maddox, G. L., & Clark, D. O. (1992). Trajectories of functional impairment in later life.*Journal of Health and Social Behavior, 33*, 114–125.

Markus, H. (1977). Self-schemas and processing information about the self. *Journal of Personality and Social Psychology, 35*, 63–78.

Markus, H. R., & Herzog, A. R. (1991). The role of the self-concept in aging. In K. W. Schaie & M. P. Lawton (Eds.), *Annual Review of Gerontology and Geriatrics* (Vol. 11, pp. 110–143). New York: Springer Publishing Company.

Markus, H. R., & Kitayama, , S. (1991). Culture and the self: Implications for cognition, emotion, and motivation. *Psychological Review, 98*, 224–253.

Markus, H. R., Mullally, P. R., & Kitayama, S. (1997). Selfways: Diversity in modes of cultural participation. In U. Neisser & D. Jopling (Eds.), *The conceptual self in context* (pp. 13–61). Cambridge: Cambridge University Press.

Markus, H., & Nurius, P. (1986). Possible selves. *American Psychologist, 41*, 954–969.

Markus, H., & Wurf, E. (1987). The dynamic self-concept: A social psychological perspective. *Annual Review of Psychology, 38*, 299–337.

Meyer, J. W. (1990). Individualism: Social experience and cultural formulation. In J. Rodin, C. Schooler, & K. W. Schaie (Eds.), *Self-directedness: Cause and effects throughout the life course* (pp. 51–58). Hillsdale, NJ: Lawrence Erlbaum.

Mirowsky, J. (1995). Age and the sense of control. *Social Psychology Quarterly, 58*, 31–43.

Pedersen, N. L., Reynolds, C. A., & Gatz, M. (1996). Sources of covariation among mini-mental state examination scores, education, and cognitive abilities. *Journal of Gerontology: Psychological Sciences, 51B*, P55–P65.

Ross, M. (1989). Relation of implicit theories to the construction of personal histories. *Psychological Review, 96*, 341–357.

Ross, C. E., & Wu, C. (1995). The links between education and health. *American Sociological Review, 60*, 719–745.

Sewell, W. H., & Hauser, R. M. (1975). *Education, occupation, and earnings*. New York: Academic Press.

Stryker, S. (1986). Identity theory: Developments and extensions. In K. Yardley & T. Honess (Eds.), *Self and identity* (pp. 89–104). New York: Wiley.

Thoits, P. A. (1983). Multiple identities and psychological well-being: A reformulation and test of the social isolation hypothesis. *American Sociological Review, 48*, 174–187.

Triandis, H. C. (1995). *Individualism and collectivism*. Boulder, CO: Westview.

Wechsler, D. (1981). *Wechsler Adult Intelligence Scale-Revised*. New York: The Psychological Corporation.

CHAPTER 9

Forging Macro-Micro Linkages in the Study of Psychological Well-Being

Carol D. Ryff, William J. Magee, Kristen C. Kling, & Edgar H. Wing

INTRODUCTION

Psychological well-being is a fundamentally micro-level construct that conveys information about how individuals evaluate themselves and the quality of their lives. In this chapter we describe a progression of scientific inquiry that initially tended to ignore social structural influences on well-being, or treat them as "noise" factors to be statistically controlled. More recently, we have incorporated macro-level influences, specifically socioeconomic standing, as part of the substantive scientific focus. In so doing, we have carried the study of positive psychological functioning beyond its disciplinary origins into sociological domains.

The ultimate vision guiding our venture is to steer clear of the "over-psychologized" nature of the person, which assumes that what is in the

This research was supported by the John D. and Catherine T. MacArthur Foundation Research Network on Successful Mid-Life Development (Orville Gilbert Brim, Director). Additional support was provided by the National Institute on Aging, Grants R01AG08979 and R01AG13613.

head (i.e., cognitive orientations, coping strategies, intellectual abilities), heart (i.e., emotions, moods, feelings), or actions (i.e., behaviors, choices) of individuals is sufficient to make sense of their well-being. The alternative "over-socialized" conception of the person (Wrong, 1961), also to be avoided, assumes that the "master variables" of the human condition are what is in the social structure, be it the invisible hand of normative guidelines contouring paths of conformity, or the strong arm of power structures controlling resource allocation and governing social organization.

We argue that both perspectives, in and of themselves, are wanting—their inadequacy is evident not only in empirical criteria (e.g., variance explained), but also in terms of theoretical scope and comprehensiveness. Individual and societal level factors are both requisite to a full understanding of human well-being, which inextricably links persons and the broader social world. The central question, thus, is not whether to bridge these realms, but how to do it. Using psychological well-being as the illustrative case, we propose that the study of well-being must simultaneously involve the assessment of social structural and individual-level variables.

More important, such inquiry must provide a conceptual and empirical formulation of the mechanisms that link these macro-micro levels of analysis. Social comparison processes will be advanced as one route through which structural and individual factors can be connected. These comparisons, we argue, follow, in part, from one's location in the social structure, and they have consequences for well-being. As such, social comparisons constitute a bridge linking macro- and micro-levels of analysis.

PSYCHOLOGICAL WELL-BEING: WHAT IS IT AND HOW HAS IT BEEN STUDIED?

We subscribe to a theory-driven, multidimensional formulation of psychological well-being (Ryff, 1989a/b, 1995a) that goes beyond absence-of-illness criteria of mental health (e.g., not being depressed or anxious). Key aspects of psychological well-being were derived from life-span developmental theories, which formulate the unfolding tasks and challenges of human growth; clinical accounts of what it means to be self-actualized, mature, fully functioning, or individuated; and formulations of positive criteria of mental health. Collectively, these formulations, sum-

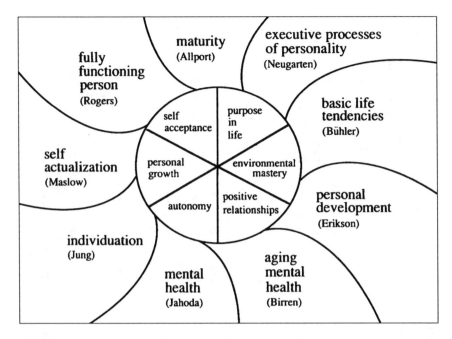

Figure 9.1 Core dimensions of well-being and their theoretical origins.

marized in the outer circle of Figure 9.1, elaborate diverse features of well-being. Points of convergence among them (see inner circle of Figure 9.1) have been the targets for empirical operationalization (Ryff, 1989b).

Definitions of the six key dimensions are provided in Table 9.1. Together, they encompass a breadth of wellness that includes positive evaluations of one's self and one's life, a sense of continued growth and development, the view that life is purposeful and meaningful, engagement and involvement in quality relations with others, the capacity to manage effectively one's surrounding world, and a sense of self-determination. Using structured self-report instruments (see Ryff, 1989b; Ryff & Keyes, 1995), these aspects of well-being have been studied in local community and national probability samples as well as in cross-sectional and longitudinal designs. Summarized below are key findings from these prior investigations.

Age and Gender Differences in Well-Being

Do people of different ages or gender report different profiles of positive functioning? The original validation sample ($N = 321$), based on commu-

Table 1. Definitions of Theory-Guided Dimensions of Well-Being

Dimension	Characteristics of a high scorer	Characteristics of a low scorer
Self-acceptance	Possess positive attitude toward self; acknowledges and accepts multiple aspects of self, including good and bad qualities; feels positive about past life	Feels dissatisfied with self; is disappointed with what has occurred in past life; is troubled about certain personal qualities; wishes to be different than what he or she is
Positive relations with other people	Has warm, satisfying, trusting relationships with others; is concerned about the welfare of others; is capable of strong empathy, affection, and intimacy; understands give-and-take of human relationships	Has few close, trusting relationships with others; finds it difficult to be warm, open, and concened about others; is isolated and frustrated in interpersonal relationships; is not willing to make compromises to sustain important ties with others
Autonomy	Is self-determining and independent; is able to resist social presures to think and act in certain ways; regulates behavior from within; evaluates self by personal standards	Is concerned about the expectations and evaluations of others; relies on judgments of others to make important decisions; conforms to social pressures to think and act in certain ways
Environmental mastery	Has sense of mastery and competence in managing the environment; controls complex array of external activities; makes effective use of surrounding opportunities; is able to choose or create contexts suitable to personal needs and values	Has difficulty managing everyday affairs; feels unable to change or improve surrounding context; is unaware of surrounding opportunities; lacks sense of control over external world
Purpose in life	Has goals in life and a sense of directedness; feels there is meaning to present and past life; holds beliefs that give life purpose; has aims and objectives for living	Lacks sense of meaning in life; has few goals or aims, lacks sense of direction; does not see purpose in past life; has no outlooks or beliefs that give life meaning
Personal growth	Has feeling of continued development; sees self as growing and expanding; is open to new experiences; has sense of realizing his or her potential; sees improvement in self and behavior over time; is changing in ways that reflect more self-knowledge and effectiveness	Has sense of personal stagnation; lacks sense of improvement or expansion over time; feels bored and uninterested with life; feels unable to develop new attitudes or behaviors

nity volunteers in a cross-sectional design (Ryff, 1989b), showed that certain aspects of well-being, such as environmental mastery and autonomy, show incremental scores with age. Personal growth and purpose in life, on the other hand, showed age decrements, particularly from midlife to old age. Self-acceptance and positive relations with others showed no significant age differences across the three age groups. Highly similar findings were evident in a second local community study ($N = 308$) (Ryff, 1991)— namely, age-incremental profiles on environmental mastery and autonomy; age-decremental profiles on personal growth, and stability profiles on self-acceptance and positive relations.

Because both investigations were conducted with community volunteers, generalizability of these findings was questionable. Thus, another investigation (Ryff & Keyes, 1995) was conducted with a national sample ($N = 1,108$). This inquiry involved a significant reduction in the number of items used to operationalize each dimension of well-being—thereby exemplifying the trade-offs in allocation of scientific resources between depth of measurement and sampling adequacy. Moreover, items for the reduced measures were selected to represent the multifactorial subdimensions of each scale, rather than to maximize internal consistency, the usual psychometric priority in large survey research.

Such decisions illustrate the compromises required to advance macro-micro linkages. What was gained by the willingness to loosen depth-of-measurement priorities of the psychologist was the opportunity to evaluate distributions of well-being in more socioeconomically diverse and representative sample. What was gained by the willingness to lessen the internal consistency priorities of the survey researcher was the possibility of carrying a theory-driven conception of psychological well-being to the realm of a national study.

Remarkably, many of the prior age patterns were replicated with these sharply reduced measures (see Figure 9.2) (Ryff & Keyes, 1995). Environmental mastery and autonomy again showed increases with age; purpose in life and personal growth showed declines with aging; and self-acceptance revealed no age differences. For positive relations, the results, contrary to prior findings of age stability, showed age increments. The consistency of the age findings across diverse samples and different scale lengths underscores the strength of the message that well-being is not uniform across different periods of the life course (or different cohorts, see below). Importantly, the strikingly recurrent incremental (environmental mastery, autonomy) and decremental (purpose in life, personal growth) age patterns from select community samples with much greater depth of measurement

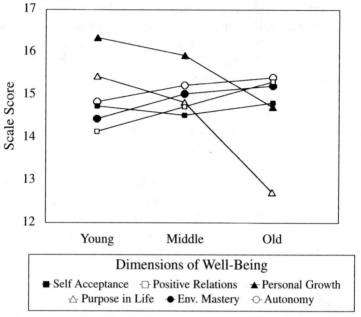

Figure 9.2 Age differences in three-item scales of well-being.

From "The Structure of Psychological Well-Being Revisited," by C. D. Ryff and C. L. M. Keyes, 1995, *Journal of Personality and Social Psychology, 69*, p. 722. Copyright 1995 by APA. Reprinted with permission.

could be generalized to larger, more diverse groups, wherein assessment procedures were much curtailed.

Longitudinal studies are needed to clarify whether these age patterns represent developmental changes, maturational changes, or cohort/historical influences. However they are to be interpreted, the findings point to diverse age trajectories in which older cohorts of adults reveal some psychological advantages (e.g., mastery), but also notable disadvantages (e.g., purpose, growth) relative to younger individuals. The replicative consistency of the latter may, in fact, be meaningfully linked to social structural influences (Ryff, 1995a). That is, lower self-ratings on purpose in life and personal growth among the aged may point to micro-level consequences of "structural lag"—namely, that social institutions currently lag behind the added years of life that many individuals now experience (Riley, Kahn, & Foner, 1994).

Gender differences in well-being have also shown replicative consistency. Women, across all studies, score higher than men on positive relations with others, and sometimes higher on personal growth as well. For the remaining dimensions, the above studies revealed no gender differences. Because women have been shown to suffer greater vulnerability to psychological depression than men (Strickland, 1992), findings on the positive side of mental functioning are particularly significant for revealing psychological strengths among women. Most recently, assessments with less educationally advantaged respondents have shown gender differences on multiple dimensions favoring men (Wing & Ryff, 1998). Thus, the most precise statement regarding gender differences in psychological well-being is that, when given opportunities for higher education, women reveal comparable, or even advantaged, profiles of well-being relative to their male counterparts.

Well-Being via Life Experience and Life Transition Studies: Where Is Social Structure?

Apart from descriptive questions about age and gender differences, initial studies of well-being also examined variation, or change, in well-being as a function of individuals' life experiences and their life transitions. Among the experiences we have studied are parenthood (Ryff, Lee, Essex, & Schmutte, 1994; Ryff, Schmutte, & Lee, 1996); health events (Heidrich & Ryff, 1993a, 1996); and community relocation (Kling, Ryff, & Essex, 1997; Ryff & Essex, 1992a; Smider, Essex, & Ryff, 1996). Across these investigations we also assess "interpretive mechanisms" which probe how people construe and give meaning to their life experiences. People make sense of their life experiences, for example, by comparing themselves to others (social comparison processes); by considering feedback from significant others (reflected appraisals); by identifying the causes of their experiences (attributional processes); by observing their own actions (behavioral self-perceptions); and by the importance they attach to particular experiences (psychological centrality) (see Ryff & Essex, 1992b, for conceptual summary).

Collectively, our studies show that considerable variance in well-being is associated not only with such life experiences/transitions but with how they are interpreted. Such assessments have included longitudinal investigations tracking change in well-being following life transitions (e.g., Kling et al., 1997; Smider et al., 1996). Social structural influences have been largely peripheral in such investigations—sociodemographic variables have typically been employed as "controls" in regression analyses predicting well-being as a function of the more proximal experiential and interpretive variables. Nonetheless, there have been hints that social structural influences are, in fact, a part of the story. We provide two examples.

Our initial investigation of the parental experience (Ryff et al., 1994) asked whether the psychological well-being of midlife adults is tied to perceptions of how adult children have "turned out." A sample ($N = 215$) of parents was asked detailed questions about the accomplishments (educational and occupational) and adjustment (psychological and social) of each of their grown (aged 21+) children. We found, not surprisingly, that multiple aspects of parents' well-being (e.g., environmental mastery, self-acceptance, purpose in life) were strongly predicted by these assessments of grown children. Consistent with our interest in "interpretive mechanisms," we asked how parents felt their adult children compared with themselves in these realms of achievement and adjustment. Again, parental well-being was predicted by these comparative assessments, net of the above effects of how well children had turned out. However, contrary to our expectation, (i.e., that parents' well-being would be enhanced by perceiving that children had done better than themselves), the direction of the social comparison effects was negative. That is, parents who perceived their children had done better than themselves had lower levels of psychological well-being.

The one exception to this pattern pertained to mothers with higher levels of education (i.e., one standard deviation above the mean) compared to mothers with lower levels of education (i.e., one standard deviation below the mean). Specifically, mothers with higher levels of education reported ever higher levels of self-acceptance and purpose in life, as they perceived their children had attained more educationally and occupationally than themselves (see Figure 9.3). Mothers with lower levels of education, however, reported lower levels of acceptance and purpose as they perceived their children had out-achieved themselves. Thus, position in the educational hierarchy appeared meaningfully linked with mothers' well-being via the perception of how they compared with children. Presumably, mothers with more education were better able to "bask in the reflected glory" of their children's achievements, whereas less educated mothers may have felt more troubled by their own lack of accomplishment and life purpose vis-à-vis marked achievement of their children. Fathers, however, showed no such interactions—those who perceived their children had done better than themselves had lower well-being, regardless of educational level.

A second example of possible social-structural influences again pertains to educational standing and its role in the experience of community relocation (Ryff, 1995b). Our prior findings (Kling et al., 1997; Ryff & Essex,

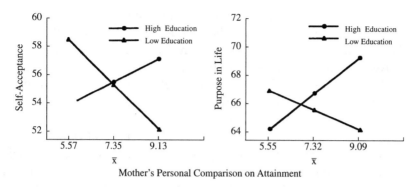

Figure 9.3 Significant interactions between mother's level of education and personal comparisons on attainment in predicting two aspects of well-being. Higher comparison scores indicate children were perceived as attaining more, educationally and occupationally, than self.

From "My Children and Me-Mid-Life Evaluations of Grown Children and of Self," by C. D. Ryff, Y. H. Lee, M. J. Essex, and P. S. Schmultz, 1994, *Psychology and Aging, 9*, p. 201. Copyright 1994 by APA. Reprinted with permission.

1992a) document the impact of interpretive mechanisms (e.g., social comparisons, reflected appraisals, psychological centrality) on post-move well-being. Education in these analyses was, however, treated as a control (noise) factor. Alternatively, when viewed as an indicator of socioeconomic standing, education may be meaningfully linked with how individuals negotiate their life transitions. Our general hypothesis was that education would exert generally salutary effects—those with more education were expected to withstand better the stresses of this transition (presumably via their access to relevant knowledge and resources).

Based on a longitudinal sample of 312 women interviewed both before and after their relocation, we found that there were significant changes in psychological well-being after the move, with respondents on average showing gains in multiple aspects of well-being. Going into the move, women with higher levels of education showed higher starting profiles of well-being, particularly self-acceptance, purpose in life, and personal growth (Ryff, 1995b). The longitudinal data also showed dynamics in interpretive mechanisms—namely, that their social comparisons (how they saw themselves relative to others) and reflected appraisals (how they thought others viewed them) also changed over time.

Regression analyses were conducted to investigate the influence of these dynamic interpretive mechanisms on respondents' changes in well-being following relocation. The findings showed that when social comparisons and reflected appraisals became more positive after the move, higher postmove levels of well-being were reported. That is, women who perceived that they compared more favorably with others (across domains of health, finances, friends, etc.) and who felt they were more positively perceived by others (across multiple domains) showed gains in psychological well-being following the move.

The targeted social-structural prediction was the following: among those women who reported negative post-move changes (i.e., less favorable social comparisons and reflected appraisals across multiple life domains after the move), we predicted higher well-being only for those with higher levels of education. That is, education was expected to cushion the effects of negative self-evaluative stresses associated with the move. This question was investigated by assessment of significant interactions between educational level and change (positive or negative) in social comparisons and reflected appraisals predicting post-move well-being.

Multiple significant interactions were found, although they were restricted to two life domains: daily activities and economics. Figure 9.4 (left side) illustrates such effects for the daily activities domain and outcomes of self-acceptance and personal growth (similar significant patterns were also obtained for purpose in life and environmental mastery). The graph represents predicted values consistent with procedures described by Aiken and West (1991). Women with higher levels of education reveal a sharper slope of the regression of psychological outcomes on positive versus negative changes in daily activities. That is, how one compared with and was perceived by others in the daily activities domain was more strongly linked to well-being among women with more education. If the move was going well (i.e., social comparisons and reflected appraisals improved following relocation), women with higher education had higher well-being. However, if the move was not going well (i.e., negative changes in comparisons and appraisals about daily activities), women with more education had lower well-being. For women with less education, there was generally a weaker relationship between social evaluations of daily activities and overall well-being.

Similar findings were evident for multiple outcomes in the economics domain (Figure 9.4, right side) graphically summarizes the patterns for purpose in life and self-acceptance). Taken together, these findings offered little support that negative post-move difficulties would be better handled by those with higher levels of education. Rather, the findings suggested that higher standing in the educational hierarchy is not uniformly an

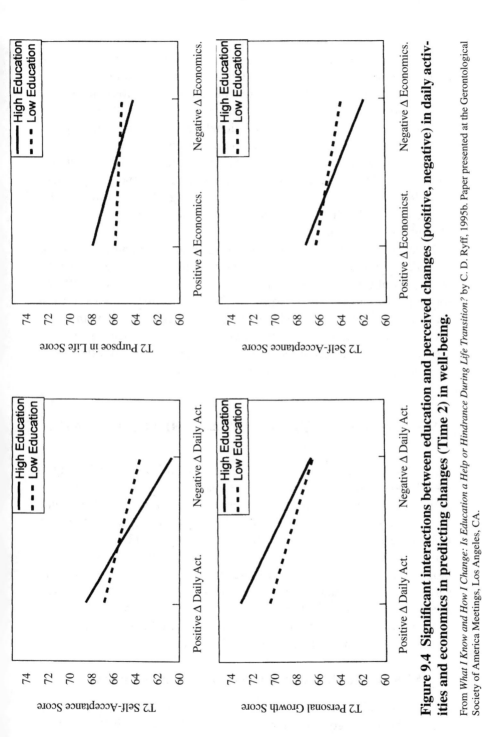

Figure 9.4 Significant interactions between education and perceived changes (positive, negative) in daily activities and economics in predicting changes (Time 2) in well-being.

From *What I Know and How I Change: Is Education a Help or Hindrance During Life Transition?* by C. D. Ryff, 1995b. Paper presented at the Gerontological Society of America Meetings, Los Angeles, CA.

advantage. Education may be a plus when life changes are going well, but not when things are going poorly (negative post-move comparisons and reflected appraisals). While these effects were specific to two of five life domains investigated, they suggest that during life transitions, higher educational levels may, paradoxically, magnify the effects of negative life changes on well-being. Higher educational standing may create expectations that one should be in control and able to prevent negative experiences. Mirowsky (1995) documents the close association between education and sense of control. Thus, violation of the general expectation that life should go well because one is knowledgeable, informed, and in charge may render the effects of negative experiences even worse in terms of impact on well-being.

In general, the preceding investigations kept social structure in the background. Its presence, nonetheless, crept in, with occasional evidence that the impact of life experiences and interpretive mechanisms were different for those with higher versus lower levels of education. Moreover, these illustrative examples revealed both benefits and costs linked with higher education. The following section addresses how the well-being agenda has recently been expanded in the direction of social structural influence by intersection with the literature on class and health.

WELL-BEING IN THE CLASS AND HEALTH AGENDA

Prior research on subjective well-being has probed a broad array of sociodemographic correlates (class, age, marital status, race, religion, geographic location) of reported happiness and life satisfaction (Bradburn, 1969; Bryant & Veroff, 1982; Diener, 1984; Diener & Fujita, 1995; Veroff, Douvan, & Kulka, 1981). These studies have employed largely atheoretical, single-item indicators of well-being, and typically examined sociodemographic variables in a descriptive manner. Such sociodemographic variables rarely account for much variance in subjective well-being (maximally around 10%). What has been distinctly missing from this literature is a formulation of intervening mechanisms and processes that connect social structural and individual levels of analysis.

SES and Health: Is Psychological Well-Being Relevant?

A growing body of evidence links socioeconomic standing to a diverse array of health outcomes (Adler et al., 1994; Mirowsky & Ross, 1989).

This literature provides impetus for linking well-being to a particular social-structural variable, namely, location in the socioeconomic hierarchy. At first glance, queries about the relationship between class and health agenda seem to do little more than document the obvious: poverty has adverse health consequences. This perception misses a key finding— namely, that there is a "social gradient" in health across the entire socioeconomic spectrum (Marmot et al., 1991). Thus, class differences in health exist even between those in middle versus upper SES strata. Why these social inequalities in health occur is not well understood.

Most extant research involves physical rather than mental health outcomes. Moreover, when investigators have gone beyond SES-related assessments of morbidity and mortality, the focus has been primarily on negative indicators of mental functioning, such as anxiety and depression (Dohrenwend & Dohrenwend, 1974; Kessler & Cleary, 1980; McLeod & Kessler, 1990). Few investigators have asked whether the prior class and health linkages also pertain to positive aspects of mental health. Such omission likely reflects the view that optimal functioning (mental or physical) is not a pressing concern relative to more grave matters of illness, disease, or dysfunction. However, dimensions of well-being may comprise powerful protective (or vulnerability) factors involved in understanding how socioeconomic status makes its way to a wider array of health outcomes. That is, the possession of core "life goods" (e.g., positive self-regard, quality ties to others, mastery, purpose) (see Ryff & Singer, 1998a) may provide critical ingredients that enable people to withstand life challenges and adversity. Moreover, there may be important "physiological substrates of flourishing" (Ryff & Singer, 1998a, 1998b) that also influence ultimate morbidity and mortality outcomes. The connection of social-structural factors to intervening biological mechanisms is another realm ripe for study of macro-micro linkages.

Integrative Evidence From Three Major Studies

The Whitehall Study of British civil servants documents a social gradient in mortality and morbidity (Marmot, Shipley, & Rose, 1984; Marmot et al., 1991): each grade of employment has higher levels of health problems and death rates than the one above it. A counterpart literature in the U.S. has been slower to accumulate, although similar inverse relationships between socioeconomic status and mortality have been documented here as well (Feldman, Makuc, Kleinman, & Cornoni-Huntley, 1989). Marmot, Ryff, Bumpass, Shipley and Marks (1997) brought together three major studies to explore class and health questions in the U.S. and Britain. The studies offered new tests of the generalizability, across diverse samples and different measures of SES, of the social gradient in health. The studies also extend the prior focus on mortality as the key outcome to new indicators of health, including psychological well-being.

Data were assembled from the Whitehall II Study of British civil servants (10,308 men and women), the Wisconsin Longitudinal Study (WLS) of midlife men and women who graduated from high school in 1957 (with over 70% of the known survivors of the original random sample of 10,317 participating), and the National Survey of Families and Households (NSFH), a national sample of U.S. adults (13,017 men and women). To determine whether the SES-health link is specific to particular measures of SES, each study used a different indicators: civil service employment grade (Whitehall), occupational status (WLS), and education (NSFH). Across four outcome measures (self-perceived health, depression, psychological well-being, and smoking), there were clear inverse relations with socioeconomic status (see Marmot et al., 1997).

The obtained SES gradients in psychological well-being are illustrated, separately for men and women, in Figure 9.5. Because each study employed somewhat different measures, well-being was operationalized across them with slightly different constructs. In Whitehall, it was assessed with a question about finding "little meaning in life"; in WLS, a 7-item version of the purpose in life scale (Ryff, 1989b) was used; and in NSFH, a 3-item version of Rosenberg's self-esteem scale was used. Each of these outcomes was dichotomized, such that relationship between well-being and particular measures of SES was expressed in terms of odds ratios. Thus, the figure illustrates the odds of reporting low meaning, purpose, or self-esteem.

The ratios are adjusted according to three models, each of which takes into account different variables possibly implicated in the class-health relationships. Model 1 includes only the SES indicator (for Whitehall only, age is also included). Model 2 then takes into account father's social class (Whitehall), or parents' education and whether one grew up in an intact family during childhood (WLS), or age and race (NSFH). Model 3 then adds a variety of other possibly intervening variables, such as work and environment and health behaviors (Whitehall), mental ability (IQ) (WLS), or parental education and intact childhood family (NSFH). The addition of variables across these models reflects the unique strengths of each study in pointing to different aspects of what might be part of class and health relationships.

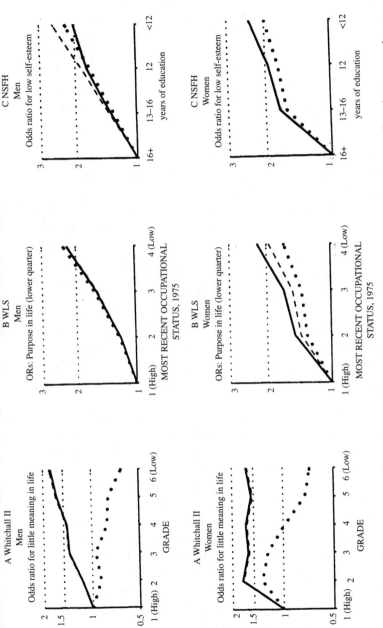

Figure 9.5 Odds ratios for predicting psychological well-being by measures of socioeconomic status in: (a) the Whitehall II Study; (b) the Wisconsin Longitudinal Study; and (c) the National Survey of Families and Households. Odds ratios adjusted according to three models (see text): ──── Model 1; ── ── Model 2; ········ Model 3.

From "Social Inequalities in Health: Converging Evidence and Next Questions," by M. G. Marmot, C. D. Ryff, L. L. Bumpass, M. Shipley, and N. F. Marks, 1997, *Social Science and Medicine, 44,* p. 905. Copyright 1997 by Elsevier Science Ltd. Reprinted with permission.

Across these models, there is a clear SES gradient in well-being for both men and women in WLS and NSFH. For Whitehall, the gradient is evident for men, although Model 3 suggests that work environment, health behaviors, etc., account for a good deal of the gradient in well-being. Although Whitehall women did not show a gradient in this indicator, both males and females in the study showed a strong gradient for affect balance (not shown). Similarly, both men and women in WLS showed a strong gradient in self-acceptance (Ryff, 1989b) (not shown). Thus, across notably different samples, distinct indicators of SES, and even diverse indicators of well-being, there was clear evidence of a socioeconomic gradient in psychological well-being. Moreover, the findings provide little support for the view that these relationships could be fully accounted for by early background or other individual factors (for example, parents' education or occupational status, nonintact family of origin, mental ability). They suggest rather that well-being is related to adult position in the social structure.

Given the usual focus on negative health outcomes, these results for positive mental health are particularly informative, because they show that lower social position not only increases the likelihood of ill health, it also decreases the chances for psychological well-being. Possessing these features of positive functioning constitutes an important window on quality of life, but more importantly, their presence may provide protective mechanisms in the face of life stresses, and their absence may create vulnerability for depression (Brown, Bifulco, & Andrews, 1990; Lewinsohn, Redner, & Steeley, 1991).

What the findings call for, however, is explanation: namely, how do these relationships come about? What are the processes that account for the fact that those at progressively higher levels in the socioeconomic hierarchy have better health (mental and physical)? Beyond the deprivations associated with poverty are numerous other likely intervening factors (e.g., health behaviors, work conditions, family life, neighborhood environments). Whitehall II has shown the import of some of these for explaining the class and health gradient (Marmot et al., 1997), and a recent U.S. survey points to an array of early background, behavioral, relational, and work characteristics to explain why people of lower socioeconomic status have worse health and lower psychological well-being (Marmot et al., in press). Beyond life conditions and behavioral actions are the ways in which individuals perceive themselves in their social contexts. Such perceptions, consistent with our prior work, address how individuals interpret themselves vis-á-vis others. These perceptions, we argue, comprise inter-vening mechanisms that link position in the social hierarchy to individual well-being.

TOWARD MACRO-MICRO INTEGRATION: EDUCATION, SOCIAL COMPARISON, AND WELL-BEING

The class and health agenda has prompted disciplinary exchange and a framework for expanding the study of well-being in new directions. As noted earlier, scholars of subjective well-being had already provided exten-sive documentation of the SES links of reported happiness and life satis-faction. What that literature neglected, however, was the intervening mechanisms that connect these macro, and micro levels of analysis. In this section, we review two recent investigations, which sharpen the class and well-being nexus by incorporating such intervening processes. Before summarizing relevant findings, we elaborate the rationale for choosing education as the primary indicator of SES standing across our studies. We also elaborate the conceptual rationale for using social comparison processes as key mechanisms of linkage.

Education as a Marker of Socioeconomic Standing

Socioeconomic status is typically defined in terms of three related, but dis-tinct, components: education, income, and occupational status. We target only one of these, education. One reason is that the other aspects of social class (income, occupational status) are, to a great extent, consequences of educational achievement, and therefore may mediate the effects of educa-tion (Hauser & Mossel, 1985; Sewell & Hauser, 1975, 1980). Sociologically speaking, education thus governs access to important future opportunities and resources. Compared to income or occupational standing, education is also a more person-specific characteristic. Wives, for example, are some-times classified according to the income or occupational standing of their husbands, but education is a variable reflecting their own SES-related status.

Psychologically speaking, we also see education as a defining feature of the self; that is, as an aspect of identity and a domain of personal achievement. In terms of the presentation of self in daily life, educational attainment is a key dimension along which people classify and evaluate others and themselves. Such assessments frequently have significant social consequences—those with high school education often exist in different social worlds (at work, at home, in the community) than college graduates. As a marker of personal knowledge and achievement, educational standing is also implicated in coping strategies, problem-solving abilities, and possibly even social supports. Further, when the three SES variables have been disaggregated and their independent influences on psychological distress have been examined, it is education, particularly among women (including homemakers and those in the labor force), that is the most important predictor of psychological distress (Kessler, 1982).

Turning to the question of educational effects on positive functioning, we also note that our prior findings on parenthood and relocation underscored the importance of educational influences. For the collective reasons described above, the remaining studies described below use educational attainment as the marker of standing in the SES hierarchy. We underscore that these studies do not address more richly textured aspects of social class such as linguistic and moral practices, lifestyles, world-views, and normative expectations (see Chapter 7, this volume).

Why Social Comparison Processes?

One rationale for targeting social comparison processes as a key intervening mechanism is continuity with our prior program of studies. Such comparisons have been included in nearly all of our investigations, although the conceptualization of them has been tied to the interpretions given to proximal life experiences, not to perceived location in the social structure. Further rationale comes from the conceptual underpinnings of our formulation of "interpretive mechanisms" (see Ryff & Essex, 1992a) as well as earlier efforts to link personality and social structure (Ryff, 1987). Rosenberg and Pearlin (1978) offered significant guidance via their efforts explain the age-related linkage between social class and self-esteem. Their query was fundamentally a challenge in how to integrate macro and micro levels of analysis.

Self-esteem, they stated, shows little connection with social class in childhood; but with age, there emerges a stronger correlation between self-esteem and social class. The reasons for this emerging linkage were tied to the changing social worlds of adolescents and young adults, i.e., transitions from the more homogeneous worlds of early childhood school and neighborhood environments to the more heterogeneous worlds of subsequent educational and occupational pursuits. What such heterogeneity catalyzed was a changing perception of self, tied fundamentally to how individuals see themselves vis-á-vis others (social comparisons), how they believe they are viewed by others (reflected appraisals), what they observe in their own behaviors (self-perceptions), and what they designate as important to them (psychological centrality). These interpretive mechanisms comprised a theoretical synthesis of numerous social psychological processes that were integrated for the purpose of explaining a particular macro- micro linkage—namely, why basic self-evaluation (self-esteem) becomes linked with SES standing as individuals age.

Of the four mechanisms, we focus primarily on social comparisons and reflected appraisals (Kling et al., 1997; Ryff & Essex, 1992a), although we have also examined psychological centrality (Kling et al., 1997). The extant literature on subjective well-being has also examined comparisons (in income) as one route to explaining variations in reported happiness and satisfaction (Diener, Sandvik, Seidlitz, & Diener, 1993; Veenhoven, 1991; see Chapter 10, this volume).

Despite their conceptual appeal, the assessment of such comparisons is neither simple nor straightforward. When asked directly, individuals frequently deny that they make such comparisons, suggesting a kind of normative climate against explicit comparative judgments. However, social comparisons can be unobtrusively probed with regard to many aspects of life (see Heidrich & Ryff, 1993b) as well as in terms of numerous referent others, some of whom may be selected, while others are imposed (e.g., friends vs. siblings). The studies we describe below draw on these distinctions to offer various alternatives for probing the social comparison domain. Findings from two investigations, both involving large and diverse samples, are summarized.

Educational Attainment and Comparison With Significant Others in Midlife

Ryff and Magee (1995) used data from the Wisconsin Longitudinal Study (WLS) to examine the linkages between educational attainment and well-being in a sample of midlife men and women. A large literature in sociology has addressed the role of education in social stratification processes; that is, how educational attainment influences subsequent occupational and economic mobility (Sewell & Hauser, 1975), or how schools serve as mechanisms for social selection and social differentiation (Karabel & Halsey, 1977). Educational systems are, depending on one's theoretical position (e.g., functionalist vs. conflict theory), viewed as structures that offer opportunities for mobility of individuals, or as mechanisms that perpetuate social inequalities (DiMaggio, 1979; Swartz, 1977).

WLS is well known for its model of status attainment that documents the prominent role of educational attainment in subsequent occupational advancements and earnings (Hauser & Mossel, 1985; Sewell & Hauser, 1975, 1980). The question we add to the inquiry is what are the individual life consequences (e.g., quality of life, mental health) of achieving different positions in the social order? Early WLS findings showed dramatic differences in educational aspirations and achievements, among children of equally high levels of ability, between those having high versus low socioeconomic backgrounds. We consider possible consequences of these different attainment profiles for psychological well-being.

In addition, we examine the influence of social comparisons about educational attainment on respondents' reported well-being. Sample members were asked to compare their own educational attainment with that of two key significant others: namely, their same-sex parent, and a randomly selected sibling. These proximal social comparisons (those within the family) are "inescapable" aspects of self-evaluation. In addition, they provide a marker for mobility processes (upward or downward) relative to one's own parents or siblings. The hypothesis was that such comparisons exert an influence on well-being, net of actual educational attainment, with those achieving more than their significant others expected to report higher well-being.

One limitation of the WLS is that although providing longitudinal assessment of educational and occupational attainment, psychological well-being did not become a part of the study until respondents were in midlife. Thus, it is not possible to track changes in well-being as a function of gains in education. However, because information was available regarding respondents' family background and early abilities, it is possible to examine the influence of educational attainment, net of these early starting resources. Parents' income could, for example, translate to material goods that enhance well-being, and selection processes could be operative whereby the more intelligent get more education. Our focus was to assess the effects of education on well-being after these influences were controlled.

All six dimensions of psychological well-being were included in the 1992/93 WLS data collection, each of which was operationalized with a 7-item scales. Social comparisons were assessed with a single-item question in which respondents rated how much better or worse they had done than their same-sex parent (or a randomly selected sibling) in getting an education. The sample for these analyses included 3,129 men and 3,609 women from the WLS on whom data were available regarding the social comparison items and well-being.

Over half of the women in WLS did not receive further education beyond their high school diploma. Another 22.3% obtained vocational training or some college, and 24.2% completed a college degree or more. For men, 34.8% completed no post-secondary education, 29.8% had vocational training or some college, and 35.4% completed a college degree or more. When education was juxtaposed with reported levels of well-being, we found that for all six measures, women with higher levels of education reported higher well-being. All combinations (but one) of mean-level differences comparing different levels of education were significant. For men, there were also differences in well-being as a function of educational attainment, but the effects were not as strong. For example, there were no educational differences in men's reported levels of positive relations with others. For the remaining aspects of well-being, significant differences were obtained, sometimes between all groups, and others just between the highest and lowest educational attainment groups.

Tables 9.2 (women) and 9.3 (men) summarize select findings from hierarchical regression analyses that tested the predictive influence of educational attainment and social comparisons on reported well-being. These analyses controlled for respondents' high school IQ, mothers' and fathers' educational, parental income, and fathers' occupational status. Education was coded as a three-level categorical variable, and high school education was the point of comparison. Thus, these analyses indicate whether there are significant differences in the prediction of well-being between those with high school degrees and the other two educational groups. Model 1 examines educational influences on well-being outcomes, net of control variables. Models 2a and 2b then show the effects of adding social comparisons, separately for same-sex parent and the randomly selected sibling.

The findings for women (Table 9.2) show that for three aspects of well-being (autonomy, purpose in life, and personal growth), the educational differences between high school graduates and the two higher educational groups remain significant after controlling for background factors. These effects drop out for environmental mastery (not shown) when background effects have been controlled. For self-acceptance and positive relations (not shown), education remains a significant predictor following controls, but only for the contrast between high school and college respondents. Subjective comparisons with mothers significantly predicted all aspects of well-being, net of actual educational attainment, and in the direction predicted. That is, women who perceived their educational attainment was

Table 9.2 Education, Social Comparisons, and Well-Being

	WLS Women					
	Model 1 (educ)		Model 2a (parent comp)		Model 2b (sib comp)	
WOMEN	beta	SE	beta	SE	beta	SE
Autonomy						
Voc/Some Coll	.13**	.04	.05	.07	.13**	.05
Degree	.13**	.05	-.04	.08	.07	.05
Parent Comp			.16***	.04		
Sib Comp					.06***	.02
Total R²	.04		.05		.04	
Purpose in Life						
Voc/Some Coll	.16***	.04	.12	.07	.17***	.05
Degree	.31***	.05	.22**	.07	.26***	.05
Parent Comp			.15***	.04		
Sib Comp					.08***	.02
Total R²	.04		.05		.04	
Personal Growth						
Voc/Some Coll	.27***	.04	.20**	.06	.26***	.04
Degree	.43***	.05	.31***	.07	.37***	.05
Parent Comp			.21***	.03		
Sib Comp					.09***	.02
Total R²	.09		.10		.10	

All models control for High School IQ, Parental Education, Parental Income, and Father's Occupational Status.
Note: Educational attainment is a three-level categorical variable (high school, vocational training/some college, college degree or higher). High school is the category of contrast.

Table 9.3 Education, Social Comparisons, and Well-Being

	WLS Men					
	Model 1 (educ)		Model 2a (parent comp)		Model 2b (sib comp)	
MEN	beta	SE	beta	SE	beta	SE
Self-Acceptance						
Voc/Some Coll	.09**	.04	.02	.06	.09	.04
Degree	.16**	.05	.05	.08	.08	.05
Parent Comp			.11**	.04		
Sib Comp					.08***	.02
Total R²	.01		.01		.01	
Purpose in Life						
Voc/Some Coll	.02***	.04	-.06	.06	.03	.04
Degree	.28***	.05	.11	.07	.18***	.05
Parent Comp			.13***	.04		
Sib Comp					.11***	.02
Total R²	.02		.03		.03	
Personal Growth						
Voc/Some Coll	.18***	.04	.13*	.06	.19***	.05
Degree	.35***	.05	.16*	.08	.25***	.05
Parent Comp			.20***	.04		
Sib Comp					.12***	.02
Total R²	.04		.04		.05	

All models control for High School IQ, Parental Education, Parental Income, and Father's Occupational Status.
Note: Educational attainment is a three-level categorical variable (high school, vocational training/some college, college degree or higher). High school is the category of contrast.

better than their mothers' had higher well-being. Moreover, such comparisons revealed mediation influences for all outcomes (except environmental mastery): i.e., effects of education in Model 1 were reduced (some to nonsignificance) when social comparisons were added to the model. Social comparisons with siblings were also significant predictors of well-being, but showed less mediating influences.

Similar but less pronounced effects were evident for men (Table 9.3). For self-acceptance and personal growth, educational differences between high school graduates and the two advanced educational groups remained significant after control variables were entered. For purpose in life, it was only the contrast between high school and those with college degrees that remained significant. Environmental mastery (not shown) revealed a similar pattern; no effects were evident for positive relations or autonomy. For all outcomes except personal growth, prior educational influences on well-being were fully mediated by social comparisons with fathers—men who perceived that educational attainment was better than their fathers' had higher levels of well-being. Comparisons with siblings were also significant predictors, but showed mediational influences only for self-acceptance. The range of variance accounted for across these models for men and women was small (1% to 10%).

In summary, these analyses from the Wisconsin Longitudinal Study elaborate the linkages between educational attainment and well-being for midlife men and women, even after controlling for background and early ability influences. Moreover, the data clarify that social comparisons, particularly with parents, are an additional influence on reported well-being, in many instances providing evidence that it is through these social comparisons that educational attainment has its influence (i.e., mediational processes). While our analyses were restricted to comparisons with significant others in one's family, such effects may also be evident in comparison with one's high school friends, or same-aged peers in adulthood.

In general, the findings were stronger for women than men, perhaps underscoring the historical changes occurring in these cohorts regarding educational opportunities for women. That is, the women of the WLS came of adult age in an era in which opportunities for continued education were expanding. Some were able to partake of these new possibilities, but many were not. Thus, the women who were able to move beyond their family of origin in educational standing may have experienced particular psychological benefits, perhaps because of the contrasts in opportunity structures available to their mothers (or their same-sex peers). Our final analysis addresses the import of educational attainment on diverse dimensions of well-being in a national sample and with an assessment of social comparisons not specific to significant others in one's family.

Education, Well-Being, and the Role of Perceived Inequalities

Wing and Ryff (1998) recently examined distributions of psychological well-being in a national survey of adults (aged 25–74, $N = 3,032$) conducted by the MacArthur Foundation Research Network on Midlife Development. These data provided an opportunity to examine the linkages between social class (marked by educational attainment) and well-being in a more representative sample. As such, the work elaborates the social gradients in health documented by Marmot et al. (1997). That study, however, had not addressed intervening mechanisms in the class/health linkage. Following on the social comparative theme, Wing and Ryff explored an interpretive process explicitly linked with social class; namely, the notion of "perceived inequalities".

The study of perceived inequalities follows from the observation that individuals live in social worlds that are thick with conspicuous symbols of class standing (e.g., occupation, car, clothing, home, leisure activities). In addition, individuals have recurrent first-hand experience of how education and income are decisive factors determining culturally valued opportunities (e.g., for interesting work, for travel, for what one can provide to one's children). The perception that one has less of the socially desired goods than others is a more expansive comparison than those that may occur with family members. Fundamentally, "perceived inequalities" probe the extent to which individuals have an awareness of an unequal distribution of life resources.

We asked about such perceptions in three life domains: how individuals compare their *work opportunities* with others (e.g., "Most people have more rewarding jobs than I do"); their ability to *provide for their children* (e.g., "I believe I have been able to do as much for my children as most other people"); and their *living environments* (e.g., "I live in as nice a home as most people"). Perceived inequalities in work, family, and home domains were tapped by three separate, 6-item scales.

Our prediction was that individuals of lower SES standing would have higher levels of perceived inequalities in all of the above domains. We also expected that perceived inequalities would constitute a key intervening process in the linkage of class and well-being. The findings showed that for five of the six dimensions of well-being (all scales except autonomy), those with higher levels of education reported significantly higher levels of well-being. In addition, as predicted, those with less education reported greater perceived inqualities across the domains of work, family, and home. Women also reported greater perceived inequalities in each of these domains than men.

Table 9.4 shows results of the regression analyses for two select dimensions of well-being: self-acceptance and purpose in life. Numerous background factors (gender, age, race, marital status, number of children, employment status, parents'education, economic background, and chronic health conditions) were included as control variables. Education is entered in Model 1, and Model 2 contains the perceived inequality variables (with analyses reported separately for each life domain). Sample sizes vary across these domains, depending on whether respondents were employed, or had children. These analyses show that education is a strong, significant predictor of both dimensions of well-being, and that the perception of inequalities across each of the three domains is also a signficant predictor of self-acceptance and purpose. While the addition of perceived inqualities did not fully mediate the prior educational influences, tests of change in the size of the SES regression coefficient from the Model 1 to Model 2 were significant (see Wing & Ryff, 1998, for details). Similar effects (not shown) were found for personal growth and environmental mastery (although only for the home domain in the latter). There was no evidence that these effects differed by gender. Parallel analyses using income as the macro-level SES variable were also conducted, and in general, these revealed that education was a stronger predictor of well-being than income.

In summary, these results from a nationally representative sample add further evidence that position in the socieoconomic hierarchy is linked with differential levels of reported well-being and underscore the role of psychosocial construal processes in bridging these macro and micro levels of analysis. The emphasis on perceived inequalities provides a class-specific operationalization of how individuals interpret their social worlds by probing the degree to which they see inequalities in their share of valued life resources relative to others. Importantly, perceived inequalities are both predicted by SES, and predictive of well-being, thereby sharpening the conceptual and empirical understanding of their role as a linking mechanism. Underscoring the importance of a multidimensional framework for the study of well-being, these findings clarify that not all aspects of positive functioning appear class-linked. Individuals' perceptions of their own autonomy (capacity to choose for themselves) is not, for example, linked to their educational attainment. Similarly, once control variables were added to the regression model, neither education nor income was a signif-

Table 9.4 Education, Perceived Inequalities, and Well-Being

	Work		Family		Home	
	B(SE)	β	B(SE)	β	B(SE)	β
Self-Acceptance						
Model 1: Education	.23(.03)	.17**	.22(.04)	.16**	.20(.03)	.14**
Model 2: Education	.15(.03)	.10**	.15(.03)	.11**	.17(.03)	.12**
Perceived Inequalities	−.40(.02)	−.40**	−.37(.03)	−.31**	−.29(.02)	−.26**
Total R^2		.25**		.19**		.18**
$\Delta\beta$[a]		−.06**		−.05**		−.02*
n	1905		1685		2789	
Purpose in Life						
Model 1: Education	.26(.03)	.18**	.31(.04)	.21**	.31(.03)	.21**
Model 2: Education	.22(.03)	.15**	.27(.04)	.19**	.29(.03)	.19**
Perceived Inequalities	−.17(.02)	−.17**	−.22(.03)	−.18**	−.21(.02)	−.18**
Total R^2		.11**		.12**		.15**
$\Delta\beta$[a]		−.03**		−.03**		−.01*
n	1905		1685		2789	

*$p<.001$; **$p<.0001$

All regression equations control for gender, age, race, marital status, number of children, employment status, parents' education (average), economic background, and chronic physical health conditions.

[a]This is the change in the standardized regression coefficient for the SES variable from Model 2 to Model 3.

icant predictor of positive relations with others. Well-being is thus a multifaceted, micro-level domain, with some components (self-acceptance, purpose, mastery, and growth) more closely linked to macro-level class variables and intervening mechanisms than others.

CONCLUSIONS AND FUTURE DIRECTIONS

Our objective in this chapter is to use the study of psychological well-being as an illustrative case for how a realm of scientific inquiry that began largely as a micro-level enterprise has been expanded to incorporate macro-level questions. We have shown that variations in well-being stem from multiple influences, including age, gender, and proximal life experiences (parenthood, health events, relocation) as well as from one's standing in the socioeconomic hierarchy, operationalized via educational standing. In addition, we have provided evidence that social comparison processes and perceived inequalities constitute intervening social psychological mechanisms that bridge the class and well-being realms.

The obtained findings were sometimes restricted to particular dimensions of well-being and reflected a primary focus on only one of three prominent components of socioeconomic standing. Neglected were thus the more complex lifestyle, world-view, linguistic meanings of social class. While the findings generally convey a message of the mental health advantages of higher educational standing, there was also evidence that having more education may sometimes hazardous, perhaps when related to a priori expectations for effective management of difficult life transitions.

The social comparison results also underscored the psychological advantages of seeing one's self doing well relative to others. However, as the work on perceived inequalities made clear, individuals with lower levels of education frequently do not have access to the life opportunities or resources that enable such positive comparisons. The study of well-being could fruitfully incorporate other intervening social psychological mechanisms (e.g., goal-setting and -seeking, coping strategies, problem-solving, optimism) that may also connect social structural influences with individual mental health outcomes.

Given the explicit aging focus of the present volume, an important future question is the extent of the cumulative impact of these structural influences and intervening mechanisms on later life health and well-being.

Ross and Wu (1996), for example, have shown that disparities in physical health and physical functioning between adults of different educational backgrounds accelerate with age. Thus, whether later life is a period in the life course when disparities in well-being become more pronounced, or are increasingly "leveled" is an important future question. Our recurrent findings of lower levels of purpose in life and personal growth among older adults, we note, were obtained even among more educationally and economically advantaged samples. The structural lag phenomenon discussed earlier may defy class distinctions, or pose even greater challenges for those at the high end of the SES hierarchy, where access to resources, opportunities, and meaningful activities may have been a more sustained and gratifying experience in earlier decades of adult life.

In promoting multidisciplinary research on well-being, we have illustrated the conceptual and empirical trade-offs sometimes required to advance scientific agendas that bridge macro and micro levels of analysis. Such integrative science requires degrees of flexibility that unfortunately are not fostered in disciplinary-specific scientific training. Future strides in linking these distant levels of analysis will thus likely rest on innovations, theoretical and methodological, that occur on the boundaries between scientific disciplines, limited as they each are to capturing but a part of the human experience. This work illustrates a scientific progression reaching toward such boundaries.

REFERENCES

Adler, N. E., Boyce, T., Chesney, M. A., Cohen, S., Folkman, S., Kahn, R. I., & Syme, S. L. (1994). Socioeconomic status and health: The challenge of the gradient. *American Psychologist, 49*, 15–24.

Aiken, L. S., & West, S. G. (1991). *Multiple regression: Testing and interpreting interactions.* Newbury Park, CA: Sage.

Bradburn, N. M. (1969). *The structure of psychological well-being.* Chicago: Aldine.

Brown, G. W., Bifulco, A., & Andrews, B. (1990). Self-esteem and depression: III. Aetiological issues. *Social Psychiatry and Psychiatric Epidemiology, 25*, 235–243.

Bryant, F. B., & Veroff, J. (1982). The structure of psychological well-being: A sociohistorical analysis. *Journal of Personality and Social Psychology, 43*, 653–673.

Diener, E. (1984). Subjective well-being. *Psychological Bulletin, 95*, 542–575.

Diener, E., & Fujita, F. (1995). Resources, personal strivings, and subjective well-being: A nomothetic and idiographic approach. *Journal of Personality and Social Psychology, 68,* 926–935.

Diener, E., Sandvik, E., Seidlitz, L., & Diener, M. (1993). The relationship between income and subjective well-being: Relative or absolute? *Social Indicators Research, 28,* 195–223.

DiMaggio, P. (1979). Review essay: On Pierre Bourdieu. *American Journal of Sociology, 84,* 1460–1474.

Dohrenwend, B. P., & Dohrenwend, B. S. (1974). Social and cultural influences on psychopathology. *Annual Review of Psychology, 25,* 417–452.

Feldman, J. J., Makuc, D. M., Kleinman, J. C., & Cornoni-Huntley, J. (1989). National trends in educational differentials in mortality. *American Journal of Epidemiology, 129,* 919–933.

Hauser, R. M., & Mossel, P. M. (1985). Fraternal resemblance in educational attainment and occupational status. *American Journal of Sociology, 91,* 650–673.

Heidrich, S. M., & Ryff, C. D. (1993a). Physical and mental health in later life: The self-system as mediator. *Psychology and Aging, 8,* 327–338.

Heidrich, S. M., & Ryff, C. D. (1993b). The role of social comparisons processes in the psychological adaptation of elderly adults. *Journal of Gerontology, 48,* P127–P136.

Heidrich, S. M., & Ryff, C. D. (1996). The self in later years of life: Changing perspectives on psychological well-being. In L. Sperry & H. Prosen (Eds.), *Aging in the twenty- first century: A developmental perspective* (pp. 73–102). New York: Garland.

Karabel, J., & Halsey, A. H. (1977). *Power and ideology in education.* New York: Oxford University Press.

Kessler, R. C. (1982). A disaggregation of the relationship between socioeconomic status and psychological distress. *American Sociological Review, 47,* 752–764.

Kessler, R. C., & Cleary, P. D. (1980). Social class and psychological distress. *American Sociological Review, 45,* 463–478.

Kling, K. C., Ryff, C. D., & Essex, M. J. (1997). Adaptive changes in the self-concept during a life transition. *Personality and Social Psychology Bulletin, 23,* 989–998.

Lewinsohn, P., Redner, J., & Steeley, J. (1991). The relationship between life satisfaction and psychosocial variables: New perspectives. In F. Strack, M. Argyle, & A. Schwarz (Eds.), *Subjective well-being: An interdisciplinary perspective* (pp. 141–169). New York: Pergamon.

Marmot, M. G., Davey Smith, G., Stansfeld, S., Patel, C., North, F., Head, J., White, I., Brunner, E., & Feeney, A. (1991). Health inequalities among British civil servants: The Whitehall II Study. *Lancet, 337,* 1387–1393.

Marmot, M. G., Fuhrer, R., Ettner, S. L., Marks, N. F., Bumpass, L. L., & Ryff,

C. D. (1998). Contribution of psychosocial-factors to socio-economic differences in health. *Milbank Quarterly, 76*, 403–447.

Marmot, M. G., Ryff, C. D., Bumpass, L. L., Shipley, M., & Marks, N. F. (1997). Social inequalities in health: Converging evidence and next questions. *Social Science and Medicine, 44*, 901–910.

Marmot, M. G., Shipley, M. J., & Rose, G. (1984). Inequalities in death—specific explanations of a general pattern? *Lancet, 1*, 1003.

McLeod, J. D., & Kessler, R. C. (1990). Socioeconomic status differences in vulnerability to undesirable life events. *Journal of Health and Social Behavior, 31*, 162–172.

Mirowsky, J. (1995). Age and the sense of control. *Social Psychological Quarterly, 58*, 31–43.

Mirowsky, J., & Ross, C. E. (1989). *Social causes of psychological distress.* New York: Aldine de Gruyter.

Riley, M. W., Kahn, R. L., & Foner, A. (1994). *Age and structural lag.* New York: Wiley.

Rosenberg, M., & Pearlin, L. I. (1978). Social class and self-esteem among children and adolescents. *American Journal of Sociology, 84*, 53–77.

Ross, C. E., & Wu, C.L. (1996). Education, age, and the cumulative advantage in health. *Journal of Health and Social Behavior, 37*, 104–120.

Ryff, C. D. (1987). The place of personality and social structure research in social psychology. *Journal of Personality and Social Psychology, 53*, 1192–1202.

Ryff, C. D. (1989a). Beyond Ponce de Leon and life satisfaction: New directions in quest of successful aging. *International Journal of Behavioral Development, 12*, 35–55.

Ryff, C. D. (1989b). Happiness is everything, or is it? Explorations on the meaning of psychological well-being. *Journal of Personality and Social Psychology, 57*, 1069–1081.

Ryff, C. D. (1991). Possible selves in adulthood and old age: A tale of shifting horizons. *Psychology and Aging, 6*, 286–295.

Ryff, C. D. (1995a). Psychological well-being in adult life. *Current Directions in Psychological Science, 4*, 99–104.

Ryff, C. D. (1995b, November). *What I know and how I change: Is education a help or hindrance during life transition?* Paper presented at the Gerontological Society of America Meetings, Los Angeles, CA.

Ryff, C. D., & Essex, M. J. (1992a). The interpretation of life experience and well-being: The sample case of relocation. *Psychology and Aging, 7*, 507–517.

Ryff, C. D., & Essex, M. J. (1992b). Psychological well-being in middle and later adulthood: Descriptive markers and explanatory processes. In K. W. Schaie & M. P. Lawton (Eds.), *Annual Review of Gerontology and Geriatrics* (Vol. 11, pp. 144–171). New York: Springer Publishing Company.

Ryff, C. D., & Keyes, C. L. M. (1995). The structure of psychological well-being revisited. *Journal of Personality and Social Psychology, 69*, 719–727.

Ryff, C. D., Lee, Y. H., Essex, M. J., & Schmutte, P. S. (1994). My children and me: Mid-life evaluations of grown children and of self. *Psychology and Aging, 9*, 195–205.

Ryff, C. D., & Magee, W. M. (1995, August). *Opportunity, achievement, and well-being: A midlife perspective.* Paper presented at the American Psychological Association Meetings, New York, NY.

Ryff, C. D., Schmutte, P. S., & Lee, Y. H. (1996). How children turn out: Implications for parental self-evaluation. In C. D. Ryff & M. M. Seltzer (Eds.), *The parental experience in midlife* (pp. 383–422). Chicago: University of Chicago Press.

Ryff, C. D., & Singer, B. (1998a). The contours of positive human health. *Psychological Inquiry, 9*, 1–28.

Ryff, C. D., & Singer, B. (1998b). Human health: New directions for the next millenium. *Psychological Inquiry, 9*, 69–85.

Sewell, W. H., & Hauser, R. M. (1975). *Education, occupation, and earnings: Achievement in the early career.* New York: Academic Press.

Sewell, W. H., & Hauser, R. M. (1980). The Wisconsin Longitudinal Study of social and psychological factors in aspirations and achievements. In A. C. Kerckhoff (Ed.), *Research in Sociology and Education* (pp. 59–99). Greenwich, CT: JAI Press.

Smider, N. A., Essex, M. J., & Ryff, C. D. (1996). Adaptation to community relocation: The interactive influence of psychological resources and contextual factors. *Psychology and Aging, 11*, 362–371.

Strickland, B. R. (1992). Women and depression. *Current Directions in Psychological Science, 1*, 132–135.

Swartz, D. (1977). Pierre Bourdieu: The cultural transmission of social inequality. *Harvard Educational Review, 47*, 545–555.

Veenhoven, R. (1991). Is happiness relative. *Social Indicators Research, 24*, 1–34.

Veroff, J., Douvan, E., & Kulka, R. A. (1981). *The inner American: A self-portrait from 1957 to 1976.* New York: Basic.

Wing, E. H., & Ryff, C. D. (1998). *Social class and psychological well-being: The mediating influence of perceived inequalities.* Unpublished manuscript, University of Wisconsin-Madison.

Wrong, D. H. (1961). The oversocialized conception of man in modern sociology. *American Sociological Review, 26*, 183–193.

CHAPTER 10

Income and Subjective Well-Being Over the Life Cycle

Richard A. Easterlin & Christine M. Schaeffer

C ross-sectional studies of the empirical relation between income and subjective well-being repeatedly find a significant positive relation between the two (Andrews, 1986; Diener, 1984; Easterlin, 1974). This suggests that the increase in material goods per person brought about by higher income leads, on average, to feelings of enhanced well-being. Over the life cycle income typically increases up to retirement; hence, the question arises whether there occurs a growth in subjective well-being like that in the cross-sectional relation. The purpose of this article is to investigate this question using cohort data on income and happiness.

One indication that the issue is not an open-and-shut one comes from studies of the happiness-income relation at the national level (Easterlin, 1995). Among countries at a point in time income and happiness are positively related, as in the cross-sectional relation within countries. However, within a country over time, happiness remains constant despite a marked up-trend in income. Thus the movement over time contradicts the association expected on the basis of cross-sectional data. Could this be true here—might happiness remain constant over the life cycle while income

The authors are grateful to Donna H. Ebata for excellent assistance and to the Andrew W. Mellon Foundation and the University of Southern California for financial support.

rises, in contradiction to the point-of-time relationship between happiness and income?

In what follows, we start with a discussion of economic theory, focusing on the micro-level foundations of the macro-level link between income and subjective well-being over the life cycle. Clearly, many other factors, such as health and family circumstances, affect subjective well-being also; the focus in the theoretical discussion here on the bivariate relation between income and subjective well-being is in accordance with the concerns of the empirical analysis. The chapter then turns to the empirical analysis proper, discussing first the concepts and data, and then the findings. As will be seen, there is the same type of contradictory outcome as is found in studies at the national level—over the life cycle, happiness does not grow as income increases, even though the point-of-time relationship between income and happiness is positive. The theoretical underpinning of this paradoxical result is the subject of the concluding section. It will be seen that a macro-micro link neglected in traditional economic theory is the key to the paradox; this link is the effect of the growth in society's income on the material norms of the individual. Thus, this paper provides a first-hand illustration from economics of macro-micro relationships of the type currently of interest in sociology and psychology (Marshall, 1993; Ryff, 1987).

THEORY

In economic theory, expectations about the macro-level relationship between income and subjective well-being are usually founded on the standard micro-level theory of subjective utility. An individual is assumed to have a set of indifference curves, I_1, I_2, , I_3, ..I_n, representing his or her subjective desires for two goods, X and Y, taken, for simplicity, to be the only two goods available (Figure 10.1). Any given indifference curve represents combinations of X and Y that yield the same subjective satisfaction; hence, these are combinations with regard to which the individual feels indifferent. As one moves outward from the origin on a ray, say OZ, an individual moves to indifference curves representing progressively higher levels of subjective well-being, because the amount of both X and Y increases.

The map of indifference curves represents a person's subjective state of mind—to what extent different combinations of X and Y yield the same

satisfaction, and how increases in both X and Y enhance subjective satisfaction. Enter, now, the "social-structural" constraints, established by market conditions. At any given time, the individual has a given amount of
income and is confronted with certain prices for the goods X and Y. The
outer limit of the possible combinations of X and Y that can be purchased
if all income is spent on X and Y is designated the "budget constraint," B_1
(Figure 10.1). The budget constraint thus delimits all combinations of X
and Y that are within reach of the individual (those on or to the left of B_1)
from those beyond the individual's reach (those to the right of B_1).

Given one's subjective preferences and the structural constraint, how
much X and Y would actually be chosen, if satisfaction is to be maximized?
The answer is given by the outermost indifference curve that is just tangent
to the budget constraint, I_2 (Figure 10.1). The tangency shows that particular consumption package (X_1, Y_1) that puts the individual on the highest
indifference curve, and thus yields the maximum possible subjective satisfaction under the externally imposed constraints of income and prices.

What will happen if income increases? The budget constraint shifts outward, say, from B_1 to B_2, indicating that the individual is able to purchase
more of both X and Y at their given prices. A new tangency with a higher
indifference curve comes within reach, and the individual moves along the
ray OZ to a new point (X_2, Y_2) consuming greater amounts of both X and
Y (Figure 10.1). Thus, according to this micro-level theory, higher income
brings about increased subjective well-being by enabling the individual to
obtain a consumption set on a higher indifference curve.

The relationship between subjective well-being and income in this
analysis can be made explicit. Imagine a third dimension in Figure 10.1
that measures the level of subjective well-being corresponding to each
indifference curve. As income increases from B_1 to B_2, one moves to a
higher indifference curve and enjoys greater subjective well-being. This is
shown by the positively sloped line cd in Figure 10.2, representing the
direct relation between income and subjective well-being.

Some economists prefer not to theorize about subjective states of mind,
as in the above, and to deal only with observed behavior. As a result, the
above analysis is sometimes replaced by what is called the theory of
revealed preference (for an excellent review of the history of utility and
revealed preference theory in economics in this century, see Lewin, 1996).
Here, the argument becomes even simpler. If an individual is observed to
buy combination X_2, Y_2 when X_1, Y_1 is also affordable at the given income
(B_2) and prices, then (based on certain axioms) the individual is deemed to
prefer X_2, Y_2 to X_1, Y_1, and hence, to be better off (Figure 10.3).

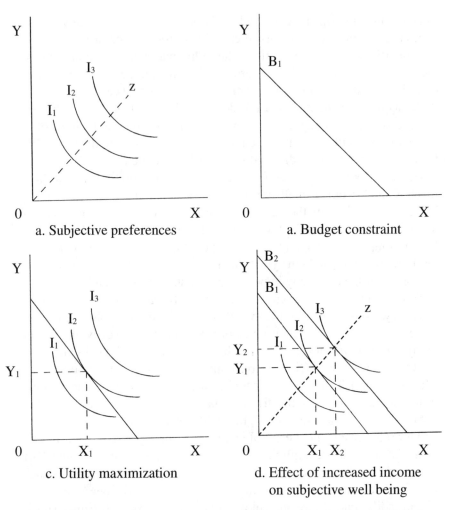

a. Subjective preferences

a. Budget constraint

c. Utility maximization

d. Effect of increased income
on subjective well being

Figure 10.1 Standard micro economic theory of subjective well-being.

One problem with this approach is that the judgment on a person's well-being is made, not by the person himself, but by an outsider who is observing the person's consumption choices. Thus, the theory of revealed preferences lends itself to a paternalistic regime, where, for example, the government sets itself up as the arbiter of individual well-being based on observed consumption behavior (Hollander, 1996). For those economists who believe that the only one who can make authoritative observations on a person's subjective well-being is the person himself, standard utility theory is superior to the theory of revealed preference.

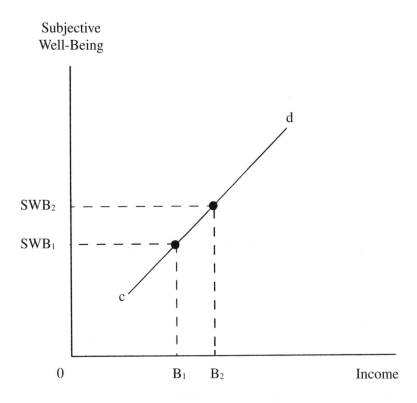

Figure 10.2 Income and subjective well-being in standard micro economic theory of subjective well-being.

Both theories, it should be noted, provide a micro-level foundation for the conclusion that an increase in the income of society as a whole would lead, other things constant, to greater well-being. Economists recognize, of course, that other things may not be constant, and that welfare depends not on material conditions alone (the quantities of X and Y obtainable), but on a variety of circumstances—family life, health, and so forth. However, if income growth is substantial, there is a presumption that for a group of persons, these other factors will tend to cancel out, yielding, on balance, a higher average level of subjective well-being (Abramovitz, 1959). At the rate of income growth typical of a modern society, real income will typically double over the working life span, yielding a material level of living at age 60 twice that at age 25. Based

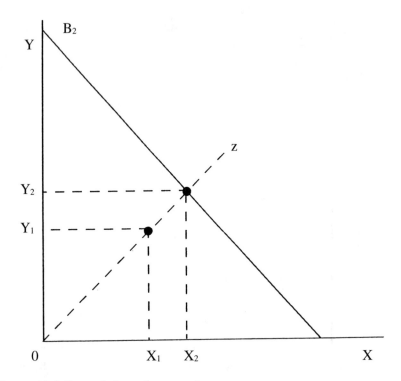

Figure 10.3 Revealed preference theory.

on economic theory, one might well expect that subjective well-being would also rise over the life cycle.

What of the empirical implementation of this theory? Is it, in fact, the case that growth in income over the life cycle brings with it greater subjective well-being? To this question, economics resolutely turns its back, falling back on the disciplinary paradigm of behavioral positivism. Subjective testimony on well-being is ruled out. A forthright statement of this methodological position, directed to noneconomists, is given by Victor Fuchs (1983, p. 14): "Economists, as a rule, are not concerned with the internal thought processes of the decision maker or in the rationalizations that the decision maker offers to explain his or her behavior. Economists believe that what people *do* is more relevant than what they say."

Do not think that economists are apologetic about this; on the contrary, they are quite militant. Here is a critic of the dominant positivist school, economist Donald McCloskey:

Unlike other social scientists, economists are extremely hostile toward questionnaires and other self-descriptions. . . . One can literally get an audience of economists to laugh out loud by proposing ironically to send out a questionnaire on some disputed economic point. Economists . . . are unthinkingly committed to the notion that only the externally observable behavior of actors is admissible evidence in arguments concerning economics. (1983, p. 514)

Empirically, then, the relation between income and subjective well-being is ruled by economics a non-issue, thanks to the disciplinary paradigm. This explains why in a survey by Diener (1984) of well over 200 studies on the measurement and determinants of subjective well-being, only two references appear to articles in economics journals. Although theorizing in economics is replete with statements relating to subjective perceptions and feelings—expectations, values, well-being—it is as if there are no data relating to these circumstances. Behavioral positivism in economics, in effect, builds a Berlin Wall that cuts off the work on these subjects by psychologists and sociologists.

There are, of course, a few who would breach this wall, and the present chapter is offered in this vein. We bring together here aggregative data on income and subjective well-being as cohorts pass through the life cycle, to ask whether the micro-level presumption of economic theory of a positive relationship between income and happiness is supported by the evidence.

PRIOR WORK

Even outside of economics, surprisingly little has been done to address this question. Although there is a voluminous literature on subjective well-being (Diener, 1984; Veenhoven, 1993), the question of the life cycle change in well-being, with or without reference to income, has been largely untouched. There are a few studies focussing on the retirement years which typically find little trend in subjective well-being (Palmore 1981). However, in the retirement years, income is declining or, at best, stable. One study that covered the full life cycle, using cohort data like that used here, reached inconclusive results, perhaps because of data incomparabilities and a small number of observations (Rodgers, 1982).

Life cycle patterns are sometimes inferred from cross-sectional data classified by age. However, studies of the point-of-time relation between happiness and age yield mixed results. Based on a survey of the literature, Linda George (1992) reports that before the 1970s older persons are less happy than younger; since then, they are happier. Subsequently, we shall return to this and other findings reported in George's valuable survey.

CONCEPTS, METHODS, AND DATA

Subjective well-being is measured here using happiness data obtained in response to the following survey question: "Taken all together, how would you say things are these days—would you say that you are very happy, pretty happy, or not too happy?" This question was asked in the General Social Survey in every year between 1972 and 1993, except 1979, 1981, and 1992.

Using such self-reports to measure happiness raises the question of comparability—if each individual has his own definition of happiness, how can happiness be compared? The essence of the answer is this: in most people's lives the dominant concerns are making a living, family life, and health, and it is these concerns that respondents chiefly report when asked what determines their happiness (Cantril, 1965; Herzog, Rodgers, & Woodworth, 1982). This is not to say that the happiness of any one individual can be directly compared with that of another, or that all individuals have identical concerns. But if one is interested in the happiness of a sizeable group of people, there turns out to be a marked similarity in what most people mention when asked about the meaning of happiness. In effect, though each individual is free to define happiness in their own terms, in practice, the kinds of things chiefly cited as shaping happiness are, for groups of people, much the same.

The preeminence in determining subjective well-being of personal economic, family, and health concerns no doubt reflects the fact that it is these matters that take up most of the time of adults at all stages of the life cycle. There is, however, some variation by age in the relative importance of these concerns. Health is relatively more important to older adults and family relationships to younger. But economic concerns are of high importance at all ages (Herzog et al., 1982).

In addition to the question of the comparability of happiness, there are other measurement issues. These relate to matters such as the reliability and validity of the replies, whether respondents are likely to report their true feelings, and possible biases resulting from the context in which the happiness question is asked. These issues have been subjected to close scrutiny in the scholarly literature, and will not be gone over here (Diener, 1984; Easterlin, 1974; Veenhoven, 1993). For our purpose, the relevant conclusion of such assessments is that measures of the type used here, though not perfect, do have substantive meaning as regards the relation between subjective well-being and income.

A birth cohort is a group of individuals born in a given year or period. Thus, the birth cohort of 1935–1939 comprises all persons born in those years. The membership of a cohort changes somewhat over the cohort's life cycle as a result of mortality and international migration, but not very greatly. We construct the life cycle experience of a birth cohort by linking appropriate age data for successive years. Thus to trace the life cycle pattern of subjective well-being of the cohort born between 1935 and 1939, we link the average happiness of those ages 33–37 in 1972 to that of those ages 34–38 in 1973, 35–39 in 1974, and so on. For comparison with the income data, which are available for years ending in 4 and 9, we compute 5-year averages of the cohort's reported happiness centered on the years ending in 4 and 9.

The happiness data span a 21-year period; hence, at best, we are able to follow any given birth cohort for only a 21-year segment of its life cycle. But since we have cohorts starting at younger, middle, and older ages, it is possible to form a reasonable impression of the pattern over the entire adult life cycle. For some cohorts the data span a smaller segment of the life cycle. The present analysis is restricted to cohorts for which data are available for at least 13 years.

Turning to the income measure, individual economic status is measured by the total money income per adult equivalent in the household in which each individual resides. The definition of income is that of the Bureau of Census' Current Population Survey—pre-tax, post-transfer money income, including public and private pension income, public assistance, other welfare payments, and alimony and child support payments. Money earnings are by far the dominant income source; income in kind is not included in the Census Bureau's survey. The money income data are adjusted for price level change from year to year.

Income per adult equivalent is computed for each household by dividing the household's total money income by the number of adult equivalents in the household. Following Fuchs (1986), the number of adult equivalents in a household is obtained by giving the first adult a value of 1.0 and all subsequent adults a value of 0.8, the first child a value of 0.4 and all others, 0.3. It would, of course, be easier to divide total household income simply by the number of persons in the household. The aim of the conversion to a per-adult equivalent basis is to obtain a better measure of differences in economic status among persons by allowing for variations among households in their size and composition, and for economies of scale in consumption. It would clearly be misleading to assume that the members of a household with a total money income of $40,000 are twice as well off in economic terms as those of a household with a total income of $20,000, if, in fact, there were twice as many persons in the former household. Conversion of household income to a simple per capita basis, by dividing total income by the number of persons per household (in effect, giving each person an adult equivalent value of one), would be similarly misleading if the proportion of adults to children differed, say, between households of the same size. This is because the economic needs or requirements of children are, on average, substantially less than those of adults. Hence there is need to take account of differences among households in both their size and adult-child composition. It is also desirable to take account of what are called "economies of scale" in consumption—the economic needs of two adults living together in one household are not as great as those of two adults, each living alone in his or her own household. The purpose of the adult equivalence scale used here is to allow in an approximate way for all of these considerations.

Every member of a given household is assigned the income per adult equivalent (IAE) of the household. The economic status of an individual is thus assumed to correspond to the average economic status of the household in which the individual resides. This is analogous to the assumption in governmental estimates of the poverty rates of persons, that an individual is in poverty if the family of which one is a member is so classified. Clearly, the allocation of income among persons within a household need not be equal, but research on intra-household income distribution has only recently begun. The economic status of a cohort at any given date is measured by averaging the income per adult equivalent of all members of the cohort.

The income data used here are from the data tapes for quinquennial years 1965 through 1990 underlying the published reports from the annual March Current Population Survey (United States Bureau of the Census, 1965–). Demographic status is measured as of March of the survey year. The reports of income refer to the previous calendar year, that is, years ending in 4 and 9. The life cycle income profile of a cohort is obtained by linking income averages for appropriate age groups from successive surveys, in the same way as for the happiness data.

RESULTS

Although there are some fluctuations in the data, the main conclusion is quite clear. On average, happiness tends to be remarkably stable over the entire course of the life cycle (Figure 10.4). At the individual level there may be trends up or down, but for the cohort as a whole, happiness tends to be constant. Economic well-being, by contrast, increases to around ages 55 to 60 and then levels off. For both happiness and economic well-being, every cohort exhibits the same pattern of change in that segment of the life cycle for which data are available. Taking all cohorts together, it appears that while a cohort manifests substantial improvement in material living level up to the retirement ages, there is no corresponding advance in subjective well-being. Nor does the leveling off of income in the retirement years appear to be accompanied by any change in average happiness. Indeed, as other studies have reported, cohort happiness continues to be remarkably stable throughout the retirement ages, despite an increased incidence of ill-health and widowhood.

The lack of a life cycle trend in happiness is supported more formally by a regression for each cohort of happiness on age (Table 10.1). Of 12 cohorts for which at least 13 annual observations are available, there is none with a statistically significant slope. Nine of the 12 cohorts have a negative regression coefficient, but none of the coefficients is significant.

There is also some suggestion in the data that the average level of happiness has decreased over time from one cohort to another, despite the fact that more recent cohorts have higher average income. This can be seen by grouping the life cycle income curves for all cohorts (Figure 10.5, top panel) and the life cycle happiness curves for all cohorts (Figure 10.5, bottom panel). In the case of income, at any given age, younger cohorts have more income than older without exception. In the case of happiness, the pattern is more mixed, but there appears to be a drift in the opposite direction—younger cohorts tending to be less happy than older. This is brought out better if the happiness curves of Figure 10.5 are replaced by regression lines based on the regressions of happiness on age for each cohort reported in Table 10.1. As Figure 10.6 shows, for more recent birth cohorts, the average level of the line is usually lower.

The result of the stable within-cohort trend in happiness and the decline in the average level of happiness from earlier to more recent cohorts is that cross-sectional comparisons of happiness and age for a given year tend to be positive, thus giving a misleading impression of the life cycle variation

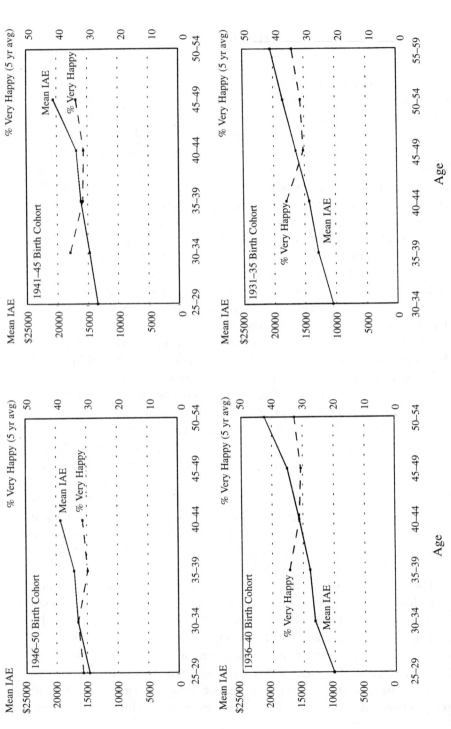

Figure 10.4 Happiness and income (in 1989 dollars) at specified ages in the life cycle for each birth cohort, 1991-95 to 1946-50

Figure 10.4 (continued)

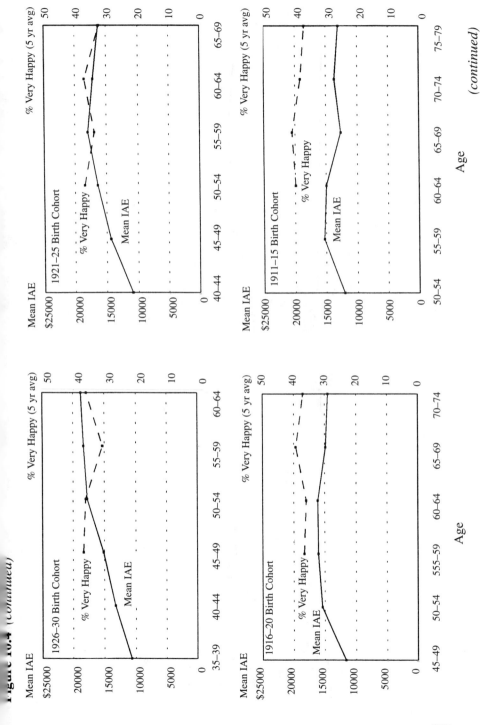

(continued)

Figure 10.4 (*continued*)

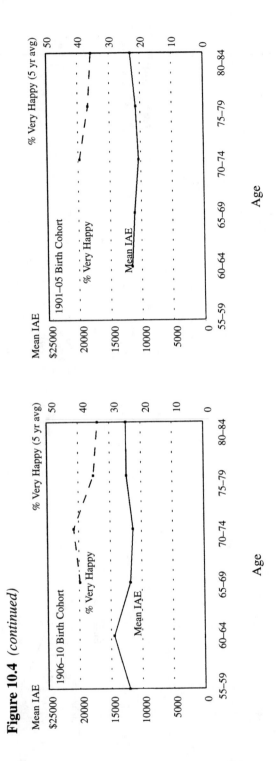

Table 10.1 Regression Statistics for Each Birth Cohort, 1901–05 to 1956–60

Birth cohort	From Regression of Percent Very Happy on Age			
	Constant term	Slope coefficient[a]	Adjusted R^2	Number of observations
1901–05	63.8	−.345	.010	14
1906–10	56.1	−.264	.026	19
1911–15	45.7	−.101	−.040	19
1916–20	36.9	−.008	−.059	19
1921–25	38.6	−.059	−.053	19
1926–30	42.2	−.140	.011	19
1931–35	40.1	−.144	−.004	19
1936–40	29.8	.062	−.049	19
1941–45	41.2	−.205	.044	19
1946–50	31.5	−.025	−.056	19
1951–55	20.1	.264	.154	18
1956–60	21.0	.334	.154	13

[a] No coefficient is significant at $p = .05$ or less.

in happiness. The results of regressing happiness on age in each year are shown in Table 10.2. Of 19 regressions, 17 have a positive slope coefficient, and seven of these are significant. This positive cross-sectional relationship is a product of the flat life cycle cohort profiles coupled with the drift toward lower average happiness for more recent birth cohorts. We have here a good example of how misleading it can be to infer life cycle patterns from cross-sectional age data.

THEORY REVISITED

To judge from the evidence, within a society at a given time, income and subjective well-being are positively related. Yet as a cohort's income increases during the life cycle, subjective well-being remains unchanged. How can one explain this paradoxical relationship?

The answer is given by adding a new macro-micro link to the standard economic theory of utility given earlier, one that connects society's level of income to one's subjective well-being via material norms. A simple thought experiment may convey the basic reasoning. Imagine that your income increases substantially while everyone else's stays the same.

Mean Income per Adult Equivalent (dollars of 1989 purchasing power)

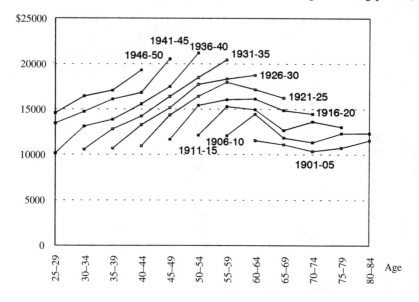

Percent Very Happy (five year average)

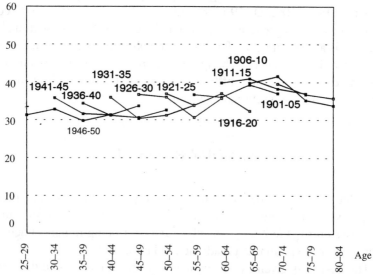

Figure 10.5 Life cycle profiles of income and happiness, birth cohorts 1901–05 to 1946–50.

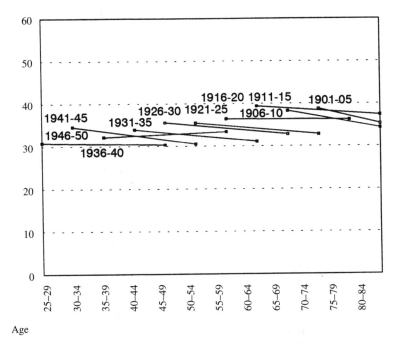

% Very Happy

Age

Figure 10.6 Regression lines of percent very happy against age, birth cohorts, 1901–05 to 1946–50.

Would you feel better off? The answer most people would give is "yes." Now suppose that your income stays the same while everyone else's increases substantially. How would you feel? Most people would say that they feel less well off. This is because judgments of personal well-being are made by comparing one's objective status with a subjective living level norm, which is significantly influenced by the average level of living of others in the society. If living levels increase generally, subjective living level norms rise. The individual whose income is unchanged will feel poorer, even though his or her objective circumstances are the same as before. Karl Marx put it this way:

> A house may be large or small; as long as the neighboring houses are likewise small it satisfies all social requirements for a residence. But let there arise next to the little house a palace, and the little house shrinks into a hut. . . . Our wants and pleasures have their origins in society. . . . Since they are of a social nature, they are of a relative nature" (Marx, 1849/1976, p. 33).

Table 10.2 Regression Statistics for Specified Year, 1972–1993

	From Regression of Percent Very Happy on Age			
Specified year	Constant term	Slope coefficient	Adjusted R^2	Number of observations
1972	29.2	.190	−.072	15
1973	32.8	.051	−.064	15
1974	25.8	.266*	.372	15
1975	23.7	.200	.131	15
1976	35.5	−.029	−.068	15
1977	27.9	.143*	.284	15
1978	32.2	.039	−.012	15
1980	26.3	.159	.150	15
1982	18.1	.270*	.374	15
1983	25.5	.123	.161	15
1984	18.9	.357*	.711	15
1985	24.2	.093	.197	15
1986	25.0	.152*	.226	15
1987	19.9	.203*	.533	15
1988	30.3	.079	.176	15
1989	32.7	.003	−.077	15
1990	36.3	−.071	−.023	15
1991	27.8	.070	.014	15
1993	22.3	.207*	.378	15

* $p = .05$ or less.

Put generally, happiness, or subjective well-being, varies directly with one's own income and inversely with the incomes of others. Raising the incomes of all does not increase the happiness of all, because the positive effect of one's own higher income on subjective well-being is offset by the negative effect of a higher living level norm brought about by the growth in society's income generally. Evidence that norms grow with society's income level is provided by Rainwater's (1990) finding that the income perceived as "necessary to get along" rose between 1950 and 1986 in the same proportion as actual per capita income.

These micro-level relationships can be represented graphically as follows. At any given time society's level of income (gdp_1) is given, and one's perception of subjective well-being varies directly with one's own income. This is the relationship expounded in the traditional economic theory of subjective well-being (Figure 10.2 above). It is shown in Figure

10.7 by the positively sloped curve, cd, relating subjective well-being to one's own income, with society's income (gdp₁) fixed. Now consider the effect on one's feelings of subjective well-being if one's own income remains fixed, but society's income increases to gdp₂. The increase in society's income raises the material norm by which well-being is judged, and causes the subjective well-being associated with any given amount of one's own income to diminish. This is shown graphically by the downward shift from cd to ef of the curve relating subjective well-being to one's own income.

The feedback from society's income level to one's subjective living level norm is the new macro-micro link that resolves the cross-sectional life cycle paradox. Consider an individual initially at the societal average whose income grows at the same rate over his or her life cycle as that of society as a whole. At any given time, he or she perceives their higher

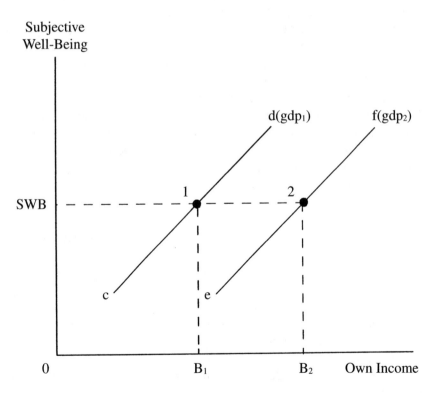

Figure 10.7 Income and subjective well-being in the relative income theory of subjective well-being.

income as bringing more well-being, because society's income and thus material norms are fixed. This is the cross-sectional relationship represented by cd, and observed in point-of-time data. But as his or her income grows over the life cycle at the same rate as society's income, the cd curve shifts downward toward ef, and the path of subjective well-being actually experienced is the horizontal one, represented in the graph by the points 1, 2. This is the life cycle pattern shown by our cohort data here.

There are models in economic theory yielding similar conclusions, although these models lie outside the mainstream (Duesenberry, 1949; Pollak, 1976). These models incorporate relativistic concepts like those stemming from the work in sociology of Durkheim (1951) and Merton (1968) on anomie and related topics, and in social psychology of Stouffer (1949) and Festinger (1957) on relative deprivation and cognitive dissonance.

In these non-mainstream economic models, the subjective well-being associated with one's preferences is not fixed over the course of the life cycle. Rather, as income and expenditure in one's reference group increase, so too do material norms. Because of this increase in norms as reference group income increases, the subjective utility yielded by a fixed amount of a person's own income declines, and an increase in personal income matching that of one's reference group is necessary simply to maintain subjective well-being at a constant level. This reasoning implies that if one's own income and that of one's reference group both increase in the same proportion over the life cycle, subjective well-being will be constant. Similarly, in the retirement years, if both reference group income and one's own income change in the same proportion, subjective well-being would remain unchanged. For elderly people the importance of such interpersonal comparisons in determining life satisfaction has been demonstrated by Liang and Fairchild (1979), Liang, Kahana, and Doherty (1980), and Usui, Keil, and Durig (1985).

Both the mainstream and non-mainstream economic theories expounded here have their counterparts in social-psychological theories of status attainment and status maintenance. If material norms are fixed, then greater economic achievement (higher income) will mean higher status attainment and greater subjective well-being. If, however, material norms rise in the same proportion as economic achievement, then status attainment, subjectively considered, remains constant, and so does subjective well-being.

In a valuable article Linda George (1992) suggests that concern with status attainment may determine subjective well-being prior to the retirement years, while status maintenance comes to the fore in retirement. However, in a model in which material norms rise up to retirement and then level off or decline (because of corresponding movements in the status of one's reference group) this distinction disappears. Adults of all ages aspire to achieve income levels that equal or exceed their norms. Status maintenance is simply that case of status attainment in which achievements just match norms. In fact, status maintenance turns out to be the nature of reality, on average, over the entire adult life cycle including both working and retirement years.

The interpretation given here of the stability in happiness over the life cycle is consistent with the conclusion of Myers and Diener (1995) that a key component of any theory of happiness is values and goals. They cite the findings of Emmons (1986) "that having goals, making progress toward goals, and freedom from conflict among one's goals" were all predictors of subjective well-being (Myers & Diener, 1995, p. 17). As was noted earlier, material concerns are typically those cited most frequently by people everywhere when asked about the factors influencing their happiness. Increased income as one moves through the life cycle means progress toward attainment of material goals. If goals were to remain fixed, happiness would grow. But since the material goals themselves increase as a function of the general growth in incomes, the positive effect on happiness of an increase in one's income is counterbalanced by the negative effect of ever-rising goals. The result is that, on balance, there is no change in subjective happiness over the life cycle, despite substantial growth in income and objective living level.

SUMMARY AND IMPLICATIONS

On average, the material living level of a cohort, as measured by its income, increases over the life cycle up to the retirement years, after which it levels off or declines. Subjective well-being, however, tends to remain constant throughout the entire course of the life cycle. This is because the change in income is, on average, matched by a corresponding change in material norms. As incomes increase generally, so too do material norms. This macro-micro feedback from the income of others to subjective norms is the key to understanding the seeming contradiction between the positive relation between income and subjective well-being in point-of-time data and the absence of such a relationship in cohort life cycle data. It is supported by research in sociology and psychology, as well as by non-mainstream work in economics.

In the body of data studied here, covering the period since 1972, there has also been a downward drift in the average level of happiness from earlier to more recent cohorts. Taken together with the flat life-cycle profile of happiness, this downward drift in average level has generated a positive cross-sectional association between happiness and age at a point in time. This positive cross-sectional relation of happiness and age gives a misleading impression of how happiness changes over the life cycle.

The downward drift in happiness from one cohort to the next and positive point-of-time relation of happiness to age should not be assumed to persist into the future. Cross-sectional studies based on data from dates earlier than those covered here typically found an inverse rather than positive association of happiness with age, implying that younger cohorts were, on average, happier than older (George, 1992). Thus, a combination of constant within-cohort trends in happiness and varying differences in the average level of happiness among cohorts may yield changing cross-sectional relations between happiness and age—positive at one time, negative or no association at another.

The present conclusions are based on bivariate analysis of a limited body of data, and there are ample opportunities for further research. There is need, for example, to incorporate other sources of happiness in the analysis, such as changing family circumstances and health. Direct evidence such as that in Rainwater (1990) on the life cycle change in material norms is also needed, along with investigation of the mechanisms shaping norms. Also, the present analysis is based on data for the noninstitutionalized population, and it would be of interest to see whether the addition of the institutional population would alter the results for those in the retirement ages as the proportion institutionalized increases. Finally, there is the need to explain why more recent cohorts have typically started with lower levels of happiness.

REFERENCES

Abramovitz, Moses (1959). The Welfare Interpretation of Secular Trends in National Income and Product. In Moses Abramovitz, Armen Alchian, Kenneth J. Arrow, Paul A. Baran, Philip W. Cartwright, Hollis B. Chenery, George W. Hilton, H. S. Houthakker, Charles E. Lindblom, Melvin W. Reder,

Tibor Scitovsky, E. S. Shaw, Lorie Tarshis, *The allocation of economic resources: Essays in honor of Bernard Francis Haley* (pp. 1–22). Stanford, CA: Stanford University Press.

Andrews, F. M. (Ed.) (1986). *Research on the quality of life.* Ann Arbor, MI: Survey Research Center, Institute for Social Research, University of Michigan.

Cantril, H. (1965). *The pattern of human concerns.* New Brunswick, NJ: Rutgers University Press.

Diener, E. (1984). Subjective well-being. *Psychological Bulletin, 95,* 542–575.

Duesenberry, J. S. (1949). *Income, savings, and the theory of consumer behavior.* Cambridge, MA: Harvard University Press

Durkheim, E. (1951). *Suicide, A study in sociology.* New York: Free Press.

Easterlin, R. A. (1974). Does economic growth improve the human lot? In P. A. David & M. W. Reder (Eds.), *Nations and households in economic growth: Essays in Honor of Moses Abramovitz* (pp. 89–125). New York: Academic Press.

Easterlin, R. A. (1995). Will raising the incomes of all increase the happiness of all? *Journal of Economic Behavior and Organization, 27,* 35–48.

Emmons, R. A. (1986). Personal strivings: An approach to personality and subjective well-being. *Journal of Personality and Social Psychology, 51,* 1058–1068.

Festinger, L. (1957). *A theory of cognitive dissonance.* Evanston, IL: Row, Peterson.

Fuchs, V. (1983). *How we live.* Cambridge, MA: Harvard University Press.

Fuchs, V. (1986). Sex differences in economic well-being. *Science, 232,* 459–464.

George, L. K. (1992). Economic status and subjective well-being: A review of the literature and an agenda for future research. In N. E. Cutler, D. W. Grigg, & M. Powell Lawton (Eds.), *Aging, money, and life satisfaction: Aspects of financial gerontology* (pp. 69–99). New York: Springer Publishing Company.

Herzog, A. R., Rodgers, W. L., & Woodworth, J. (1982). *Subjective well-being among different age groups.* Ann Arbor, MI: Institute for Social Research, University of Michigan.

Hollander, H. (1996). *On the validity of utility statements: Standard theory versus Duesenberry's.* Unpublished paper, Universität Dortmund, Dortmund, Germany.

Lewin, S. (1996). Economics and psychology: Lessons for our own day from the early twentieth century. *Journal of Economic Literature, 34,* 1293–1323.

Liang, J., & Fairchild, T. J. (1979). Relative deprivation and perception of financial adequacy among the aged. *Journal of Gerontology, 34,* 746–759.

Liang, J., Kahana, E., & Doherty, E. (1980). Financial well-being among the aged: A further elaboration. *Journal of Gerontology, 35,* 409–420.

McCloskey, D. N. (1983). The rhetoric of economics. *Journal of Economic Literature, 21,* 481–517.

Marshall, V. (1993). *The micro-macro link in the sociology of aging.* Paper presented at the Images of Aging II Conference, Sierre, Switzerland.

Marx, K. (1976). Wage-labour and capital. In K. Marx (Ed.), *Wage-labour and capital and value, price, and profit* (pp. 5–48). New York: International Publications. (Originally published 1849).

Merton, R. K. (1968). *Social theory and social structure.* New York: The Free Press.

Myers, D. G. & Diener, E. (1995). Who is happy? *Psychological Science, 6,* 10–19.

Palmore, E. B. (1981). *Social patterns in normal aging.* Durham, NC: Duke University Press.

Pollak, R. A. (1976). Interdependent preferences. *American Economic Review,* 66, 309–320.

Rainwater, L. (1990, October). *Poverty and equivalence as social constructions.* (Luxembourg Income Study Working Paper 55). Paper presented at the Seminar on Families and Living: Observations and Analysis, European Association for Population Studies, Barcelona.

Rodgers, W. (1982). Trends in reported happiness within demographically defined subgroups, 1957–78. *Social Forces,* 60, 826–842.

Ryff, C. D. (1987). The place of personality and social structure research in social psychology. *Journal of Personality and Social Psychology,* 53, 1192–1202.

Stouffer, S. A., Suchman, E. A., DeVinney, L. C., Star, S. A., & Williams, R. M. Jr., (1949). *The American soldier: Adjustment during wartime life* (Vol. 1). Princeton, NJ: Princeton University Press.

United States Bureau of the Census, 1965–(annually). *Current Population Reports.* Series P-20, Population Characteristics, and Series P-60, Consumer Income.

Usui, W. M., Keil, T. J., & Durig, K. R. (1985). Socioeconomic comparisons and life satisfaction of elderly adults. *Journal of Gerontology,* 40, 110–114.

Veenhoven, R. (1993). *Happiness in nations, subjective appreciation of life in 56 nations 1946–1992.* Rotterdam, Netherlands: Erasmus University.

PART 3

Contexts of Self and Society: Work and Family

Structure and Agency in the Retirement Process: A Case Study of Montreal Garment Workers

Julie A. McMullin & Victor W. Marshall

INTRODUCTION

In Canada, public pension eligibility rules have constructed age 65 as the marker that defines the "normal" age of retirement (Marshall, 1995b). Yet, the average retirement age in Canada is 62 (Lowe, 1992). The contradiction between the "normal" retirement age and work exit practices points to the complexities of retirement processes and suggests that, while retirement is framed within the context of the power and control held by

This chapter draws on a case study by the Issues of an Aging Workforce Project, Institute for Human Development, Life Course and Aging, University of Toronto, funded by the Innovations Fund of Human Resources Development Canada to V. W. Marshall, Principal Investigator. The case study received cooperative support from the International Ladies' Garment Workers' Union (now, UNITE), Mr G. Roy, Canadian Director, and the Québec Fashion Apparel Manufacturer's Guild, Mr S. Purcell, Executive Director. Our appreciation also to J. Wineman, Director, Retiree Services Department of UNITE, and to the garment workers, company owners and union officials in Montreal who took part in the study. The research team included J. Edwardh, A. Ford and S. LeBlanc, as well as McMullin and Marshall.

governments, employers, and unions, it also falls within the realm of individual agency.

Historically the study of retirement focussed on individual level characteristics and the subjective experience of retirement among men (Palmore, Burchett, Fillenbaum, George, & Wallman, 1985). Recognizing the neglect of issues relating to social structure in this literature, researchers have attempted to integrate structural and individual level characteristics in assessments of "on-time" and early retirement (McDonald, 1996). Yet, missing from recent accounts of retirement are the assessments of meaning and subjective experience that were common in the early work. Although we know that individual level characteristics and social-structural characteristics both play a role in determining retirement outcomes, we know little about how workers make retirement timing decisions or what their subjective views of these decisions are. We know little of how human agency—the way in which individuals interpret and act within their worlds—interacts with the social structure in framing retirement processes.

We begin this chapter by discussing what is meant by social structure among age stratification and political economy researchers. We then explore some of the ways in which human agency has been handled in aging research. From there we turn to a theoretical discussion of the intersection of human agency and social structure by examining the work of Berger and Luckmann (1966) and Giddens (1979). In our analysis we explore how the institution of retirement is established by a dialectic between agency and structure at the industrial and state levels. We then examine how the views of retirement held by employed, displaced, and retired garment workers in Montreal are shaped by the structural circumstances of their work and in turn, how these views serve to reproduce the structure of retirement itself. In particular, we are interested in retirement timing and the relationship between job exit and financial circumstances.

SOCIAL STRUCTURE IN AGING RESEARCH

When researchers discuss social structure, they are generally referring to the enduring, orderly, and patterned relationships among the elements of society. Yet, there is considerable disagreement over what the key elements of society are and how these elements are related; and there is additional disagreement as to the extent, if any, to which analyses of social structure can be related to analyses of the individual (Layder, 1994). To illustrate, in the following paragraphs we discuss what is meant by social structure in two well established theoretical traditions in gerontology—the age stratification and political economy perspectives; and we then turn in the following section to consider the individual.

The development of a formal statement of the age stratification perspective was foreshadowed in the late 1950s and early 1960s by Leonard Cain (1959, Marshall, 1995c), but Matilda White Riley and her colleagues are responsible for the formalization and subsequent elaborations of the theory. Notably, Riley now refers to her work as "the aging and society paradigm", which reflects her concerns about the overly static nature of the term stratification (Riley, 1994).

Riley and her colleagues conceptualize age as both a process and a structure. At the structural level, similar aged individuals form strata that may be defined on the basis of either chronological age or biological, psychological, or social stages of development (Riley, Johnson, and Foner, 1972). Age strata differ from one another in size and composition as well as the relative contributions that each makes to society. Age is also established in the social structure as a "criterion for entering or relinquishing certain roles" (Riley et al., 1972, p. 7), and thus is used as a marker through which age-appropriate behavior is gauged.

Riley and her colleagues refer to structure in a structural-functionalist way. According to this perspective, society is the all-encompassing social structure that may be decomposed into several specialized structures. Examples of these are the economic, the political, and the educational structures of society. From this point of view, the elements of social structures include social institutions (work organizations, political institutions), and patterns of social roles (Grabb, 1990; Parsons, 1951). Roles are the building blocks of institutions that are, in turn, the building blocks of society (Riley et al., 1972). Role is the concept in this theoretical apparatus that makes a place for the individual, and role occupancy is the means of integration of the individual and society. The individual in this construal disappears, being viewed solely as role occupant or as a bundle of roles (the sense in which this is so is our major theme).

Hence, elements of the social structure are either viewed as social institutions (families, schools, work organizations, and nations) (Riley, 1994; Riley & Riley, 1994), or as patterns of social roles (Riley et al., 1972). People (population structure) and roles (role structure) are differentiated by an age structure (Riley et al., 1972), the elements of which include age strata, age-related acts, age structure of roles, and age-related expectations and sanctions. Age strata with their related roles, expectations, and sanctions are considered necessary to the functioning of society. However, this approach tends to assume that there is widespread agreement in a society as to the content of age roles, and to thereby neglect the conflict that may occur if normative age-based roles are violated.

Like other structural functionalist positions, this perspective stands in opposition to the idea, informed by Marxist sociology, that social relations are the fundamental elements of the social structure. This view of social structure is generally employed by political economy of aging researchers.

Political economy theorists seek to explain the relative situation of older individuals by focussing on the interrelationship between the economy, the polity, and the ideological structures that these systems of domination construct and reconstruct. Rather than explaining the problems that older people face as a result of their inability to adjust to retirement or aging (as indicated by adequate role performance in the role of retired person or old person), or to their naturally diminishing physical or mental capacities, political economists attribute the problems of older people to structural characteristics of the state, the economy, and to inequalities in the distribution and allocation of resources that these institutions create (Estes, 1979; Guillemard, 1983; Myles, 1989; Phillipson, 1982; Walker, 1981).

Crucial to the political economy of aging approach is the concept of social class. Like Marx (1867/1967), political economy of aging researchers place emphasis on the relations of production in their conceptualization of social class and specifically on the relations between those who own the means of production and those who do not (Guillemard, 1982, 1983; Myles, 1989; Phillipson, 1982; Walker, 1981). Thus, according to Guillemard (1982), "the traditional Marxist definition, which analyzes the class structure of the capitalist mode of production by basically contrasting the two antagonistic classes—capitalist and proletarian—must be upheld" (p. 228). Among political economy of aging researchers, this understanding of social class is generally enhanced by the work of more recent Marxist scholars like Poulantzas (1975) who stresses the effects of economic, political, and ideological structures in class relations, or Wright (1985), who places emphasis on the control as well as on the ownership of property and resources (see Estes, Swan, and Gerard, 1982; Guillemard, 1982; Walker, 1981).

Our view of structure lies closer to that of the political economy approach than the age stratification approach. In general, we view social relations as fundamental elements of the social structure that are charac-

terized by conflict rather than consensus. However, whereas political economy researchers place emphasis on class relations, in this chapter, we propose that age relations, class relations, gender relations, and ethnic
relations are all crucial elements of the social structure. The structural significance of these sets of relations refers to the manner in which they produce enduring, orderly, and patterned social systems. By taking this
approach we do not mean to imply that social roles, normative expectations, socialization processes, and role sanctions are unimportant. Rather,
we suggest three related things: first, that these dimensions of social life
are grounded in social relations that are characterized more by conflict
than by consensus; second, that, social structure does not stand outside of
the human, social behavior that produces it yet, it nevertheless takes on
properties that transcend the behavior of those who construct it; and third,
that while these properties of durability constrain and limit the agency of
the individual, they never do so completely. In critiquing structural-
functionalism, Dennis Wrong (1961) has referred to this as the "oversocialized conception of man in modern sociology" (p. 183). The problem in
political economy approaches has been more in simply ignoring the individual in focussing the analytical gaze on macro-level social structures.
Thus, we are arguing for a theoretical position in which the constraining
effects of social structure are recognized, but in which the freedom or
agency of the individual is simultaneously celebrated.

There is a notable lack of human action in each of the theories discussed above. This is not a problem if one adheres to the assumptions of
functionalist theory which suggest that properties and characteristics of
societies are entirely separate from, and the dominant influence over, individuals and their behavior (Durkheim, 1982; Parsons, 1951). Nor is it a
problem if the subject of theory becomes the place in the social hierarchy
that individuals occupy or the social relations that they bear, as is the case
in some branches of structuralism and Marxism (see Giddens, 1979).
However, the neglect of human action in conceptual development or theory does become a problem if one assumes, as in the symbolic interactionist and interpretive tradition (e.g., Goffman, 1959; Mead, 1934), that
social life is "an active accomplishment of purposive, knowledgeable
actors" (Giddens, 1979, p. 50). It is also a problem if there is a theoretical
emphasis on the integration of not just the macro and micro levels of
analysis (for this can be done in many ways that do not necessarily recognize either human agency or the role of such agency in creating structure),
but an emphasis on the linking of structure and agency (Berger & Luckmann,
1966; Giddens, 1979; Layder, 1994).

HUMAN AGENCY IN AGING RESEARCH

The French sociologist Alaine Touraine (1988) draws on both Weber and Marx in his analyses of social movements. In calling for a sociology of social action, he recognizes that "actors do not limit themselves to reacting to situations but actually produce situations. They define themselves both by their cultural orientations and by the social conflicts in which they are engaged" (p. 26). This recognition of the importance of true human action flies in the face of most research and theorizing in social gerontology.

In research formulated within the modernization theory of aging, for example, older people as individuals are hardly present. The individual is not a self, but a kind of cypher recognizable only through role occupancy. The modernization theory of aging can be summarized as an argument that macro-level changes in the economy (as characterized by industrialization and a shift from human and animal forms of power to mechanical forms of power, by urbanization, and increases in education, literacy, and medical technique), produce inexorable changes in the number and importance of roles occupied by the aging individual, with a resulting loss of status (personal authority, power, and prestige) (Cowgill & Holmes, 1972). Variables are present in this formulation, such as rates of urbanization and average levels of education or income, but real people are absent. In failing to focus on the experience of modernization by individuals, modernization theorists have tended to rely on an ad hoc or post hoc social psychology to explain why it is, for example, that peasants or rural villagers will respond to the growth of urban-based technology by migrating to the city.

In the age stratification perspective, there is a rudimentary social psychology, drawing on structural-functionalist foundations, which views the individual in terms of the roles he or she is occupying. The link between the individual and society is through the two processes of role allocation and socialization. Role allocation refers to formal or informal processes that assign individuals as eligible to hold certain (age-stratified) status positions, or withdraw such eligibility. Socialization refers to a social process, again formal or informal, that "serves to teach individuals at each stage of the life course how to perform new roles, how to adjust to changing roles, and how to relinquish old ones" (Riley, et al., 1972, p. 11; for an elaboration of the premises concerning socialization, see Riley, Foner, Hess, & Toby, 1969). The general thrust of this framework downplays a notion of human agency (Giddens, 1993; Turner, 1988).

Agency is also not well addressed in most sociological aging research focussed at the micro level of analysis. During the 1960s and much of the 1970s, the focus on adjustment of the aging individual, particularly in the debate between activity (Palmore, 1968) and disengagement theorists (Cumming & Henry, 1961; Williams & Wirths, 1965) was cast largely in the language of Parsonian structural-functionalism (Marshall, 1994), subject to the criticisms we have noted above. While the individual in disengagement theory is viewed as "voluntarily disengaging", this voluntarism is seen as universal and inevitable, a triumph perhaps of socialization over agency. In any event, disengagement theorists and activity theorists are interested not in the agentic self but, at most, in the self as object and, in particular the extent to which the self as object is satisfied. The self in disengagement theory is subject to the same criticism that Meyer (1986) has made about life course research in general: with socialization viewed as a major link between the individual and society, the self is no longer seen as choosing and acting, but as reflecting the wider sociocultural system. Describing Parsons' structural-functionalist perspective, Anderson (1998, p. 211) puts it thus: "Actors, he [Parsons] believed, were not individuals per se, but specifications of broad cultural patterns that entered into role relationships and identities through socialization"; and he notes Parsons' failure in not producing a compelling account of "action as such, that is, of concrete, living, breathing actors making their way through time and space" (Alexander, 1998, p. 212).

Some sociological aging research has, however, emphasized human agency. Theorists drawing on symbolic interactionist and phenomenological theory and on the Weberian tradition of interpretive sociology have stressed that older people struggle to make their way through life, that this struggle seeks to preserve some sense of continuity between past, present, and future selves (Atchley, 1982, 1989) , and that doing so is a fundamentally social process (Bielby & Kully, 1989). As Hendricks (1992, p.1) puts it, "Through negotiation with those around us, we realize who we are and launch ourselves toward who we want to become".

In her study, *The Ageless Self: Sources of Meaning in Late Life*, Kaufman (1986) explicitly asks whether identity is socially structured. This is a focus on the organization of selves as objects, and Kaufman finds that major historical events such as the two world wars and the depression have little impact on the narratives of her respondents. This may be because their generational cohort placement meant that most of them were not subject to active military service in either war, and most were placed in the workforce prior to the start of the depression. They led, then,

generationally favored lives, and might not have developed any genera-
tionally-based consciousness because of the relative unimportance of these
historical events in shaping their life chances. One might argue that their
consciousness, in the form of a lack of generational consciousness, is in
fact structured by their generational placement. This, however, was not the
purpose of Kaufman's study, and could not be tested by her research
design. But Kaufman does find that other social-structural factors such as
their income security in their early lives, their education, ethnic background, and early family life have played a part in shaping the meaning
of their identities in later life. This does not occur, however, in an automatic way:

> Certain structural factors appear to hold meaning for many members of the
> group as a whole, reflecting their common cultural background. But exactly
> what meaning a given factor yields varies widely from one individual to
> another, depending on how it interacts with other factors in a person's life.
> Structural factors in the life story do not in themselves illuminate fully the
> dynamic relationship between identity and cultural context, but they do illu-
> minate one key aspect: the limitations and opportunities a person has faced,
> the choices made accordingly, and the meaning drawn from those choices
> as it emerges in themes (Kaufman, 1986, p. 87).

The influence of social structure on the self is dynamic: "Certain structural factors are, generally speaking, more meaningful than others: they
represent the conditions that these people with a common cultural background have all responded to. But within that shared framework, the content and intensity of meaning drawn from a given factor by an individual
are highly idiosyncratic" (Kaufman, 1986, p. 113).

Kaufman's approach, which is close to our own, is unusual. For the
most part, research in social gerontology has taken a micro-sociological
approach that does not link selves to the larger social structures in
which human lives are lived. Unlike research that places emphasis on
the social structure over and above the actor, we (like Kaufman) do not
start with the assumption that structure ultimately or fully determines
individual action. Individuals are not passive objects who conform to
structural forces in their day-to-day lives (Mead, 1934; Wharton, 1991).
Nor do we start with the assumption that individuals act freely in a
world that is left untouched by structural pressures. Indeed, the options
that are available to individuals vary, and are constrained by a host of
structural factors.

How then does an integrative approach to structure and agency proceed? The issues are complex and have been much discussed and debated among sociologists (Alexander, 1998; Barnes, 1995; Layder, 1994; Smelser, 1997). We develop this understanding by focussing on two theoretical sources, each of which has attempted to be integrative of other solutions linking structure and agency, and each of which we consider to have made a valuable contribution.

THE INTERSECTION OF AGENCY AND STRUCTURE

Berger and Luckmann (1966) approach the relationship between structure and agency in dialectic terms. According to them, reality is socially constructed through three dialectical processes in which "subjective meanings become objective facticities" (Berger & Luckmann, 1966, p. 18). The first of these processes is externalization. In this process individuals create their social worlds through their own actions. Social order is the result of past human activity and the reproduction of this social order is only possible through this action.

The second, objectivation, process refers to the views that individuals share about social reality, such that they see this reality as something independent of themselves, something existing prior to their own reality-construction activities. The term "facticity" refers to "the quality or state of being a fact" (Webster's Dictionary, 1986) and its use may be intended by Berger and Luckmann to emphasize that social reality is objective and not merely in the subjective consciousness of actors. In the objectivation process, individuals come to understand that everyday life is ordered and prearranged. Objectification and reification of the social order occur when individuals forget that human activity created the social order in the first place.

The third process is called internalization, the process by which the "objectivated social world is retrojected into consciousness in the course of socialization" (Berger & Luckmann, 1966, p. 61). Social order is legitimized and reinforced in this stage. Elements of socialization are apparent in this stage whereby individuals learn what is expected of them, often forgetting that this knowledge is learned, and behave accordingly. However, as Smelser (1988) has observed, objectivated reality "acts back" upon individuals not solely through socialization, but through a number of "reality maintenance" devices which are processual and often involve the use of language and ritual, with institutional and physical traces of these processes as well.

When individuals engage in the social process by conforming to the existing social order, they are also reproducing that social order. An example from previous work that builds on Berger and Luckmann's approach is in order, as this point is crucial for our subsequent analysis. The ways in which people face impending death—their own, or that of others—in our society are shaped by cultural beliefs and social practices that originated during an earlier era. Until recently, death could quite easily occur at any stage of the life course. Its cultural meaning was somewhat capricious; and religious meaning systems evolved to play a major role in "explaining" or making sense of death. Moreover, social practices around care of the dying and treatment of the dead provided an institutionalized framework to manage death and dying, in a form described by Blauner (1966) as the "bureaucratization of death". Thus, a set way of dying and managing death came to be institutionalized in our society, and in turn this social institution came to be seen as the appropriate, typical, and morally normal way to die and manage dying and death. Every time another person's death followed the pattern of this institutionalization, that pattern became more objectivated, more real. In Berger and Luckmann's terminology, this describes first the production through externalization of a social institution, then the objectivation of it, and finally the internalization of it as people learned that there was an appropriate way to die.

However, the placement of death in contemporary modernized societies is now much more predictably in the later years of old age. People "normally" die at the end of a long life. Older systems of meaning seem to be inadequate to provide an explanation of death as completion of life, as opposed to death as capricious interruption of life. The socially constructed reality of the institutionalization of death and dying confronts the individual as an external fact that, today, is not so well suited to guide people's behavior or to render it meaningful. Not surprisingly, as has been well documented by Lofland (1978), active efforts at constructing new meanings and behavior patterns around death and dying have occurred (Marshall, 1996). While the fact that people die is inevitable and transcends human agency, the experience of dying is shaped by the collaborative social processes of meaning construction and the active efforts of dying individuals and those around them to shape that experience.

In Berger and Luckmann's (1966) approach to social life, individuals are treated as active participants. They are able to evaluate the social structure and respond critically to it. However, they are not viewed as unconstrained in their action, or as all equal in their ability to act either in conformity with or opposition to the objectivated social order. Some actors and institutions have more power than others to develop, sustain, and enforce social realities. Thus, this approach recognizes that many actors feel that their choices are limited, and that others will have their choices limited but lack awareness of these limitations. This said, there is nevertheless in Berger and Luckmann a tendency to emphasize the dynamics of the individual actor rather than those of social structure. Their theoretical perspective recognizes that it is in the interests of some individuals or groups to maintain the existing social order and to limit the choices available to others (e.g., Berger & Luckmann, 1966); but, by locating limited choice within the realm of individual responsibility, they discount the importance of power relations as fundamental, structural elements of social life.

Alternatively, power relations are fundamental to Giddens' integrative approach to structure and agency. Like Berger and Luckmann (1966), Giddens (1979) believes that action and structure are dialectically related. However, recognizing that action and structure "presuppose one another" requires the rethinking of these concepts and others that are linked to them (Giddens, 1979, p. 53). To make a case for the integration of agency and structure, Giddens (1979) evaluates and expands upon research that has considered action, structures, systems, and power. To this end Giddens develops a theory of structuration that involves

> the duality of structure which relates to the fundamentally recursive character of social life, and expresses the mutual dependence of structure and agency. By the duality of structure I mean that the structural properties of social systems are both the medium and the outcome of the practices that constitute those systems. (Giddens, 1979, p. 69)

According to Giddens, action refers to a continuous flow of conduct by an actor, or the activities of an agent. But agency itself "refers not to the intentions people have in doing things but to their capability of doing those things in the first place (which is why agency implies power. . . . Agency concerns events of which an individual is the perpetrator, in the sense that the individual could, at any phase in a given sequence of conduct, have acted differently" (Giddens, 1984, p. 9). Acting differently can mean either doing something else or not acting at all. Action can bring about consequences that are not intended as well as consequences that are intended.

Involved in action, therefore, are issues relating to its purposive or intentional processes, its human accountability, its unintended consequences, and the unacknowledged conditions under which it takes place. By accountability is meant that people are able to give reasons for their actions and to justify them in terms of norms. People are seen as using norms to account for their actions; this is quite distinct from a functionalist view that sees people as acting in accordance with norms. By unintended consequences is meant that, in realizing their projects through social structure, actors also reproduce the social structure. Layder summarizes this as follows (Layder, 1994),

> Giddens emphasises that what he means by "structure" in social life has to be seen as both the medium and outcome of social activity. . . . The rules and resources we draw on are the medium of our activity in the sense that they enable us to do things and to have intentions. At the same time, they also represent the outcome or consequence (largely unintended) of our activities insofar as we endorse their value by using them, and therefore contribute to their further continuance (p. 94).

To understand Giddens' theory of structuration, his use of the terms "structure" and "system" must also be clarified. According to Giddens, structure is comprised of rules and resources that are organized as properties of social systems. Rules are the norms and practices of a given society and resources are bound to power relations. In fact, resources are the bases of power that comprise the structures of domination. Social systems are systems of social interaction that reproduce relations between actors or collectivities and have structural properties. The theory of structuration seeks to explain "the ways in which that [social] system, via the application of generative rules and resources, and in the context of unintended outcomes, is produced and reproduced in interaction" (Giddens, 1979, p. 66).

In this approach, structure is involved in the production of action, but structure is not thought to place deterministic or fixed limits on action. Giddens (1979) suggests that "rules and resources are drawn upon by actors in the production of interaction but are thereby also reconstituted through such interaction. Structure is thus the mode in which the relation between moment and totality expresses itself in social reproduction" (p. 71). According to Giddens, the assumption that structure is involved in the production of action stands in opposition to the view that structure places limits on action:

Structure must not be conceptualized as simply placing constraints upon human agency, but as enabling. This is what I call the duality of structure. Structure can always in principle be examined in terms of its *structuration*. To inquire into the structuration of social practices is to seek to explain how it comes about that structure is constituted through action, and reciprocally how action is constituted structurally (Giddens, 1993, p. 169).

The assumption that structure is involved in the production of action is not to oppose the view that structure places limits on action; the distinction is more subtle. Structure is simultaneously enabling and constraining. Giddens himself invokes Marx on this point, and he is worth quoting at length here:

The production of society, I have argued, is always and everywhere a skilled accomplishment of its members. While this is recognized by each of the schools of interpretative sociology that I have discussed . . . . they have not managed successfully to reconcile such an emphasis with the equally essential thesis, dominant in most deterministic schools of social thought, that if human beings make society, they do not do so merely under conditions of their own choosing. In other words, it is fundamental to complement the idea of the production of social life with that of social reproduction. Giddens, 1993, p. 133)

In fact, Giddens' discussion of power points to the subtleties, not the opposition, of the distinction between a structure that produces action and one that constrains it. Giddens rejects notions of power that treat it as a phenomenon of intended action. He also rejects views of power that locate it within the social structure as a medium whereby group interests are realised. According to Giddens, Lukes comes closest to the correct consideration of power. Lukes (1974) suggests that

A person or party who wields power could have acted otherwise, and the person or party over whom power is wielded, the concept implies, would have acted otherwise if power had not been exercised. 'In speaking thus, one assumes that, although the agents operate within structurally determined limits, they none the less have a certain relative autonomy and could have acted differently' (cited in Giddens, 1979:91).

Giddens argues that by suggesting that structure places limits on agency, this approach is "unable satisfactorily to deal with structure as implicated in power relations and power relations as implicated in structure" (Giddens, 1979, p. 91). The only way this problem can be alleviated is "if the resources which the existence of domination implies and the exercise of power draws upon, are seen to be at the same time structural components of social systems. The exercise of power is not a type of act; rather power is instantiated in action, as a regular and routine phenomenon." One aspect of power is that it exists in one modality in the absence of action—it is the capability to act, "the capacity of the agent to mobilize resources" and *"transformative capacity"* (Giddens, 1993, pp. 116–117).

For Giddens it is important to consider the dialectic between action and structure in discussions of power. As he puts it,

> Resources are the media whereby transformative capacity is employed as power in the routine course of social interaction; but they are at the same time structural elements of social systems as systems, reconstituted through their utilisation in social interaction (Giddens, 1979, p. 92).

Thus, the subtle difference between the view that structure limits action and that structure produces action lies in Giddens' dialectical assumption that one mutually creates the other.

In our view structure produces action but the particular action that is produced lies largely within the realms of the structure itself. Only under exceptional circumstances does human agency push structural barriers to the extent that the structure itself is substantially changed in a short period of time (as is the case in revolutions and, to a lesser extent, protests and lobbying movements). Rather, routine social action reproduces and reifies those patterns of action that we call structure and leads to slight modifications in the short term but nevertheless can lead to important changes in a more long-term evolutionary sense.

The study we now describe is not concerned with exceptional events; nor is it a study of long-term social change. Rather, its focus is on the day-to-day lives of garment workers who live and work in Montreal. Thus, for the purpose of this analysis, we start with Lukes' assumption that agents have a certain relative autonomy and could have acted differently even though they operate within structurally determined limits. In doing so, we examine how the dialectic between human agency and social structure shapes the institution of retirement and the process of retirement timing.

METHODOLOGY

This chapter employs data from a case study of the Montreal Garment Industry. This is one of seven case studies that comprise the project entitled *Issues of an Aging Workforce: A Study to Inform Human Resources Policy Development* (IAW) which was conducted by CARNET: The Canadian Aging Research Network. This project addresses theoretical issues of aging and retirement in a life course context, including the ways in which work experiences intersected with education and training, health status, and family relationships, and the ways in which changes in human resources policies and practices in a firm or industry influenced the retirement experience. These theoretical interests therefore emphasize the significance of, not only individual experiences of working and retiring, but the structural changes in the working life course and the factors shaping that life course (Marshall, 1995a; 1998).

The evidence gathered in this case study consists of archival data, key informant interviews, focus group discussions with employed, retired, and displaced garment workers, and a small survey of industry owners and representatives (the latter data source is not used in this chapter). Between May 1994 and March 1995, 12 focus group discussions were conducted in Montreal: two with retired workers, three with displaced workers, and seven with employed workers. The focus group discussions were relatively unstructured. However, the focus group mediator followed a list of guidelines developed by the IAW research team and always asked several questions relating to the key themes of the project—career mobility, health, retirement, technology, and family.

The focus groups ranged in size from four to ten people. Five of the focus groups were comprised of employees who worked together in five different shops. Two of these shops were relatively large by industry standards, employing between 80 and 100 people. Two of the shops were of average size (about 50 people) and one was small (about 20 people).[1] These discussions were held on work time and the IAW project paid these employees for their time away from their jobs. Participants either volunteered to participate in a focus group at the request of the shop's union official, or the union official chose who would participate. In the other two employee focus groups, union officials asked workers who were not

---

1. To preserve anonymity and confidentiality, focus group participants and the garment shops are referred to by pseudonyms, which were chosen to reflect the ethnicity of the participants (see Snell, 1993).

necessarily employed at the same shop to participate in the IAW study. These focus groups were held at the union headquarters outside of normal working hours.

The retiree focus groups were comprised of members of the union's retiree club. The retirees get together every Thursday at the union head-quarters to participate in activities such as playing cards. Occasionally, the club plans special activities for the Thursday meetings. The IAW focus groups were planned as one of these special activities. Those who chose not to participate in the focus group discussions carried on (in another room) with their regular Thursday activities. The IAW project contacted displaced workers through the union as well. Again, a union official asked for volunteers among employees who were currently looking for work.

STRUCTURE, AGENCY, AND
RETIREMENT PROCESSES

How does the dialectic between structure and agency shape the retirement processes of garment workers in Montreal? It is important to recognize that this dialectic operates at several levels of analysis. At the industrial level, employees or their representatives negotiate pension schemes that tend to reinforce the rules established by the state. At the level of the state, government officials establish and develop pension schemes and retire-ment regulations that take into account the views of many lobbying groups, some of which are more powerful in their influence than others. Private pension programs are developed within the context of public pen-sions, and issues such as the normal age of retirement or ideal income replacement ratios are often reinforced. Yet, agency is demonstrated in the variations from the state-established retirement norms that emerge. Industries and organizations, for instance, are likely to establish pension guidelines based, in part, on the nature of work within their particular field. In turn, these negotiations produce a structure of retirement that is specific to a particular industry or organization. Thus, for instance, the process of retirement is likely quite different for auto workers than it is for university professors.

Beyond the levels of the state, industry, and organization, the dialectic between agency and structure works at an individual level as well. Individuals shape their own retirement experiences by assigning subjec-tive meaning to them, by developing strategies that make the structural circumstances of retirement work to their advantage, and simply by accepting the retirement structure as it stands. Hence, the social order of retirement is reproduced by the policies and negotiations that transpire at multiple levels of analysis (state, industrial, organizational) with actors producing and reproducing the social order at each level. Below we outline how these processes work within the Montreal Garment Industry.

Retirement Policy in the Montreal Garment Industry

The focus group participants in this study are unionized employees, and the relations between The Guild and The Union fundamentally shape their benefits and working conditions. The Quebec Fashion Apparel Manufacturers' Guild is a nonprofit organization that represents 40 companies in Quebec. It has a board of directors and various other committees that act within the Guild to make decisions on issues as they arise. The Guild serves as the shop owner's liaison with the government and the union. It lobbies and negotiates with the government over issues of trade or any other activity that pertains to the women's clothing industry, and it negotiates with the union over the collective agreements and other labor issues.

The International Ladies Garment Workers Union (I.L.G.W.U.)[2] is a voluntary, nonprofit, unincorporated association which attempts to act in the best interest of its members. Its membership is comprised of persons who are employed by Guild members. The key objective of the Union is to negotiate a collective agreement with the Guild that will ensure reasonable benefits and working conditions for unionized employees.

In negotiating benefits, representatives of The Union and The Guild act with the interests of their members in mind. Each organization is engaged in a bargaining process whereby they use their power to achieve their goals. This results in a collective agreement which outlines the specific benefits and working conditions that are to be adhered to in unionized shops. With respect to retirement, the collective agreement states that retirees of the union are entitled to certain pension benefits if they meet the rules of eligibility.

Prior to 1987 a retiring union member had to meet the following requirements to receive a full pension: 1) be age 65 or older; 2) be a union member for at least 20 years, the last 10 of which must be continuous; and 3) be continuously employed in a contributory shop for the last 10 years,

---

2. During our study (July, 1995) the I.L.G.W.U. merged with the Amalgamated Clothing and Textile Workers' Union to form the Union of Needletrades, Industrial and Textile Employees (UNITE).

except for periods of lay-off, illness and the like (I.L.G.W.U., 1986). The minimum pension for retiring members who met these criteria was $200.00 per month. An extra $1.50 for each year of service to a maximum of $30.00 per month was provided for those who had worked more than 20 years.

A key problem with this structure of retirement benefits is that it places workers who have had discontinuous employment histories at a disadvantage, thereby reproducing social hierarchies of inequality. Thus, women are at a disadvantage relative to men because they are more likely to have leaves from paid employment due mainly to family responsibilities. And among garment workers, older employees are disadvantaged relative to younger ones because they are more likely to have had breaks in their employment due to management attempts to eliminate highly paid employees from their shops (McMullin & Marshall, 1997). By actively establishing pension benefit regulations that penalize workers who have had discontinuous work histories, the social order, in which certain groups are disadvantaged relative to others, is reproduced through the institution of retirement. Notably, this structure of retirement was actively established by the collective agencies of The Union and The Guild and could have been established differently. However, we must recognize that these negotiations take place within an established social structure that limits the choices that are available to groups with less relative power. Relative to The Guild, The Union tends to have less power and, not incidentally, it is likely within the best interests of the Guild to limit and restrict pension payments. Further, both The Guild and The Union work within a social structure that takes social hierarchies of inequality for granted. Hence, within the logic of a capitalist system that is driven almost entirely by a quest for profit, it makes sense that persons who have discontinuous work histories are penalized in retirement.

Retirement benefits are not negotiated within a vacuum. Rather, they are one part of a large collective agreement that covers issues such as wages, hours of work, and health benefits, and the agreement itself is bargained within the context of market conditions that influence the relative power of The Union and The Guild. During the late 1980s, market conditions deteriorated in the Montreal Garment Industry as free trade agreements were ratified. These trends, combined with significant job loss, resulted in The Union having substantially less bargaining power than was true throughout the 70s and in the early 80s (McMullin, 1996).

One might hypothesize that collective agreement negotiations under these conditions would lead to reductions in pension and retirement benefits. However, the changes to the pension plan and its eligibility requirements that came into effect on January 1st, 1987, better accommodate persons who have had discontinuous employment histories. Future pensions (for service after January 1, 1987) were to be based on pre-retirement incomes and directly on the contributions that an employer makes to an employee's account. Pensions were now vested (a vested pension is an acquired right to a pension after 2 years of employment in a contributory shop) and a bonus system was established, whereby future increases in individual pensions could result from profitable fund investments. The pensions of union members who worked prior to January 1, 1987 but who will retire after that date will be calculated based on a combination of these two plans.

The post-1987 pension entitlement is quite straightforward. It is 25% of the total amount of the contributions made to the fund by an employer on behalf of an employee after January 1, 1987. This amount is divided by 12 to convert to a monthly pension. Assume that an employee started work in the garment industry in 1987, expects to work for 20 years, and that the expected contributions made by this person's employers will be $16,800. Assuming that the contributory rate stays the same (4%), this person earned an average of about $10.00 per hour, or approximately $1,750 per month over the last 20 years. Upon retirement at age 65, this person is entitled to a yearly pension of $4,200 (25% of 16,800) or $350 per month. If this person retires between the ages of 60 and 65 the pension will be reduced by ½% for each month by which the age at retirement is less than 65. For example, if an individual wants to retire at age 62, their pension will be reduced by 18% (36 months X 1/2%). Likewise, if a person decides to retire after age 65, their pension will be increased by 1/2% for each month by which the age at retirement is over 65.

Union members who have not had contributions made to their pension accounts for the past 36 consecutive months are considered terminated members. If these employees have had at least 24 months (not necessarily consecutive) of contributions made to the pension on their behalf, they are entitled to a "vested pension". This pension will be calculated based on the rules outlined above and will be payable as a deferred pension for life, starting at age 65. The trustees of the fund make every effort to collect all contributions owing to the fund, but no compensation is made to an employee whose employer fails to contribute to the pension on their behalf.

Thus, even within the context of poor market conditions, a system of retirement emerged that provided more benefits for employees even if their employment history had been considerably disrupted. The data collected for this study do not specifically address why the pension scheme was improved in 1987. One possible explanation is that The Union lost its power to negotiate over the key aspect of the collective agreement, wages. In fact, average wages within the Montreal garment industry have declined since the mid-1980s (McMullin, 1996). As a concession for limited and nonexistent wage increases, The Union may have pushed hard for changes to the pension regulations, and The Guild may have yielded some of its power to meet these demands.

Nonetheless, the structure of retirement is still based on liberal notions of equal opportunity, which place women, older, and ethnic workers at a disadvantage. For example, this system perpetuates gender- and ethnic-based inequalities into later life by basing pension incomes on pre-retirement incomes. Furthermore, because women and older workers are more likely to have interrupted employment histories, the amount of money that they can contribute to their pension is substantially reduced. There are no provisions under the new pension system that allow for childrearing or periods of unemployment. Thus, although substantially improved, the current pension regulations still reproduce a structure of inequality that is based on class, age, gender, and ethnicity.

Retirement Policy in Quebec

At the outset of this section, we noted that industry policy regarding retirement transpires within the context of state regulations. How do state policies influence pension and retirement regulations in the Montreal garment industry? Monies received from government sponsored retirement and pension programs comprise a significant proportion of most seniors' incomes (Myles, 1989). Generally, public pension structures have either been based on pre-retirement incomes, or on the idea of a national minimum benefit. In the first instance, pensions perpetuate class-, gender-, and ethnic-based structures of inequality in older age by "graduating" pension incomes according to pre-retirement income. In the second instance, income equality among older people is sought because the same sum of money is paid to everyone based on citizenship only (flat benefit structure).

Most Western capitalist nations have pension structures that combine flat and graduated pension schemes (Myles, 1989). In Canada, for instance, Old Age Security (OAS) has traditionally guaranteed a flat, per-month benefit, based on a minimum residency requirement, to all people aged 65 and over. For the purposes of the current chapter, we focus on Quebec's graduated pension scheme.

The similarities between the pension regulations in the Montreal Garment Industry and the Quebec Pension Plan (QPP) are striking. The QPP represents a graduated scheme whereby employees and employers pay into the plan according to the employee's pre-retirement income. The QPP is a compulsory social insurance plan that was established in 1965. In 1991, employees and employers were required to pay 2.3% of an employee's wage (up to a maximum wage of $30,500) to the QPP. The normal qualifying age for QPP benefits is 65. Flexible provisions were added to the plan in 1984 that would allow a worker to retire between the ages of 60 and 70. Based on age 65 as the normal retirement age, the pensions of persons who retire between the ages of 60 and 64 are reduced by 1/2% for each month that they retire before age 65. Likewise, for those who retire between the ages of 66 and 70, their pensions are increased by 1/2% for each month that they retire after age 65 . Although there is no minimum investment necessary to be eligible for benefits, an individual is required to have contributed for at least 1 year to be eligible for the QPP.

The annual pension is 25% of the average adjusted pensionable career earnings received during the contributory period. In calculating the QPP, the assumption made is that individuals will work between the ages of 18 (or from 1966 for those who were over the age of 18 at that time) and 65. Thus, average pensions are calculated based on a numerator that reflects the contributions that an individual has made to the plan and on a denominator of 47 years, regardless of the number of years that the individual has actually contributed to the plan. The denominator is adjusted for people who have had periods of unemployment or low earnings by calculating a maximum dropout time that equals 15% of the contributor's months in the plan prior to age 65 provided that the total remaining time is not less than 10 years. The denominator is also adjusted for childrearing responsibilities. The plan allows a parent to drop out for up to seven years after their child is born (in other words the denominator is reduced by up to 7 years). Pensions are also adjusted based on a cost-of-living expense.

On first glance, the QPP appears to be sensitive to the retirement needs of women because it takes childrearing responsibilities into account. Women who take time off from paid employment to work at home caring for their children do not receive yearly wage increases and often re-enter the labor market with lower salaries than they were previously making. Adjusting the QPP to cover a 7-year absence from work does not consider the wage reductions and limited saving power that is associated with taking a leave from paid employment. Further, because the QPP does not adjust for other structural inequalities within labor markets that determine the wage, inequalities associated with ethnic- and gender-based segregated occupational practices are perpetuated into older age.

The structure of union- and state-based pensions also produces and reproduces inequalities on the basis of age. It is assumed that older, retired people only require a small proportion of their income to meet their needs. While this assumption may be reasonable for middle-class male workers, most garment workers cannot afford to have their incomes reduced. Further, because chronological ages are established as a basis of rules of eligibility, some workers are disadvantaged relative to others according to their age.

In this section we have shown that through the actions of Union and Guild representatives, social hierarchies of inequality are reproduced by establishing pension regulations that mimic the state's. Yet, we have also shown that the pension regulations established in collective agreements do not represent a static structure. Rather, the system evolves as individuals lobby for changes that would either make the structure of retirement more or less equitable, depending on one's point of view. Hence, we have illustrated some of the ways in which the dialectic between structure and agency work at the state and industry levels. In the next section, we demonstrate that this dialectic also operates at the individual level, as garment workers negotiate and assign meaning to their own retirement.

Retirement Timing Among Garment Workers

Within the context of state and industry policy, there are several structurally defined retirement timing options available for garment workers in Montreal. Workers could retire as early as age 60 with a reduced pension, or as late as age 70 with an enriched pension. Given that the nature of work within the garment industry is very difficult, one might expect workers to retire as early as pensions schemes would allow. On the other hand, because the work is so poorly paid, one might expect that financial necessity would require that workers continue working until their 70th birthday.

Currently Employed Garment Workers

When we asked currently employed garment workers when they would like to retire, most of them, regardless of their current age, indicated that some time before age 65 would be ideal. Their wish to retire early stemmed from a view of work, prevalent among many, that was captured by phrases like "I've had enough" or "I'm fed up". In fact, this theme emerged in each of the employee focus group discussions.

As Jo-elle puts it, "I joined the union in '57. I've always been working. So, I'm fed up, I've had it (laughing)." In the same focus group Margariette echos this sentiment, saying "I've been working nearly 25 years in the garment industry, and I started here [at this factory] in '87. And, me too, I'm anxious not to go into retirement, but to take early retirement. I'm really fed up now."

If social life was shaped entirely by the social structure, the question of retirement timing itself would not make sense, because everyone would take the retirement age of 65 for granted. Only in a world in which structure and agency work together simultaneously would one be able to formulate a response to this question, and the workers we talked with responded loud and clear—early retirement for them would be wonderful. Yet, choice is the operative word in the question of retirement timing, and as we will see below the ability to retire early is severely constrained by financial limitations among these workers. The paradox is such that the structure of garment work simultaneously limits the retirement choices that are available to workers while influencing their desire to retire early and the meaning of early retirement. Thus, unlike many middle class workers who have less physically demanding jobs and who may shudder at the thought of retiring early, these workers are tired, "fed up", and suffer from industrial health problems that make them want to quit working.

Although garment workers dream of early retirement, most choose to work until they are 65 years old because their structurally defined alternatives are bleak. Financial concerns influence this choice, which suggests that dreams of early retirement cannot be divorced from the ability to afford it. The following discussion highlights the relationship between the desire for early retirement and financial issues.

Angela[3]: Are you going to leave at 60?
Several: All of us are ready to leave.
Unknown: It depends on your pay.
Another: I've come to that decision.
Denene: We don't have huge pension plans. It's not big.
Angela: Do you receive any pension from the union?
Denene: Yes, but it's not a lot.
Jo-elle: I joined the union at the age of 14, then after that, I came back in 57. Now, I'm 58. So, I will get approximately a $500 pension from the union.

---

3. Angela is the focus group moderator.

Angela:	Have you been . . . able to put money aside by yourselves for the old age?
Jo-elle:	Well, I bought a house for myself, but I said to myself, when I'll stop working, I'll sell the house and I'll be able to eat (others laughing). It's the only way I could see it; that's it.

This discussion points to two related sources of retirement income that are influenced both by agency and structure. At the industry level, policies are negotiated in the collective agreements between the owners and the union that dictate how much money garment workers earn and what percentage of earnings go toward pensions. These policies are tied to the relations of production, and they disadvantage some groups of people relative to others on the basis of gender, age and ethnicity.

Another source of retirement money comes from individual savings. How much one saves for retirement is largely dependent upon the wage, but also varies according to marital status, parent status, and the employment status of one's spouse. Further, given similar wages, some are able to save more than others, and workers use different strategies to save money for retirement. Some of the focus group participants simply said that they did not make enough money to live on, which made saving impossible. However, a more common response to our queries about saving money for retirement was, "Not a lot remains". As one worker bluntly states, saving is difficult because "We're working here since ages and we still don't make $25 per hour."

There was a general belief among workers that the ability to save is linked to marital status and the employment status of one's spouse. Many noted that because they were not married and did not live in a two-income household they could not save money. Others suggested that if their husbands were working it would be easier to save. As Celine puts it,

If my husband was working, it would be different. Well, I know I have to go on [working] till 65. It's like I tell you, I save up money too, but I say to myself even at that point, if there were a shutdown of the shop, in that case, I won't be able to buy RRSPs [Registered Retirement Savings Plans] anymore.

Even when workers are able to put money aside for their retirement, a crisis like unemployment might arise, making it necessary to draw on savings. As Francesca describes, "You put money aside and then it goes. My husband isn't working and we have to eat."

For those who were able to save for retirement, some of the focus group participants chose to buy a house as a means of investing money. Others invested their money in Registered Retirement Savings Plans (RRSPs), which are a government regulated, tax-deductible savings mechanism, but those who did so invested only small amounts. Clarece is 57 years old and says that she is lucky because she was working at a factory where other older workers advised her to buy RRSPs. In her words,

> I started, with $1,000 . . . in the end I had the opportunity to collect a small amount, perhaps $15,000, in a RRSP. But, now it's more difficult . . . You know you can't put money aside, because actually when you're working, your wages are just enough to live decently, you just make it, you hardly make it.

The preceding analysis shows that although the ability to save varies somewhat from individual to individual, low wages make saving difficult for everyone and, for those who do put some money away, it is a small amount. Missing from the previous account is that certain groups of people have less saving power than others because they are segregated into low-paying jobs. Structural characteristics in place within the garment industry segregate women and ethnic groups into lower-paying occupations and shops, thus reducing their potential savings. Company closures, which disproportionately affect older workers, make saving impossible for the unemployed workers that are affected. The limited saving power among garment workers in general, and women, ethnic, and older workers in particular, highlights the importance of state and union pensions to the financial security of retired garment workers.

In summary, the ability to save for early or on-time retirement among garment workers is severely limited by the structural circumstances of their lives. Yet, these workers make choices about their savings, and devise investment strategies within the realm of the barriers that constrain them financially. They talk among themselves about buying RRSPs and do so rather than simply putting their savings into a bank account. Some buy houses as an investment rather than buying RRSPs. Most choose to save "a little bit" but others choose not to save at all.

Retired Garment Workers and Displaced Garment Workers

Most of the retired workers we talked with worked until they were 65, even though they found their jobs difficult and unfulfilling. As Nicole, who retired at age 65, said, "I was planning for my pension for a long time. I said I have 6 years left, 5 years left. Yes, I counted the days." Likewise, most of the displaced garment workers would prefer to take an "early retirement" than to go back to work. However, the preference for early retirement among displaced workers is influenced by their inability to afford retirement, on the one hand, and the difficulties they experience in trying to find work on the other. In fact, none of the displaced workers felt that they could afford "early retirement" on their own, and all of them have applied for special financial assistance from the government.

For displaced garment workers who lose their jobs before they reach age 65, the dream of early retirement is soured by grave financial difficulties. Nonetheless, these workers assign meaning to their unemployment by redefining it as early retirement. They do so because they are faced with a paradox of being too old to find work and too young to receive full retirement benefits (public or private). For these workers, the transition to retirement comes quickly, without warning and with considerable fears regarding money.

Indeed, the formally retired and displaced garment workers we talked with found it difficult to make ends meet on the income that they received from state- and union-based pension programs. When the issue of having enough money to live on in retirement was discussed, several workers made reference to the fact that they would have to sell their houses in order to have money to eat. Angelina sums up the continuing financial difficulties that garment workers face once they are out of the labour force when she bluntly says, "In retirement, no money". Likewise, a group of retired workers discussed their financial hardships in relation to the so called, "golden years" of older age. As they put it,

Madeline: There's no question that this [retirement and older age] isn't golden.
Mary-Jade: I missed the golden age.
Carmen: We don't have the means to pay for it.

The financial hardships of retired and displaced garment workers vary according to their age. Workers who lose their jobs through displacement or retirement at age 65 are able to collect Old Age Security (OAS) and their Union and Quebec Pension Plan (QPP) benefits with no penalty. Sixty- to 64-year-olds in similar employment circumstances are not eligible for OAS but could apply for QPP and their Union pension with a penalty. Yet, even within these structural boundaries that limit the financial options that are available, some workers devise strategies that allow them retire early. One such strategy is for workers to quit work at the age of 64 and then collect unemployment insurance for the year that they are not entitled to collect a pension or old age security. As one worker put it, "I decided (laughter) I've had it . . . Yes, I will receive my unemployment insurance and I could ask for my Quebec return afterwards." Hence, although the nature of retirement timing is structured by chronological age, which establishes the age of pension eligibility, individuals actively devise strategies that allow them to manipulate this age structure so that their best financial interests, however minimal these may be, are realized.

In other instances, persons who are under the age of 60 and who lose their jobs are not eligible for any state or union pension benefits, and must deplete their savings and sell their homes before they are eligible for social security (see LeBlanc and McMullin, 1997a). Josée, for instance, is a 53-year-old woman who had worked as a foreperson at the same shop for 25 years. The factory she worked in closed, and she collected unemployment insurance for 1 year. After that year she worked for a couple of months at a factory that was far from her home and, with the stress of the work and the commuting, she became ill with a serious virus. She describes her situation as follows:

> So I got sick, I stopped working, but I don't have any income. Since then, I'm not working. I have no income. I'm not entitled to anything. I don't have unemployment insurance. I'm not entitled to anything, so, I'm living on my money [savings].

Workers believe that they are faced with a contradictory financial situation. On the one hand, they feel that because they are old they cannot find work. On the other hand, because they are young, they are not entitled to OAS, a full union pension, or a full QPP. The following comments highlight this contradiction. According to Maralisa, a 56-year-old displaced worker, "[Employers] always look for somebody younger." Theresa agrees, saying,

> You go somewhere, they ask your age, and after they say, ah! ah! For the application, they say yes; then, after they say ah, no, no, no. We have no work. Come back next week. We'll see, maybe.

Later in the discussion Maralisa talks about her situation, which reflects the despair that many of these working-class women feel:

I don't work and my husband doesn't work, unemployment finishes in a month and two weeks. It's a very bad time for me, it's bad because, it's bad. There's no money coming in. You don't take no pension, there is no work.

In summary, although garment workers would prefer to retire early, class, age, gender, and ethnicity limit the retirement timing options that are available because of the financial barriers they produce. In turn, the difficult nature of garment work, which is also shaped by class, age, gender and ethnicity, influence the perceptions and desires of these workers about their retirement timing; garment workers dream of early retirement because they have had enough of their work. The circumstances of these garment workers clearly stand in contrast to the experience of workers in many white-collar jobs or better-paid blue-collar jobs (e.g., the insurance industry) where in some cases early retirement may be viewed in a positive light and where the dream of early retirement can be realized financially (for an automobile industry case in which most workers resisted early retirement, see Hardy, Hazelrigg, & Quadagno, 1996) or in other cases whereby the work is enjoyable and early retirement would be perceived negatively.

One possible interpretation of the preceding analysis is that garment workers are powerless in their retirement timing decisions and that garment workers lack agency because of their structurally defined circumstances. However, this explanation masks the complexities of the dialectic between agency and structure. Garment workers do make choices. Recall, for instance, that garment workers could wait until they reached age 70 to retire with higher pensions. Yet, most garment workers choose to retire at age 65, thereby reproducing the institutionalized "normal" age of retirement. And for the few workers who choose to retire before age 65, they actively devise strategies that would allow them to do so financially.

DISCUSSION AND CONCLUSIONS

We have argued that social research in aging and the life course has not adequately addressed the problem of linking self and social structure. We argued that attempts to develop a theoretical perspective to address the ways in which individual lives and social structures are mutually implicated should seek to conceptualize both self and society in terms that respect the importance of human agency. Micro-sociologies of aging and the life course have tended to view the individual as reactive, rather than as intentional and voluntaristically proactive or agentic. Macro-sociologies have tended to assume that social structure exists without any requirement for it to be constituted, on a continuous, ongoing basis, by patterns of action; and the further assumption runs through many of the macro-sociologies that social structure has an impact on individuals (it structures their behavior into patterns) in some automatic or inexorable manner. While it is quite possible to describe both social structure and individual behavior in this way—as the history of the field of aging and the life course demonstrates—we find this unsatisfactory.

We have recommended the theoretical approach of interpretive sociology, particularly as evidenced in the work of Berger and Luckmann and Giddens, to address the self-society linkage. These theorists provide a language that can accommodate both self and social structure, and their linkage through co-constitutive social structuration. At this point we can note that Giddens himself said that his "structuration theory" is not an "interpretative sociology", in that it does not see society as the creation of individual subjects (Giddens, 1984, p. *xxvi*). We are not using the term "interpretive" sociology in this narrow sense, which presumably refers to subjectivist schools of theory that reject any notion that there is such an entity as society independent of those who construct it (see Layder, 1994). We refer to a broad tradition of theorizing drawing on Weberian, phenomenological, and symbolic interactionist sources that emphasizes the importance of human agency and the social construction of reality. Giddens and Berger and Luckmann clearly fall within this tradition.

To illustrate some of the insights of this theoretical approach, we drew on a case study of Montreal garment industry workers and the industry in which their lives are shaped. A number of points about the conceptualization of self and society linkages are evident in this illustration. Both owners in the industry and workers can be viewed as actors, acting within a broader social environment, to be sure, yet mutually constructing the social conditions which structure the lives of these garment workers. Thus, the workers are co-producers of their lives.

Owners make active use of legislative loopholes to exercise their power over employees. Representatives of The Guild use poor market conditions to enhance their power in negotiating the collective agreement. Clearly, in the sense of power as capacity, owners have more power resources than their employees, and these resources include provincial government legislative loopholes that allow the dissolution of their businesses, with declared bankruptcy followed by a resurrection of a new business with conditions less advantageous to labor.

Social factors such as class, age, gender, and ethnicity act to structure the lives of garment workers by limiting and conditioning choices. Interestingly, if you take the first letter of these bases of inequality, you come up with the word CAGE. There is a lot of imagery that comes to mind when one hears the word CAGE—and for the purposes of the garment workers, much of it is probably quite accurate. Why then do we not make more of this metaphor? Because it is too deterministic. Within a structuration framework, it is necessary to speak of choices, however constrained and choice is constrained for the garment workers. For example, they have dreams of early retirement, but are frustrated in realizing these dreams because of their low incomes and marginalised labor force histories. Their choices concerning retiring or continuing to work are nevertheless active, involving knowledge of the range of options before them, calculation of which of these options is feasible and desirable, and, at times, the development of innovative strategies (such as using unemployment insurance or other government assistance programs) to facilitate an economically viable retirement. Further, at the industrial level collective agency is evident, as union representatives actively negotiate retirement policies that serve the interests of workers.

It is also clear that these strategies are social—they are discussed in a strategic way not only in our focus groups but, almost certainly, in the everyday work lives of these garment workers and at the collective level between union and guild representatives. Thus, their identities are socially constructed. Their identity construction is not only strategic with respect to behavior, but it involves active and social meaning construction in which, for example, job displacement may be reinterpreted as retirement.

Agency thus runs through the lives of these individuals, and this agency is engaged socially in the lives they share with their co-workers. Agency also is manifest at the collective action level through their union involvements, for the union is an important and close-at-hand vehicle through which the workers in these small manufacturing institutions seek to exercise some control over their lives.

One could not give a satisfactory account of the lives of these garment workers by focussing on agency—for their agency is indeed constrained and, more than constrained, constituted by their embeddedness in social structure. And the structuration processes which shape their identities and their life courses involve complex interweaving of the influences of age, gender, social class, ethnicity, and marital and family relationships. On the other hand, one could not fully understand the lives of these women if agency were ignored. Their lives are not influenced by these social structural factors in a uniform or automatic way, but in terms of what they themselves make of these social relationships that are so constitutive of their lives.

The garment industry discussed in this chapter is an example of an industry in which workers are extremely marginalized through their exploitation and oppression. Agency, although apparent here, is perhaps constrained among the workers in this industry by structural factors more than it would be in another. Thus it is important for future research to consider how the dialectic between agency and structure shapes retirement processes in other industries and organizations. In industries and organizations where the power balance between management and employees is relatively more equal, the retirement processes, financial constraints, and timing decisions are likely quite different. Compare, for instance, the likely retirement experiences of lawyers with retail service clerks. More research needs to be done in this regard, keeping in mind the structural nature of the CAGE and the agency of the actors within it.

REFERENCES

Acker, J. (1988). Class, gender and the relations of distribution. *Signs, 13*, 473–97.

Alexander, J. C. (1998). After neofunctionalism: Action, Culture, and civil society (Chapter 9). In J. C. Alexander (Ed.), *Neofunctionalism and after* (pp. 210–233). Oxford: Blackwell.

Atchley, R. C. (1982). The aging self. *Psychotherapy: Theory, Research and Practice, 19*(4), 388–396.

Atchley, R. C. (1989). A continuity theory of normal aging. *The Gerontologist, 29*(2), 183–190.

Barnes, B. (1995). *The elements of social theory*. Princeton: Princeton University Press.

Berger, P. L., & Luckmann, T. (1966). *The social construction of reality*. New York: Doubleday.

Bielby, D. D., & Kully, H. S. (1989). Social construction of the past: Autobiography and the theory of G.H. Mead. *Current Perspectives on Aging and the Life Cycle, 3*, 1–24.

Blauner, R. (1966). Death and social structure. *Psychiatry, 29*, 378–394.

Cain, L. (1959). The sociology of aging: A trend report and bibliography. *Current Sociology, 8*, 57–133.

Cowgill, D. O., & Holmes, L. D. (Eds.) (1972). *Aging and modernization.* New York: Meredith Corporation.

Cumming, E., & Henry, W. E. (1961). *Growing old: The process of disengagement.* New York: Basic.

Durkheim, E. (1982). *The rules of sociological method.* (Steven Lukes, Ed.). New York: Free Press.

Estes, C. L. (1979). *The aging enterprise.* San Francisco: Jossey-Bass.

Estes, C. L., Swan, J. H., & Gerard, L. E. (1982). Dominant and competing paradigms in gerontology: Towards a political economy of ageing. *Aging and Society, 12*, 151–164.

George, L. K. (1990). Social structure, social processes, and social-psychological states. In R. H. Binstock & L. K. George (Eds.), *Handbook of aging and the social sciences* (3rd ed., pp. 186–204). San Diego: Academic Press.

Giddens, A. (1979). *Central problems in social theory.* London: Macmillan.

Giddens, A. (1984). *The constitution of society: Outline of the theory of structuration.* Berkeley and Los Angeles: University of California Press.

Giddens, A. (1993). *New rules of sociological method* (2nd ed.). Stanford, CA: Stanford University Press.

Goffman, E. (1959). *The presentation of self in everyday life.* New York: Doubleday.

Grabb, E. (1990). *Theories of social inequality: Classical and contemporary perspectives* (2nd ed.). Toronto: Holt, Rinehart, and Winston of Canada.

Guillemard, A. M. (1982). Old age, retirement, and the social class structure: Toward an analysis of the structural dynamics of the later stage of life. In T. K. Hareven & K. Adams (Eds.), *Aging and the life course transition: An interdisciplinary perspective* (pp. 221–243). New York: The Guildford Press.

Guillemard, A. M. (1983). The making of old age policy in France. In A. M. Guillemard (Ed.), *Old age and the welfare state* (pp. 75–99). Beverly Hills CA: Sage.

Hardy, M. A., Hazelrigg, L., & Quadagno, J. (1996). *Ending a career in the auto industry: "30 and Out".* New York: Plenum Press.

Hendricks, J. (1992). Learning to act old: Heroes, villains or old fools. *Journal of Aging Studies, 6*(1), pp. 31–47.

International Ladies Garment Workers Union (I.L.G.W.U.) (1986). *Your new, improved, pension plan: Quebec Fashion Industries Retirement Fund, I.L.G.W.U.*

Kaufman, S. (1986). *The ageless self: Sources of meaning in late life.* Madison: University of Wisconsin Press.

Kohli, M. (1986). Social organization and subjective construction of the life course. In A. B. Sorensen, F. Weinert, & L. Sherrod (Eds.), *Human development: Multidisciplinary perspectives* (pp. 271–292). Hillsdale, NJ: Erlbaum.

Layder, D. (1994). *Understanding social theory.* London: Sage.

LeBlanc, L. S., & McMullin, J. A. (1997a). Falling through the cracks: Addressing the needs of individuals between employment and retirement. *Canadian Public Policy, 23*(3), 289–304.

LeBlanc, L. S., & McMullin, J. A. (1997b). *Understanding the growing complexity of retirement: The role of institutional pathways in the transition to retirement.* Unpublished manuscript.

Lofland, L. (1978). *The craft of dying: The modern face of death.* Beverly Hills: Sage.

Lowe, G. S. (1992). *Human resource challenges of education, computers and retirement.* (Catalogue number 11-612E, no. 7). Ottawa: Statistics Canada.

Lukes, S. (1974). *Power, a radical view.* London: Macmillan.

Marshall, V. W. (1994). Sociology, psychology, and the theoretical legacy of the Kansas City studies. *The Gerontologist, 34*(6), 768–774.

Marshall, V. W. (1995a). The next half-century of aging research—and thoughts for the past. *Journal of Gerontology Social Sciences, 50B*(3): S131–S133.

Marshall, V. W. (1995b). Rethinking retirement: Issues for the twenty-first century. In E. M. Gee & G. M. Gutman (Eds.), *Rethinking retirement* (pp. 31–50). Vancouver: Gerontology Research Centre, Simon Fraser University.

Marshall, V. W. (1995c). The state of theory in aging and the social sciences. In R. H. Binstock & L. K. George (Eds.), *Handbook of aging and the social sciences* (4th ed., pp. 12–30). San Diego: Academic Press.

Marshall, V. W. (1996). Death, bereavement, and the social psychology of aging and dying. In J. D. Morgan (Ed.), *Ethical issues in the care of the dying and bereaved aged* (pp. 57–75). Amityville, NY: Baywood.

Marshall, V. W. (1998). Commentary: The older worker and organisational restructuring: Beyond systems theory. In K. W. Schaie & C. Schooler (Eds.), *Impact of work on older adults* (pp. 195–206). New York: Springer Publishing Co.

Marx, K. (1967). *Capital* (Vol. 1). New York: International Publishers. (Originally published 1867.)

McDonald, L. (1996). The casualties of Canada's dualist pension policy. In V. Minichiello, N., Kendig, C. H. & Walker, A. (Eds.), *Sociology of aging: International perspectives* (pp. 304–327). International Sociological Association, Research Committee on Aging. Melbourne: THOTH.

McMullin, J. A. (1996). *Connecting age, gender, class, and ethnicity: A case study of the garment industry in Montreal.* Doctoral dissertation, Dept. of Sociology, University of Toronto.

McMullin, J. A. & Marshall, V. W. (1997, August). *Age relations: A basis of inequality in the garment industry in Montreal.* Paper presented at the 92nd Annual Meeting of the American Sociological Association, Toronto.

Mead, G. H. (1934). *Mind, self and society.* Chicago: University of Chicago Press.

Meyer, J. W. (1986). The self and the life course: Institutionalization and its effects. In A. B. Sorenson, F. E. Weinert, & L. R. Sherrod (Eds.), *Human development and the life course: Multidisciplinary perspectives* (pp. 199–216). Hillsdale, NJ: Erlbaum.

Myles, J. F. (1989). *Old age in the welfare state: The political economy of public pensions.* Kansas: The University Press of Kansas.

Palmore, E. B. (1968). The effects of aging on activities and attitudes. *The Gerontologist, 8*, 259–263.

Palmore, E. B., Burchett, B. M., Fillenbaum, G. G., George, L. K. & Wallman, L. M. (1985). *Retirement: Causes and consequences.* New York: Springer Publishing Co.

Parsons, T. (1951). *The social system.* New York: The Free Press.

Phillipson, C. (1982). *Capitalism and the construction of old age.* London: Macmillan.

Poulantzas, N. (1975). *Classes in contemporary capitalism.* London: New Left Books.

Riley, M. W. (1994). Aging and society: Past, present and future. *The Gerontologist, 34*, 436–446.

Riley, M. W., Foner, A., Hess, B., & Toby, M. L. (1969). Socialization for the middle and later years. In D. Goslin (Ed.), *Handbook of socialization theory and research* (pp. 951–982). Chicago: Rand McNally.

Riley, M. W., Foner, A., & Waring, J. (1988). Sociology of age. In N. J. Smelser (Ed.), *Handbook of sociology* (pp. 243–290). Newbury Park, CA: Sage.

Riley, M. W., Johnson, M., & Foner, A. (Eds.) (1972). *Aging and society: Volume 3. A sociology of age stratification.* New York: Russell Sage Foundation.

Riley, M. W., & Riley, J. W. Jr. (1994). Age integration and the lives of older people. *The Gerontologist, 34*, 110–115.

Smelser, N. J. (1988). Social structure. In N. J. Smelser (Ed.), *Handbook of sociology* (pp. 103–119). Newbury Park, CA: Sage.

Smelser, N. J. (1997). *Problematics of sociology: The Georg Simmel Lectures, 1995.* Berkeley: University of California Press.

Snell, J. G. (1993). The gendered construction of elderly marriage, 1900–1950. *Canadian Journal on Aging, 12*, 509–523.

Touraine, A. (1988). *Return of the actor: Social theory in post-industrial society.* (M. Godzich, Trans.). Minneapolis: University of Minnesota Press. (Originally published 1984.)

Turner, J. H. (1988). *A theory of social interaction.* Stanford, CA: Stanford University Press.

Walker, A. (1981). Towards a political economy of old age. *Ageing and society, 1*, 74–94.

Wharton, A. (1991). Structure and agency in socialist-feminist theory. *Gender and Society, 5*, 373–389.

Williams, R. H., & Wirths, C. G. (1965). *Lives through the years.* New York: Atherton.

Wright, E. O. (1985). *Classes.* London: Verso

Wrong, D. (1961). The oversocialized conception of man in modern sociology. *American Sociological Review, 26*(2), 183–193.

CHAPTER 12

Gender and Distress in Later Life: The Importance of Lifelong Employment and Familial Experiences

Lorraine Davies

The efforts of sociologists to theorize and analyze the connections between macro and micro "levels of reality" are central to our understanding of the complexities underlying social life (Marshall, 1995). Although theories illustrating these linkages have contributed much to our knowledge of aging, (see for example, Elder, 1991), they share the same limitation as theories of aging generally in that they fail to consider the relationship between gender and age relations (McMullin, 1995). Indeed, as McMullin (1995) has pointed out, aging theorists have devoted surprisingly little attention to the impact of gender as an organizing feature of social life.

The conceptualization of gender as a socially created component of structural arrangements can be attributed to feminist scholarship (see Acker, 1992) and is only recently infiltrating all aspects of sociological thought. Viewing gender as a social construction rejects the more com-

I am grateful to Dale Dannefer, Donna McAlpine, Victor Marshall, Julie Ann McMullin, Carol Ryff, and Clint Wilson for their comments on earlier versions of this work.

monly held belief that gender, based on sex, is located only within the individual, and can best be conceptualized as an individual attribute or role assessed by the dichotomous variable gender. Indeed, social constructionists argue against an essentialist notion of gender, rejecting the premise that at the core of "gender" are immutable biological differences between women and men, differences from which "gender" springs (see Fausto-Sterling, 1992; Kessler & McKenna, 1978; Lorber, 1994).

Beliefs about essential differences between women and men, however, are a central component of gender, and infiltrate both the structural arrangements of society and the actions and behaviours of individuals. Ideological systems, social structures, and individual interactions are constantly in flux and are interconnected, created by and simultaneously creating the gender arrangements specific to the historical time and cultural setting one is studying. Intertwined within these gender relations are power dynamics which distribute opportunities and rewards differentially, in favor of men as a group over women.[1]

With the recognition that gender, conditioned by historical and cultural contexts, is a component of both the macro and the micro levels of society, the social creation of gender emerges as a useful framework within which one can explore the linkages between the structural arrangements of society and individual characteristics. Although there is no explicit reference to age relations within this theory of gender, its attention to micro- and macro-level forces and the recognition that gender is a process rather than a variable make it a useful framework within which we can theorize about how gender relations are implicated with age relations to shape inequality in later life. The examination of gender inequality, then, provides an opportunity to explore the connections between and among the broader organization of society and the reality of life at the individual level.

This chapter is motivated by the lack of attention in the aging literature to the gendered nature of marriage in older age. Indeed, there is an assumption that as they age, women and men become more alike, thereby decreasing the relevance of gender as an organizing feature of marriage (Hagestad, 1987; Szinovacz, 1986–87). In an effort to challenge this premise, I strive to illuminate the gendered nature of marriage in later life by examining gender differences in psychological distress, and then by exploring how paid work and familial arrangements over the life course

---

1. While I recognize that multiple hierarchies of inequality, such as race, class and sexuality shape social life, I focus here on gender and age.

are related to distress among older wives and husbands. Although researchers have persuasively argued that gender inequality is manifested in higher rates of psychological distress among women than men generally (Horwitz, 1982; Mirowsky & Ross, 1989; Rosenfield, 1989, 1992), the relationship between gender and distress among elderly married persons has not been examined within the context of recognizing gender inequality in older age.

To the extent that marriage has been studied in later life, it has largely been disconnected from the biographies and historical circumstances that importantly influence marital relations over the life course. Consequently, it remains unclear how paid work and familial history shape the mental health of elderly persons. The results presented here rely on U.S. cross-sectional data and as such provide only a glimpse into the complexities of social life. Before turning to these results, I draw attention to the gendered nature of marriage, showing how the organization of the broader systems in society, particularly the labor force, shape and are shaped by inequities between husbands and wives. Then I show how age relations are also implicated and affect the operation of gender within marriages, drawing attention to the connections between historical and life course factors and the nature of marriage. This is followed by a discussion of how these factors might shape the psychological distress of husbands and wives in later life. I draw on both U.S. and English Canadian examples to illustrate the gendered nature of social life historically, in an attempt to capture general patterns within North American society.[2]

THE GENDERED NATURE OF MARRIAGE

Feminist scholarship has been instrumental in identifying the inequities inherent within the institution of marriage, and their connection to broader systems of male domination in society generally (e.g. Delphy, 1984; Lorber, 1994). To put simply, gender relations within marriage represent unbalanced power relations, deriving in part from women's and men's relationship to productive and reproductive relations. For example, decisions that women make about employment are constrained both by cultural expectations concerning their futures as mothers and wives and by

---

2. It is beyond the scope of this chapter to analyze the ways in which the gendered nature of social life differ between U.S. and Canada.

the reality that "women's jobs" are typically low paying, with little status (Arber & Ginn, 1995).

Resistance to a more equitable distribution of paid and unpaid work reflects adherence to traditional norms concerning the "proper" roles of wives and husbands, as well as entrenched beliefs about the meaning of gender (Ferree, 1990; West & Zimmerman, 1987). Therefore, it may appear as if women and men make unconstrained choices about work and family based on their individual desires and abilities; it may appear as if the patterns that emerge reflect "natural outcomes" of biological predispositions. In reality, however, gender "differences" in work and family responsibilities are outcomes of multiple interlocking systems of female disadvantage (Frye, 1983; Gerson & Peiss, 1985; Lorber, 1994). The rationalization of these work arrangements as "natural" and therefore "inevitable" deflects attention away from broader institutional inequities, central to which are the connections that exist between the disadvantaged status of women within and outside of the home (Lorber, 1994).

While documenting the dimensions of inequality inherent within marriage and their connections to the broader institutions in society is important, perhaps the most compelling motivation for understanding the gendered nature of social life can be found in its manifestations in differential mental health consequences by gender. Higher rates of psychological distress among wives have been attributed, in part, to these gender inequities in marriage. Lower status, or less power, among wives is evidenced by lower income, different employment experiences, greater childcare responsibilities, and greater role overload. Rosenfield (1992) argues that not-employed women "suffer from lower power in terms of prestige and resources relative to men" (p. 213); meanwhile, employed women are also disadvantaged by lower status and less rewarding work, and this contributes to greater domestic demands, and has consequences for psychological distress.

Viewed within a social constructionist framework, then, we see that gender is both a component of the labor market and a component of marriage. Assumptions about differences between women and men, and therefore about "gender", shape and are shaped by the organization of structural arrangements, and ultimately affect individual actions, interactions, and choices. While agency is constrained by larger systems, human agency has the capacity to reinforce and/or challenge social structure (Connell, 1987). We thus see that the pervasiveness of gender as it orders, and is ordered by, social life extends far beyond the individual.

GENDER, MARITAL, AND AGE RELATIONS

Interestingly, there is an assumption in the sociology of aging literature that the gendered nature of marriage may become less evident or less relevant over the life course. It has been argued that the reduction in work and childcare responsibilities in later life reduces the salience of gender and therefore female disadvantage among older married women. Furthermore, as couples age, fewer parenting and employment responsibilities may narrow the gap between women's and men's roles and create similarities instead (Hagestad, 1987). Others describe a process whereby women become more assertive and men more affiliative as they age, suggesting that similarities between women and men increase in later life as a result (Gutman, 1977). Such a convergence in gender roles implies harmony rather than conflict, equality rather than power. This view of gender is also reflected in studies documenting an improvement in marital quality over the life course, although there is some evidence that men are more satisfied than women (Quirouette & Gold, 1992). Thus, when one compares the analysis of gender in marriages of working aged adults to those of elderly persons, it seems as if gender may lose much of its relevance in later life marriage.

Yet the assumption that gender is not a relevant organizing feature of social life in older age runs counter to feminist contributions that conceptualize gender as inextricably embedded in all social relations, including class, race, and marriage (Acker, 1989; Smith, 1987). Indeed, gender as an element of structural arrangements constantly changes shape so that the form taken alters even though the consequence—gender inequality—is continually reproduced (Acker, 1989). For example, compared to their female counterparts, married elderly women are in the most financially secure position (Ballantyne & Marshall, 1995). But marriage provides a false sense of security; with limited employment histories, elderly wives' economic situation is largely dependent upon the survival of their husbands (Logue, 1991). Meyer (1990) reports that in the U.S. in 1988, married older women's median income (as separate from their husband's) was only 43% of married men's income. Indeed, in Britain, women who are or who have been married receive the lowest pension income of all elderly women (Arber & Ginn, 1991). Economic dependency, accumulated over the life course, structures power relations in favour of the husband, even in older age.

The death of their husbands thus puts many married women in a precarious financial position; this reflects the gendered nature of the society in which they grew up. These women had to manoeuvre through a world set up for, and dominated by, men (Smith, 1987). Ironically, while the loss of a spouse brings about a substantial reduction in their standard of living for many women, it is also the first time that they can spend money freely and without restriction (Ballantyne & Marshall, 1995; McMullin & Ballantyne, 1995). The constraining ties of marriage for women continue into later life.

These gendered relations are clearly historically situated—constructed, in part, through meanings and events that are rooted in the social conditions of the early 20th century. The experience of being a spouse represents a trajectory that is influenced by the political, economic, and social climate throughout the marriage. Within this trajectory may be various transitions, for example, the addition and departure of children, the acquisition or loss of jobs, as well as a host of other life events. It is important to understand how gender arrangements within the broader social context combine with individual biographies and characteristics to shape marital relations, and therefore mental health, in older age.

GENDER, HISTORICAL FACTORS, AND THE LIFE COURSE

Throughout their lives, current elderly women were subject to a societal resistance to female equality masked in an essentialist view of gender that infiltrated all aspects of society, including individual belief systems and behaviours. Biological differences between girls/women and boys/men were emphasized to justify the notion of separate spheres, which dictated that women's place was naturally in the home, while men were best equipped for the public life of employment. This division was embedded in institutions like the legal and economic systems. For example, it was not uncommon for employed women to be fired once they became married (Jones, Marsden, & Tepperman, 1990; McLaughlin et al., 1988).

Strong-Boag (1993), focussing on English Canada between 1919 to 1939, describes how from birth "individuals and institutions of every sort, from the mother to the police magistrate, from the family to the school, regarded and treated girls differently from boys (p. 8)." From the "little mother" badges that girls could earn in Girl Guides, to restrictions against young women applying for university awards, to advertisements proclaiming the importance of femininity and attractiveness for women's marital success, girls and young women were "prepared" for their "destiny" of marriage and children, and therefore their duties of wife and mother (Strong-Boag, 1993).

Restricted employment opportunities further reinforced images of difference; available positions were low-paying, offered few benefits, and were confined to "female" or "light" jobs (Jones et al., 1990; McLaughlin et al., 1988; Milkman, 1987). In fact, beliefs about the primacy of marriage justified lesser wages and job restrictions for women (who didn't really "need" more), and higher wages and job opportunities for men (who "had to" support a family) (Kessler-Harris, 1990). Therefore, the organization of society reflected an image of women as nurturers and caregivers, and ensured that this "choice" would be met with the least resistance. The movement of the majority of women into marriage and motherhood justified and recreated these structural arrangements, supporting the image of women as "best suited" for this lifestyle.

As a result of the gendered organization of structural arrangements and belief systems, married elderly women's employment trajectories were disjointed, being closely tied to their familial circumstances. Moen (1994, pp. 153, 154) describes wives' employment and family responsibilities as "sequential". Paid work was typically engaged in before and sometimes after raising a family; if it was necessary to combine the two, employment did "not seriously conflict with their principal homemaking responsibilities" (Moen, 1994, p. 154). Indeed, often in the form of taking in boarders, or doing laundry, or sewing, married women's labor was almost rendered invisible (Strong-Boag, 1993). The interdependence of work, marriage, and parenthood was such that familial commitments overshadowed the primacy of paid work (Elder, 1988). Although it was neither common nor easy for these women to work consistently throughout their lives, many were employed before they got married and had children; many more moved into the workforce in midlife (Bianchi & Spain, 1986).

World War II opened up employment opportunities for married women with and without children (McLaughlin et al., 1988), and provided a more specific example of how historical settings serve as opportunity structures (Elder & O'Rand, 1995) for gender equality. The fact that during the war years women successfully entered into "men's" jobs with minimal training and no experience attests to the socially constructed nature of sex-typing in the workplace (Milkman, 1987). Jobs that were previously defined as "male", such as welding and rivetting, were performed by women whose previous job options included housecleaning and menial factory and clerical work. For this to happen in a socially acceptable way, however, jobs were actively "feminized" to justify lower wages for women, thereby protecting men's wages and reducing the threat of segregation. Milkman's (1987) analysis of this process reveals that the redefinition of sex-typing (from "heavy" to "light" jobs) was not consistent among the auto and electrical industries across the U.S., challenging a categorical view of gender which promotes certain jobs as being intrinsically male or female (Milkman, 1987; Reskin & Roos, 1991).

The erosion of women's gains in the workplace after World War II can only be understood with attention to the particular "economic, political and social forces operative" during this time (Milkman, 1987, p. 157). Many of today's elderly women experienced this unique period of history where better paying, often more challenging "men's" jobs briefly opened up to them, only to close after the war. This phenomenon was largely successful in recreating and reinforcing the expectation that women should be mothers and wives, and also therefore in justifying the exclusionary practices that prevented more viable choices, thus reinstating a labor force segregated by traditional divisions of labor. Yet, despite the mobilization of forces aimed at returning women to "the family" after the war, many of them, particularly widowed, minority and lower-class women, desired and needed to continue working (McLaughlin et al., 1988).

Especially for minority and lower-class married women, employment was an economic necessity as well as a reality for most of their lives. Black and White women's job opportunities varied considerably during the early decades of the 1900s, with Black women mostly confined to domestic work (Bose, 1987). For example, in the United States, it was only after 1966 that restrictions limiting clerical jobs for women of color were reduced, although minority groups continue to be over-represented in "lower-level clerical jobs" (Ferree, 1987, p. 329). For lower-class and minority women, paid work experiences reflected a common, necessary, and particularly important contribution to family life (Ferree, 1990). Rather than representing these women as passive recipients of the opportunities provided by society, attention to race and class reveals them as actively engaged in the struggle to improve their family's circumstances, as well as, and despite, the oppressive economic conditions thrust on them (Ferree, 1987; Glenn, 1987).

More recently, another relevant historical period shaping women's employment experiences occurred after the 1960s, a time of reduced social constraints for women generally. For many of today's elderly, this was a period of mid-life, and it offered more opportunities for participation in paid work (Bianchi & Spain, 1986). Decisions about labor force involvement, however, appeared to depend, in part, upon health and financial necessity (Clausen & Gilens, 1990). Thus, we see the importance that historical conditions and individual resources have in shaping the labor force participation of married women.

IMPLICATIONS FOR MENTAL HEALTH IN LATER LIFE

Based on this review, I now ask how might the gendered employment and familial experiences characteristic of the life course of current elderly wives and husbands shape their present level of mental health? In other words, how can we understand the lives of older persons "in terms of their dynamic organization and reorganization across time"? (Pearlin & Skaff, 1996, p. 246). Connidis (1982) argues that a lifetime of combining family and employment careers ultimately benefits married women in later life. "Constant modification in female careers [work and family roles] over the life cycle leaves women better equipped to cope with change generally, including the adjustment to old age" (p. 23). Thus, juggling work and family may in the long run increase flexibility and coping strategies for women. Indeed, research finds that, compared to women who have never participated in the labor force, women with the experience of employment over the life course show increased self-confidence, assertiveness and intellectual investment (Clausen & Gilens, 1990). It is possible, then, that the experience of competing work and family demands throughout the life course increases one's capacity to adapt to life change, ultimately enhancing feelings of control as well as power within marriage (c.f. Spitze, Logan, Joseph, & Lee, 1994). These factors should have a positive impact on their well-being in later life.

The mental health benefits of combining employment and familial responsibilities throughout the life course may not be uniform for all married women, though. As was discussed above, work patterns vary considerably among this cohort (Connidis, 1982; Moen, 1991; Pienta, Burr, & Mutchler, 1994), and are shaped by a variety of factors including economic necessity and structural opportunities. Therefore, although the lifelong experiences of juggling work and family demands may positively impact on their mental health, it seems reasonable to expect that variations in employment patterns, in relation to family demands, may differentially shape this outcome. Therefore, the lifelong employment experiences of elderly married women vary depending upon factors like amount of part-time and full-time employment, number of interruptions, and proportion of life worked. While it seems likely that the combined experiences of paid work and family will have general long-term benefits for women, less clear is whether these benefits hold regardless of how they have been combined.

To more clearly understand the gendered nature of these connections, it is important to perform comparative analysis on men. While we would not expect the combined impact of paid work and family to be similar for women and men, less clear is how they might differ. A study by Pavalko, Elder, and Clipp (1993) is insightful in this respect. Relying on life history data from a sample of middle-class men followed from 1922 to 1992, they found that work history is consequential for mortality. Most noticeably, men whose worklife patterns consist of several different jobs experience a greater likelihood of mortality (Pavalko et al., 1993). Although they did not examine consequences of work history for psychological distress, their results do suggest that discontinuous work experience may have a negative impact on mental health among men. Thus, perhaps men with work histories that most conform to the image of a stable, continuous employee, and by implication a good "family man", will experience the greatest mental health benefits over the life course.

Methods

The sample used in this study is based on the National Survey of Families and Households[3] conducted by James Sweet, Larry Bumpass and Vaughn Call between 1987–1988. The data for this study are drawn from a national multi-stage probability sample of 13,017 households, including 9,643 adults (one adult randomly selected per household), and 3,374 persons who are either their spouse or cohabiting partner (Sweet, Bumpass, & Call, 1988). This study uses the representative sample, and draws from it a sample of 592 married elderly persons for whom data are most complete.

The dependent variable, psychological distress, is assessed by a version of the Center for Epidemiologic Depression Scale (CES-D) (Radloff, 1977). This scale typically includes 20 items that assess affective depressive symptomatology in the general population. Depressive symptomatol-

---

3. The National Survey of Families and Households was funded by a grant (HD21009) from the Center for Population research of the National Institute of Child Health and Human Development. The survey was designed and carried out at the Center for Demography and Ecology at the University of Wisconsin-Madison under the direction of Larry Bumpass and James Sweet. The field work was done by the Institute for Survey Research at Temple University.

ogy refers to depressive feelings that fall short of clinical depression. This data set includes the 12-item version of the scale reflecting depressed mood. This version has been shown to differentiate between clinically depressed persons and those without clinical depression (see Ross & Mirowsky, 1984). Responses range from 0 to 7, according to the frequency of occurrence of depressive symptoms in the last week, with a total scale range of 0 to 84.

Three variables assess lifelong work experience. First, "percentage of life employed" is based on a sum of the number of years in a respondent's life where she or he worked more than 6 months, and divided by the respondent's current age. Percentage of life worked during and following childbearing years was also assessed. Percentage worked during childbearing years was computed by dividing the number of years worked between the ages of 18 and 45 years, by 27 (total number of possible years worked). Percentage worked after childbearing years was computed by dividing the number of years worked after age 45 by the respondents' age minus 45. Respondents were also characterized by their lifelong employment status and the number of periods in their life that they worked. Lifelong employment status is operationalized here as: never employed; always employed part-time; employed both part-time and full-time; always employed full-time. Number of work periods is a continuous variable ranging from 0 (never worked) to 10 (worked during 10 different periods).

In addition to looking at employment indicators, family demands were also assessed through the number of children born. Along with age and race, the other demographic variables include education (number of years of schooling completed) and income (total couple income). Missing values on the income variable were substituted by the mean of the similar gender and work status group. Finally, given the documented association between physical and mental health among older persons, self-assessed health was included as a control in the multivariate analyses. This item asks, "Compared with other people your age, how would you describe your health?" Responses range from very poor to excellent.

Results

As Table 12.1 demonstrates, the married elderly persons in this sample are overwhelmingly White, middle-class, and young-old. Not surprisingly, the men on average spent approximately 59% of their lives employed, while women were employed 25%. Greater workforce participation among men than women also occurs during and after childbearing years. For the variable number of work periods, women and men do not significantly differ; the average number of work periods is approximately 1 1/2 for each.

With respect to employment status, women are more likely than men to report never having been employed (14.8% versus 1.8%). Women are similarly more likely than men to be employed always part-time and both part- and full-time, while men are more likely to report always working full-time. Among women, 54.3% always worked full-time. In comparison, the majority of men worked either full-time (81%) or both full- and part-time (16.4%). On average, both women and men had 2.6 children.

Finally, women report significantly higher distress scores than men ($\bar{x}$ = 15.2 vs 10.8). Whether the different characteristics and patterns of work differ for women and men, and consequently matter differently for their mental health, is still unclear. Among certain subgroups of the sample, work patterns may interact with family conditions to result in different patterns of distress by gender.

To focus more closely on this issue, Table 12.2 presents regression coefficients separately for ever-employed women and men of distress on each employment characteristic individually, controlling for age, income, education, race, and health. Among women, the percentage of one's total life spent in paid employment is positively associated with current levels of distress (b = .19, p <.05). That is, among employed women, the greater the percentage of their life spent employed, the higher their level of depression in older age. In order to assess whether this association holds for employment generally or is specific to time employed during different periods of one's life, percentage of life worked was broken down into the amount of time worked during, and after, childbearing years. As Table 12.2 reveals, both percentage of life worked during and after childbearing years are positively associated with level of depression. Work periods, the next characteristic of lifelong employment, is not significantly related to distress.

The final lifelong employment characteristic, work status, is significantly related to distress for women. Specifically, women who have worked both full-time and part-time throughout their lives experience more distress than women who have always worked full-time. This suggests that the negative consequences of duration spent in employment on distress in later life may not be uniform across all types of work; variations in employment trajectories by work status may also shape patterns of distress in later life. These lifelong work variables are not mutually exclusive, but rather are interrelated, and should therefore be examined in combination.

In this regard, Table 12.3 examines the relationship between percentage of life worked, domestic demands and distress by work status (i.e., "both

Table 12.1 Descriptive Characteristics by Gender

Variables	Women		Men
Demographics			
White (%)	94.9		94.0
Education ($\bar{x}$) (s.d.)	11.4 (2.7)		11.2 (3.8)
Age ($\bar{x}$) (s.d.)	71.2 (5.4)	*	72.1 (5.7)
Income ($\bar{x}$) (s.d.)	27901.1 (24616.5)		28106.5 (26909.4)
Health ($\bar{x}$) (s.d.)	3.7 (.88)		3.8 (.90)
Employment			
Percent Employed:			
Total Life	25.0	*	58.8
Childbearing Years	31.9	*	85.3
Middle Years	20.3	*	43.4
Number of Work Periods ($\bar{x}$) (s.d.)	1.6(1.1)		1.5(.9)
Employment Status:			
Never (%)	14.8	*	1.8
Always Part-time (%)	6.6	*	.7
Both Full & Part-time (%)	24.2	*	16.4
Always Full-time (%)	54.3	*	81.0
Family Demands			
Number of Children ($\bar{x}$) (s.d.)	2.6 (2.0)		2.6 (1.8)
Psychological Distress			
C-ESD ($\bar{x}$) (s.d.)	15.2 (18.9)	*	10.8 (13.6)
n	256		336

* $p \leq =.05$

full- and part-time" and "always full-time") for women, controlling for demographic variables. Model I for each group indicates that while the relationship between percentage of life worked and distress is significant for women who have combined full- and part-time employment ($b = .42$, $p < .05$), it is not significant for those who have worked full-time ($b = .14$ n.s.). It appears, then, that the negative impact of percentage of life spent in paid work on distress is limited to those women whose employment trajectories are characterized by both full- and part-time jobs. For these women, the more time spent working is associated with greater distress in later life.

Model II for each group assesses the impact of domestic demands on the relationship between employment and distress by adding the variable

Table 12.2 Regression Coefficients of Distress on Employment Characteristics,[1] Controlling for Demographic Variables,[2] by Gender

	Women b (se[b])	Men b (se[b])
Percent Employed: Total Life	.19* (.06)	.03 (.06)
Percent Employed: Childbearing Years	.09* (.04)	.02 (.04)
Percent Employed: Middle Years	.18* (.06)	.02 (.05)
Employment Periods	1.42 (1.28)	1.71*(.81)
Work Status[3]:		
Always Part-time	−1.29 (4.60)	−9.13 (7.40)
Both Full and Part-time	5.38*(2.76)	2.27 (1.87)
n	217	329

[1] Sample excludes never employed.
[2] Each work variable entered separately, controlling for age, race, education, income and health.
[3] Reference category—Always full-time
* $p \leq .05$

"number of children". For women who have worked both full- and part-time, the amount of time employed continues to be a significant predictor of distress ($b = .32, p < .05$). Moreover, the number of children is also significant, but it is negatively associated with distress ($b = −3.90, p < .05$). Thus, the more time one has spent in full- and part-time jobs the greater distress reported, yet the more children one has, the less distress reported. In order to look more closely at this, Model III explores the interaction term of time worked and number of children. The interaction term is significant, ($b = −.23$), suggesting that the effect of proportion of time worked on distress is conditional upon the number of children. For women with few children, the relationship between proportion worked and distress is stronger than for women with many children. Interestingly, then, for women with few children, more time in the workforce is associated with greater distress. Yet as the number of children increases, more time spent in the workforce is not associated with greater distress.

Among women who worked full-time, although neither the percentage of time worked nor the number of children has a main effect on distress, the interaction term of time worked and number of children is positive and significant ($b = .09, p < .05$). This also suggests that the impact of propor-

Table 12.3 Regression Coefficients of Distress on Employment and Family Characteristics for Women, by Work Status[1]

| | Both Full- and Part-Time | | | | | | Always Full-Time | | | | | |
| | Model I | | Model II | | Model III | | Model I | | Model II | | Model III | |
	b	se[b]	b	se[b]	b	se[b]	b	se[b]	b	se[b]	b	se[b]
Percent of life employed	.42*	.16	.32*	.15	.94*	.28	.14	.08	.16	.08	–.05	.12
No. of children			–3.90*	1.62	3.51	3.30			.99	.82	–1.48	1.39
Percent of life employed X No. of children					–.23*	.09					.09*	.04
R²	.17*		.23*		.30*		.10*		.11*		.13*	

[1] Each model controls for age, race, education, income and health.
*p≤.05

tion worked on distress is conditioned by the number of children, but differently from those who worked both full- and part-time. The relationship between time in the workforce and distress is not significant for those women who worked full-time and had few children. For those with many children, the more time spent in employment, the greater the level of distress in later life.

Finally, the amount of variance explained in the models for women who have worked "both full- and part-time" is greater than that for women who have worked full-time. This suggests that the variables of time employed and number of children have more explanatory power for women who have combined full- and part-time employment than for women who have always worked full-time. Thus, the nature of one's work status appears to be an important differentiating factor among women, and points to the need to look more closely at variations in work patterns among women.

To return to Table 12.2, and to follow a similar logic of analysis for men, we see that, among husbands, only number of employment periods is significantly related to distress. So, for men, the more discontinuous their lifelong work periods, the higher their current levels of distress. Table 12.4 assesses the impact of distress on work periods, family demands, and the interaction of work periods and family demands.

Model I re-iterates the significant impact of employment, or work periods, on distress. Model II introduces the impact of family demands, which are not significant for men. In Model III, the interaction term indicates that the distressing impact of work periods is conditioned by number of children, so that for men with fewer children, number of work periods translates into distress at a greater rate than for men with more children. Thus, for men, discontinuous work histories are associated with higher distress in later life. Moreover, this effect is shaped by family conditions, being most pronounced for men with fewer children.

DISCUSSION AND CONCLUSIONS

Unique sociohistorical, gendered structural arrangements, and conditions characterize the lives of older wives and husbands, shaping their employment patterns, their experience of family demands and their level of mental health. For the most part, the employment experiences of elderly women occurred within a societal ideology that endorsed the primacy of childcare and spousal duties over employment responsibilities for women.

Table 12.4 Regression Coefficients of Distress on Employment and Family Characteristics for Men[1]

	Model I		Model II		Model III	
	b	se[b]	*b*	se[b]	*b*	se[b]
No. of work periods	1.79*	(.78)	1.78*	(.78)	3.98*	(1.34)
No. of children			.16	(.39)	1.49*	(.77)
No. of work periods × No. of children					−.81*	(.40)
R^2		.17*		.16*		.17*

[1] Each model controls for age, race, education, income and health.
* $p \leq .05$

Therefore, compared to current cohorts of young women, these women were much less likely to have expected to work outside of the home. Nonetheless, the overwhelming majority of these women did work outside of the home at some point in their lives, both for reasons of financial necessity and for personal gratification (Kessler-Harris, 1990). For men, their responsibilities as providers for their family were clear, and structural arrangements greatly facilitated this role (Kessler-Harris, 1990). The degree to which work arrangements responded to familial conditions is a basic difference between the lives of married women and men.

Drawing on the life course perspective, which argues that individuals' current circumstances partly reflect the accumulation of their life experiences (Moen & Forest, 1995), I attempted to more closely examine the impact of gendered work arrangements over the life course on levels of distress in later life. I interpret the finding that elderly wives report significantly higher rates of psychological distress than husbands as an indication that gender inequality continues to exist in later life. Rather than examine the current ways in which marital arrangements impact on psychological distress, I instead explored the linkages between the broader context of one's life and one's current mental health. The recognition that inequities in marriage are rooted in historical circumstances serves as an important stepping stone upon which future research should elaborate. I tried to show that age relations are gendered, and both age and gender shape marital relations in later life. As women and men move through the life course, or age, their opportunities are constrained and enabled by a world that is not gender-neutral. Thus, gender and age, in all of their complexities, order social life.

Considering the serious limitations imposed by the cross-sectional sample design, the fact that significant associations emerged among lifelong family demands, employment conditions, and current levels of psychological distress attests to the strength of the connections among these factors. That lifelong employment characteristics are related to distress in later life differently for women and men is not surprising, given the gendered nature of the means of production and reproduction. Normative expectations for men were that they conform to full-time, long-term employment with minimal work interruptions, in the expectation that this best enabled them to provide for their wives and children. The analysis presented here suggests that men who did not conform to this pattern experience greater distress in older age. Moreover, this relationship is most pronounced among those with fewer, as opposed to many children. A selection effect may also be operating, however, in that distressed husbands may have been more likely to hold many jobs during their lifetimes and they may have had fewer children.

Another central question was whether the lifelong experience of juggling paid work and family has psychological benefits for women in later life. Examined in the context of women's employment patterns over the life course, juggling "work and family" could take on several different forms and meanings, ranging from the simultaneous experience of employment and familial responsibilities to the absence of paid work during times of high family demands, with considerable variation of movement in and out of the labor force in between these two extremes. The results reveal that most women worked either full-time or combined full- and part-time jobs. Very few women reported that they had worked mostly part-time throughout their lives or were not employed at all. Moreover, variation exists both in duration of time spent in employment and in number of jobs.

That employment duration did not affect distress among women who worked full-time throughout their lives, although it did among women who combined full- and part-time employment, suggests that work conditions between these groups may differ. The jobs held by women who describe their work patterns as consisting of both full- and part-time employment may have been characterized by fewer opportunities for promotion, fewer benefits, intrinsic rewards, or less control, all of which have been found to benefit mental health (Lennon and Rosenfield, 1992).

My results also alert us to the importance of recognizing the interconnections between employment and familial relations, and to the necessity of exploring how they operate throughout the life course to shape distress.

Finding that the impact of employment duration on distress is conditioned by the number of children, and is conditioned differently depending upon whether women's paid work trajectory is always full-time or both full- and part-time, highlights the different ways in which the public and private domains overlap, but leaves to speculation the processes through which these strategies result in different mental health consequences. Connidis' (1982) premise that women who were more likely to juggle family and paid work responsibilities would benefit in older age was not supported, at least when looking at mental health benefits. The relationship between the intersection of paid work and family responsibilities appears to be much more complex. For those who worked both full- and part-time, children reduce the negative impact of work duration, so that for those with few children, work duration translates into distress at a greater rate than for those with more children.

That the opposite effect was found among women who always worked full-time could be suggestive of the long-term implications of work over-load. Working full-time while rearing children was most typical for working-class women. Greater financial strain, fewer resources, and little recognition for or assistance with the difficulties of combining paid and unpaid work may have a lasting, negative impact on mental health.

There appears to be a substantive difference between the impact of work histories on distress for those who always worked full-time and those who included part-time employment, with the impact of each on distress depending on the amount of time worked and the number of children involved. A more comprehensive study of the processes behind these associations would better illuminate the patterning of these events within individual trajectories, and the importance of economic and social resources—as well as the more gendered, cohort-specific cultural and historical context—in shaping decisions about paid work and family.

IMPLICATIONS FOR THE MICRO/MACRO LINKAGE

Structural arrangements are not neutral in their treatment of women and men, and such differential or inequitable treatment has health implications. Behavior at the individual level reflects choices constrained by macro-level forces. The fact that women and men differ in their orientations toward paid and unpaid work needs to be understood as emerging from largely invisible, interlocking systems of inequality that are embedded in social structures which reflect and reinforce beliefs about essential differences between women and men. These belief systems infiltrate individual perceptions about gender, serving to deflect attention away from the power inequities inherent in the way we "do gender" at both the macro and micro levels (West & Zimmerman, 1987).

Indeed, individuals are also active participants in the creation of gender, serving both to reinforce and challenge these broader systems. Thus, it is important to recognize that the components of gender include the individual as an active agent with the potential to change and challenge existing systems. This is why the gendered nature of social life is continually in flux, and is therefore more appropriately viewed as a process rather than as a variable. Gender relations, however, do not exist in isolation, but rather function as part of other systems of inequality like race/ethnicity, class, and age (McMullin, 1996). While the focus of this chapter has been on the intersection of age and gender relations, we should recognize that individuals are dominated or privileged depending upon these other central axes of inequality as well, none of which exists alone. Questions about the mechanisms linking macro and micro levels of reality are ultimately also questions about change. Identifying the means through which structures influence individual outcomes, and individual negotiations modify structural arrangements, helps us understand social change as a whole. For the women in this sample, the decisions they made about entering the workplace, albeit constrained by the larger historical, structural, and ideological systems at play, made possible greater opportunities for future generations of women because they negotiated a new terrain of paid work and family for younger women to tread upon, just as previous generations of women did for them.

REFERENCES

Acker, J. (1989). The problem with patriarchy. *Sociology, 23*, 235–240.

Acker, J. (1992). Gendered institutions: From sex roles to gendered institutions. *Contemporary Sociology, 21*(5), 565–569.

Arber, S., & Ginn, J. (1991). *Gender and later life: A sociological analysis of resources and constraints.* London: Sage.

Arber, S., & Ginn, J. (1995). The mirage of gender equality: Occupational success in the labour market and within marriage. *British Journal of Sociology, 46*(1), 21–43.

Ballantyne, P., & Marshall, V. W. (1995). Wealth and the life course. In V. W.

Marshall, J. A. McMullin, P. J. Ballantyne, J. F. Daciuk, & B. T. Wigdor (Eds.), *Contributions to independence over the adult life course* (pp. 49–83). Toronto: Centre for Studies of Aging, University of Toronto.

Bianchi, S. M., & Spain, D. (1986). *American women in transition*. New York: Russell Sage Foundation.

Bose, C. E. (1987). Dual spheres. In B. B. Hess & M. M. Ferree (Eds.), *Analyzing gender: A handbook of social science research* (pp. 267–285). Newbury Park, CA: Sage.

Clausen, J. A., & Gilens, M. (1990). Personality and labor force participation across the life course: A longitudinal study of women's careers. *Sociological Forum, 5*(4), 595–618.

Connell, R. W. (1987). *Gender and power: Society, the person and sexual politics*. Cambridge: Polity Press.

Connidis, I. (1982). Women and retirement: The effect of multiple careers on retirement adjustment. *Canadian Journal on Aging, 1*(3), 17–27.

Delphy, C. (1984). *Close to home: A materialist analysis of women's oppression*. Amherst, MA: The University of Massachusetts Press.

Elder, G. H., Jr. (1988). Foreword. In S. D. McLaughlin, B. D. Melber, J. O. G. Billy, D. M. Zimmerle, L. D. Winges, & T. R. Johnson (Eds.), *The changing lives of American women* (pp. xii–xvi). Chapel Hill, NC: The University of North Carolina Press.

Elder, G. H. Jr. (1991). Lives and social change. In W. R. Heinz (Ed.), *Theoretical advances in life course research* (pp. 58–86). Weinheim: Deitscher Studien Verlag.

Elder, G. H., Jr., & O'Rand, A. M. (1995). Adult lives in a changing society. In K. Cook, G. A. Fine, & J. S. House (Eds.), *Social perspectives on social psychology* (pp. 452–475) New York: Allyn and Bacon.

Fausto-Sterling, A. (1992). *Myths of gender*. New York: Basic Books.

Ferree, M. M. (1987). She works hard for a living: Gender and class on the job. In B. B. Hess & M. M. Ferree (Eds.), *Analyzing gender: A handbook of social science research* (pp. 322–347). Newbury Park, CA: Sage.

Ferree, M. M. (1990). Beyond separate spheres: Feminism and family research. *Journal of Marriage and the Family, 52*, 866–884.

Frye, M. (1983). *The politics of reality: Essays in feminist theory*. Freedom, CA: The Crossing Press.

Gerson, J. & Peiss, K. (1985). Boundaries, negotiation, consciousness: Reconceptualizing gender relations. *Social Problems, 32*, 317–31.

Glenn, E. N. (1987). Gender and the family. In B. B. Hess & M. M. Ferree (Eds.), *Analyzing gender: A handbook of social science research* (pp. 348–380). Newbury Park, CA: Sage.

Gutman, D. (1977). The cross-cultural perspective: Notes toward a comparative psychology of aging. In J. E. Birren & K. W. Schaie (Eds.), *Handbook of the psychology of aging* (pp. 303–326). New York: Van Nostrand Reinhold.

Hagestad, G. O. (1987). Able elderly in the family context: Changes, chances, and challenges. *The Gerontologist, 27*(4), 417–422.

Horwitz, A. V. (1982). Sex-role expectations, power, and psychological distress. *Sex Roles, 8*(6), 607–623.

Jones, C., Marsden, L., & Tepperman, L. (1990). *Lives of their own: The individualization of women's lives.* Toronto: Oxford University Press.

Kessler, S. J., & McKenna, W. (1978). *Gender: An ethnomethodological approach.* Chicago: The University of Chicago Press.

Kessler-Harris, A. (1990). *A woman's wage: Historical meanings and social consequences.* Lexington, Kentucky: The University Press of Kentucky.

Lennon, M. C., & Rosenfield, S. (1992). Women and mental health: The interaction of job and work conditions. *Journal of Health and Social Behavior, 33*(4), 316–327.

Logue, B. J. (1991). Women at risk: Predictors of financial stress for retired women workers. *The Gerontologist, 31*(5), 657–665.

Lorber, J. (1994). *Paradoxes of gender.* New Haven, CT: Yale University Press.

Marshall, V. W. (1995). The micro-macro link in the sociology of aging. In C. Hummel & C. J. L. D'Epinay (Eds.), *Images of aging in Western societies* (pp. 334–371). Geneva: Centre for Interdisciplinary Gerontology, University of Geneva.

McLaughlin, S. D., Melber, B. D., Billy, J. O. G., Zimmerle, D. M., Winges, L. D., & Johnson, T. R. (1988). *The changing lives of American women.* Chapel Hill, NC: The University of North Carolina Press.

McMullin, J. A. (1995). Theorizing age and gender relations. In S. Arber & J. Ginn (Eds.), *Connecting gender and aging: A sociological approach.* Milton Keynes, England: Open University Press.

McMullin, J. A. (1996). *Connecting age, gender, class and ethnicity: A case study of the garment industry in Montreal.* Unpublished doctoral dissertation, University of Toronto, Toronto, Ontario, Canada.

McMullin, J. A., & Ballantyne, P. (1995). Employment characteristics and income: Assessing gender and age group effects for Canadians aged 45 years and over. *Canadian Journal of Sociology, 20*(4), 519–555.

Meyer, M. H. (1990). Family status and poverty among older women: The gendered distribution of retirement income in the United States. *Social Problems, 37*(4), 551–563.

Milkman, R. (1987). *Gender at work: The dynamics of job segregation by sex during World War II.* Urbana, IL: University of Illinois Press.

Mirowsky, J., & Ross, C. E. (1989). *Social causes of psychological distress.* New York: Aldine de Gruyter.

Moen, P. (1994). Women, work, and family: A sociological perspective on changing roles. In M. W. Riley, R. L. Kahn, & A. Foner (Eds.), *Age and structural lag: Society's failure to provide meaningful opportunities in work, family and leisure* (pp. 151–170). New York: Wiley.

Moen, P. (1991). Transitions in mid-life: Women's work and family roles in the 1970s. *Journal of Marriage and the Family, 53*, 135–150.

Moen, P., & Forest, K. B. (1995). Family policies for an aging society: Moving to the twenty-first century. *The Gerontologist, 35*(6), 825–830.

Nolen-Hoeksema, S. (1987). Sex differences in unipolar depression: Evidence and theory. *Psychological Bulletin, 101*(2), 259–282.

Pavalko, E. K., Elder, G. H., Jr., & Clipp, E. (1993). Worklives and longevity: Insights from a life course perspective. *Journal of Health and Social Behavior, 34*, 363–380.

Pearlin, L. I., & Skaff, M. M. (1996). Stress and the life course: A paradigmatic alliance. *Gerontologist, 36*(2), 239–248.

Pienta, A. M., Burr, J. A., & Mutchler, J. E. (1994). Women's labor force participation in later life: The effects of early work and family experiences. *Journal of Gerontology, Social Sciences, 49*(5), S231–S239.

Quirouette, C., & Gold, D. P. (1992). Spousal characteristics as predictors of well-being in older couples. *International Journal of Aging and Human Development, 34*, 257–269.

Radloff, L. S. (1977). The CES-D scale: A self-report depression scale for research in the general population. *Journal of Applied Psychological Measurement, 1*, 385–401.

Reskin, B. F., & Roos, P. A. (1990). *Job queues, gender queues: Explaining women's inroads into male occupations.* Philadelphia: Temple University Press.

Rosenfield, S. (1989). The effects of women's employment: Personal control and sex differences in mental health. *Journal of Health and Social Behavior, 30*, 77–91.

Rosenfield, S. (1992). The costs of sharing: Wives' employment and husbands' mental health. *Journal of Health and Social Behavior, 33*, 213–225.

Ross, C. E., & Mirowsky, J. (1984). Components of depressed mood in married men and women. *American Journal of Epidemiology, 119*, 997–1004.

Smith, D. E. (1987). *The everyday world as problematic: A feminist sociology.* Toronto: University of Toronto Press.

Spitze, G., Logan, J. R., Joseph, G., & Lee, E. (1994). Middle generation roles and the well-being of men and women. *Journal of Gerontology, 49*(3), S107–S116.

Strong-Boag, V. (1993). *The new day recalled: Lives of girls and women in English Canada 1919–1939.* Toronto: Copp Clark Pitman Ltd.

Sweet, J., Bumpass, L., & Call, V. (1988). *The design and content of the National Survey of Families and Households* (Working Paper NSFH-1). Madison, WI: Center for Demography and Ecology, University of Wisconsin-Madison.

Szinovacz, M. (1986–87). Preferred retirement timing and retirement satisfaction in women. *International Journal of Aging and Human Development, 24*(4), 301–317.

West, C., & Zimmerman, D. H. (1987). Doing gender. *Gender and Society, 1*(2), 125–141.

CHAPTER 13

The Caregiving Context: The Intersection of Social and Individual Influences in the Experience of Family Caregiving

Marsha Mailick Seltzer & Jan S. Greenberg

INTRODUCTION

In this chapter, we consider how the experience of family caregiving is conditioned by both contextual and individual influences. We summarize a program of research which examines how specific elements of the caregiving context exert important influences on the psychological well-being

We acknowledge the significant contributions of our colleagues Marty Wyngaarden Krauss of Brandeis University and Lydia Li of the University of Wisconsin to the research described in this chapter. Support for the research was provided by grants from the NIMH (R03 MH46564), and the National Institute on Aging (R01 AG08768 and R01 AG09388), and from the Waisman Center at the University of Wisconsin and the Starr Center, Heller School, Brandeis University.

of caregivers, above and beyond the objective demands of providing care. The two contexts of caregiving we examine are 1) the type of disability of the care recipient, and 2) the kinship relationship between the caregiver and care recipient, which we address sequentially in this chapter.

Most past studies of caregiving have examined two questions. The first concerns the extent to which the objective demands of giving care to a relative with health problems or disabilities negatively affect the well-being of the person providing care. The stresses of caregiving are notable and there is now considerable evidence that such stresses take a toll on the well-being of the caregiver psychologically, physically, financially, and socially (Aneshensel, Pearlin, Mullan, Zarit, & Whitlach, 1995; Brody, 1985; Kiecolt-Glaser, Dura, Speicher, Trask, & Glaser, 1991; Lawton, Moss, Kleban, Glisksman, & Rovine, 1991; Pruchno, Peters, & Burant, 1995).

However, there is also evidence that the caregiving role is not experienced uniformly, and that there is great heterogeneity in its effects on the caregiver. In fact, for many caregivers, there are positive consequences of assuming this role, such as feelings of gratification that emanate from helping a loved one or a renewed sense of purpose in life. Such positive consequences exist side by side with the more negative outcomes that predominate (Kramer, 1997; Lawton et al., 1991). This leads to the second question that has been addressed in research on caregiving, namely what are the factors that explain the heterogeneity of response of caregivers? For this second line of research, many studies have used a stress and coping model which posits that the effects of a potentially stressful situation, such as family caregiving, are dependent on the adequacy of personal and social resources, such as an individual's ability to cope with challenges and the social supports that are available to aid in this endeavor (Pearlin, Lieberman, Menaghan, & Mullan, 1981). Many studies have shown that productive coping lessens the negative impact of the stresses of caregiving (Haley, Levine, Brown, & Bartolucci, 1987; Pratt, Schmall, Wright, & Cleveland, 1985), as does having an adequate network of supportive relationships (George & Gwyther, 1986; Zarit, Reever, & Bach-Peterson, 1980).

In most family caregiving research, social factors are conceptualized as background variables which need to be controlled. However, theoretical perspectives on the stress process call attention to how social factors provide the context for understanding individual responses to stress (George, 1993; Mattlin, Wethington, & Kessler, 1990; Pearlin, 1989; Ryff, 1987; Thoits, 1995). In other words, the larger social context in which the stress occurs affects the success of one's coping efforts and the usefulness of social support in mitigating the effects of stress. For example, as Thoits

(1995) points out, gender conditions the stress and coping process; women are generally more vulnerable to interpersonal stresses, whereas financial and job-related stresses seem to take a greater toll on men. Folkman (1984) has made a similar observation about coping, noting that the controllability of the stressful situation (which often is a function of one's social status) will affect the success of various coping efforts.

We think there is a need to expand the focus of caregiving research to investigate how larger social factors may determine the extent to which personal and social resources (such as coping and social support) are helpful in reducing the stresses of caregiving. We have designed our research to bring aspects of the caregiving context that are closely linked to macro social processes from the background into the foreground. Our program of research includes three longitudinal studies of caregiving. In two, we are studying aging mothers who provide care to an adult child with a chronic disability—either mental retardation or mental illness. In the other study, wives who provide care to their elderly husband are contrasted with adult daughters who provide care to their elderly parent. Thus, in our research, the caregiving context is defined both by variations in the type of disability of the care recipient—mental retardation, mental illness, the problems of old age—and by variations in the kinship relationship of the care provider to the care recipient—mother, daughter, or wife.

We focus on the type of disability and kinship relationship as dimensions of the caregiving context because of their connection to larger social factors that shape the individual's experience of caregiving. Regarding disability, the adequacy of community-based services varies considerably depending on the nature of the disability. Society has developed a more comprehensive system of services for persons with mental retardation and for the elderly than for those with psychiatric disorders. Persons with mental illness confront a considerably more depleted service menu, and are at much greater risk of having no services and even to be homeless (Rossi, Wright, Fisher, & Willis, 1987). The differential responsiveness of communities in meeting the service needs of persons with different types of disabilities may reflect underlying cultural beliefs and attitudes about the etiology of these disabilities. For years, parents of persons with mental illness have been blamed both by professionals and the general public for their child's condition. In contrast, the causes of other types of disabilities, such as mental retardation and Alzheimer's disease, have not been viewed as the fault of the family, and society, in general, and service providers, in particular, have responded with greater understanding and support.

In a similar vein, wife caregivers may experience the service system differently than daughters who provide care, and the service system may have different expectations of them. Wives and daughters, in turn, may have different expectations regarding the extent to which they need social and health services to enable them to provide the needed care. Thus, daughters may define the boundaries of the public-private caregiving partnership differently than do wives (Hooyman & Gonyea, 1995). Daughters are more likely than wives to have multiple role demands, given their earlier stage in the life course, and may expect supportive services to help them deal with parental needs so that they can continue to meet their other role expectations. Wives, in contrast, may be more reluctant to interact with the service system, both because caregiving is a natural extension of the wife role and because of cohort-specific attitudes regarding formal services. Thus, the nature of the disability and the kinship relationship are linked to larger social factors that influence caregiving role expectations and behaviors, and determine access to community resources and supports to cope with the challenges of caregiving.

There is some past research that has examined both of these elements of the caregiving context. Although several studies have found no differences between caregivers for care recipients with different types of disabilities or health problems (Cattanach & Tebes, 1991; Dura, Haywood-Niler, & Kiecolt-Glaser, 1990; Rabins, Fitting, Eastman, & Fetting, 1990), a larger number of studies revealed differences in the level of caregiver's well-being depending on the type of disability of the care recipient (e.g., Clipp & George, 1993; Haley et al., 1987; Holroyd & McArthur, 1976; Karlin & Bell, 1992; Kiecolt-Glaser et al., 1991; Pruchno, Patrick, & Burant, 1996; Seltzer, Krauss, & Tsunematsu, 1993; Sistler, 1989).

Another body of research has questioned whether the type of kinship relationship of the caregiver and the care recipient affects the well-being of the caregiver. Most studies have found differences between wife and daughter caregivers. In general, wife caregivers report more burden (Cantor, 1983; Harper & Lund, 1990) and have poorer physical and psychological well-being than daughter caregivers (George & Gwyther, 1986; Quayhagen & Quayhagen, 1988). Aneshensel and colleagues have shown that the type of kinship relationship may be related to feelings of role overload, role captivity, and loss of intimate exchange (Aneshensel et al., 1995).

These studies have shown that both type of disability and kinship relationship affect the caregiver's well-being. Few, however, have addressed the question of whether personal and social resources operate differently depending on these elements of the context of caregiving (Pruchno et al.,

1996). This is an important distinction. Whereas the former questions whether a family member caring for a person with cancer, for example, differs in well-being from a family member caring for a relative with Alzheimer's disease, or whether a wife caring for her husband differs in well-being from a daughter caring for her aging parent, the latter line of research questions why such differences exist. In the latter tradition, we question whether the caregiving context alters the effectiveness of coping efforts and the impact of social support.

DESCRIPTION OF OUR PROGRAM OF RESEARCH

Our three studies are designed similarly. The first is an investigation of aging mothers of adults with mental retardation (Seltzer & Krauss, 1994). The second is a study of aging mothers of adults with mental illness (Greenberg, 1995). The third contrasts wives providing care to an elderly husband with adult daughters providing care to an elderly parent (Seltzer & Li, 1996). In all three, the primary respondent is a woman who is providing care to a close relative. We collect data via personal interviews conducted with the caregiver, augmented by self-administered questionnaires. All three studies are longitudinal, although in this chapter we present only cross-sectional analyses.

The three studies share similar conceptualizations of the stress of caregiving, focusing on the demands for direct care due to the functional limitations of and the behavioral problems manifested by the care recipient. We also look to similar personal resources of the caregiver that can buffer or otherwise modify the effect of these stressors, namely coping and social support. In addition, all of our studies employ a multidimensional conceptualization of caregiver well-being. However, in this chapter we focus on one dimension, namely depressive symptoms. Among family caregivers, there is a higher frequency of depressive symptoms (Dura, Stukenberg, & Kiecolt-Glaser, 1990). Also, as caregiving involves loss and deprivation, the use of effective coping strategies and the receipt of social support can promote feelings of control and self-worth that counteract depressive symptoms (George, 1989; Haley et al., 1987; Stoller & Pugliesi, 1989).

Thus, our program of research consists of three similarly conceptualized and similarly designed studies of different caregiving contexts, which provide us with the opportunity to address the question of whether the caregiving context affects mechanisms by which personal resources, such as coping and social support, counteract the negative effects of caregiving stress. In this chapter, we begin by examining how the type of disability of the care recipient defines the caregiving context, contrasting aging mothers of adults with mental retardation and aging mothers of adults with mental illness. We investigate whether the same coping strategies have different effects on maternal depressive symptoms, depending on whether the care is provided to an adult child with mental retardation or mental illness. Next, we examine how the type of kinship relationship between caregiver and care recipient defines the caregiving context, contrasting wives caring for their elderly husband with adult daughters caring for their elderly parent. In this analysis, we examine whether social support operates differently for caregiving wives than for daughters in this role. Finally, in the last segment of this chapter, we consider next steps in this line of inquiry and implications for theories of the stress process.

THE CAREGIVING CONTEXT AS A FUNCTION OF THE TYPE OF DISABILITY

Similarities and Contrasts Between Mental Retardation and Mental Illness

We selected mental retardation and mental illness to highlight how the disability of the care recipient affects the caregiving context because older parents whose child has one of these types of disabilities face overlapping, yet distinct, sets of stressors. Their experiences are similar with respect to their feelings of loss and grief associated with the realization that their child will not experience a normal life. Both mental retardation and serious mental illness are chronic conditions that limit an individual's capacity to function independently in the community without support. In addition, a common history of deinstitutionalization in the 1960s and 1970s has increased the importance of the caregiving role of the family in the lives of adults with mental retardation and mental illness. Finally, parents of both groups experience similar worries about their child's future when they, the parents, are no longer able to provide the needed care or supervision.

There are also distinct differences in their caregiving experiences. First, whereas mental retardation is ordinarily diagnosed at birth or within the first few years of the child's life, the onset of mental illness generally occurs during adolescence or young adulthood. Thus, the period of family caregiving extends considerably longer for parents of persons with mental retardation than persons with mental illness.

Second, the course of mental illness is less stable than the course of mental retardation. The behavioral problems of mental illness create a situation in which parents experience considerable uncertainty and distress regarding how their adult son or daughter will react in everyday interactions. In contrast, most adults with mental retardation show comparatively few behavior problems, and stability in their functional and cognitive abilities (Eyman & Widaman, 1987).

Third, there are many differences in the mental retardation and the mental health service delivery systems. In particular, community-based services for adults with mental illness historically have been less well-developed than such services for persons with mental retardation, with a greater burden consequently falling on the family. Although persons with mental retardation vary in the extent to which their service needs are met, in general they have access to a more differentiated array of publicly-funded supports and services (Braddock, Hemp, Bachelder, & Fujiura, 1995).

In addition, whereas professionals have often turned to parents as allies in the care of adults with mental retardation (Turnbull, Turnbull, Bronicki, Summers, & Roeder-Gordon, 1989), parents of adults with mental illness have often felt excluded from the treatment process because laws surrounding confidentiality lead mental health professionals to be reluctant to share information about the treatment process with them (Francell, Conn, & Gray, 1988; Hatfield, 1988). By restricting information from the family members who are responsible for providing care, professionals may intensify the family member's distress by eroding his or her sense of mastery over the caregiving context (Holden & Lewine, 1982; Riebschleger, 1991).

Lastly, there is a greater societal acceptance of mental retardation than of mental illness, which carries considerably more stigma. In a study of mental health professionals who themselves had family members with mental illness, Lefley (1987) found that 74% were reluctant to speak openly with their colleagues about mental illness in their own families. Similarly, the stigma of mental illness is evident in medical insurance policies that narrowly limit mental health care, placing a considerable financial burden on families.

These similarities and differences allow us to separate out processes that have parallel effects across different caregiving contexts from those that are specific to the nature of the disability.

Mental Health of Caregiving Mothers

In light of the differences in the caregiving context of mothers of adults with mental retardation and mothers of adults with mental illness, it is not surprising that we have found striking differences in their mental health profiles. In our past research, we have found that there is a higher risk of depressive symptoms among mothers of adults with mental illness than among their counterparts whose adult child has a diagnosis of mental retardation (Seltzer, Greenberg, & Krauss, 1995). Also, mothers of adults with mental illness report considerably higher levels of subjective caregiving burden (Greenberg, Seltzer, & Greenley, 1993). In addition, mothers of adults with mental illness report feeling more pessimistic about their child's future than mothers of adults with mental retardation (Greenberg, Seltzer, Krauss, & Kim, 1997). Thus, mothers of adults with mental illness evidence a psychological profile more likely to be characterized by feelings of depression, burden, and pessimism about the future than that of mothers of adults with mental retardation.

Based on these differences in the caregiving context and maternal psychological well-being, our analysis examines whether the types of coping strategies used and the effects of coping are similar or different in mothers of adults with the two types of disabilities. In essence, we are aiming to elucidate whether differences in the caregiving context are associated with differences in the likelihood that coping will maintain the psychological well-being of aging women who care for their adult child with disabilities.

Methods Used to Investigate the Influence of Disability and Coping

Our ongoing studies of aging mothers of adults with mental illness ($n = 107$) and aging mothers of adults with mental retardation ($n = 461$) share many common features. In both studies, families met two criteria when initially recruited: the mother was age 55 or older, and the adult with disabilities lived at home with her. Both groups of sample members were recruited for the research via the same strategies. For the majority, recruitment was accomplished with the assistance of the state or county agencies responsible for providing services to persons with either mental retardation or mental illness, and the state agency on aging. Others were referred by service providers, and still others were nominated by participating sample members. All sample members were volunteers.

All adults with mental illness had a diagnosis of a serious mental illness, including schizophrenia (72%), bipolar disorder (17%), major depression (9%), or other psychiatric diagnosis (2%). The adults with mental retardation had primarily mild (38%) or moderate (41%) retardation, while the remaining 21% had severe or profound retardation. Forty percent had Down syndrome.

Participants in the study of mothers of adults with mental retardation are interviewed in the mother's home every 18 months. All mothers also complete a set of self-administered standardized measures. In total, eight "waves" of data will be collected, one every 18 months between 1988 and 2000. The data used in this analysis are from the second wave of data collection and included a subset ($n = 389$) of the full sample. Excluded were those who had placed their son or daughter out of the home prior to the second wave of data collection, families in which either the mother or the adult with retardation had died during the interval between Waves 1 and 2, and those for whom there were any missing data on variables used in this analysis.

Participants in the study of mothers of adults with mental illness have been interviewed twice, 36 months apart. The first point of data collection was approximately the same point in time as the second wave of the mental retardation study, and hence it was selected for analysis here. The same data collection procedures were used with mothers of adults with mental illness as with mothers of adults with mental retardation. Of the 107 mothers, two cases were excluded from the present analysis because of missing data.

The two samples of aging mothers have highly similar profiles of demographic characteristics, which strengthens the investigation of the possible differences in their caregiving experiences. Specifically, we have found the two groups of mothers to be similar in age, level of education, marital status, health, and family income. (See Table 13.1.) They are in their mid-sixties, on average, and most are high school graduates. The majority are married, although widowhood is an increasingly common experience. They rate their own health as "good" on a scale that ranges from "poor" to "fair" to "good" to "excellent." Their family incomes place them in the middle- to lower-middle class category. The adults with disabilities are similar in age, about 35 years old. One marked difference between the two groups is the gender of the adult with the disability. Only about 45% of the adults with mental retardation, but fully 70% of the adults with mental illness, are male. Hence, with the exception of the gender of the adult with disabilities, individual-level demographic characteristics are not sources of great variation between these two groups of families who experience a substantially divergent context of care.

Table 13.1 Characteristics of the Samples of Mothers of Adults With Disabilities

Characteristic	Mothers of adults with			
	Mental retardation	Mental illness	t	χ^2
Maternal characteristics				
Age	66.78	65.73	1.43	
Level of education[a]	2.15	2.22		2.77
Marital status[b]	0.63	0.57		1.15
Health[c]	2.83	2.99		3.16
Family income ($)	28,129	26,414	1.07	
Characteristics of the adult with disabilities				
Age	34.58	35.61	1.27	
Gender[d]	0.46	0.70		20.21***

[a] 1 = less than high school, 2 = high school graduate, 3 = some college.
[b] 0 = not married, 1 = married.
[c] 1 = poor, 2 = fair, 3 = good, 4 = excellent.
[d] 0 = female, 1 = male.
***$p < .001$.

As we noted earlier, the dependent variable in this analysis is depressive symptoms, measured by the Center for Epidemiological Studies-Depression Scale (CES-D; Radloff, 1977). For each of 20 depressive symptoms, the CES-D asks the respondent to indicate how often during the past week the symptom was experienced (0 = never; 3 = 5–7 days). Scores range from 0 to 60, and a score of 16 or higher is generally considered to be an indicator of an elevated risk of clinical depression.

We included two measures of caregiving stress: caregiving demands and behavior problems. Caregiving demands was a count of the number of everyday living tasks for which the mother provided help or care to her adult child with disabilities, from a list of 11 personal and instrumental activities of daily living. The measure of behavior problems of the adult with disabilities yielded a count of up to eight maladaptive behaviors (Bruininks, Hill, Weatherman, & Woodcock, 1986) such as behavior that is harmful to self, destructive, or disruptive to others.

Carver, Scheier, and Weintraub's (1989) multidimensional coping inventory was used to assess the different ways mothers respond to stressful situations or events. Of the 13 subscales in the measure, we used 7 for this analysis. Three were indicators of problem-focused coping (active coping, planning, positive reinterpretation and growth) and four were indicators of emotion-focused coping (focus on and venting emotions, denial, behavioral disengagement, and mental disengagement). Additional details regarding the methods used in this analysis can be found in Seltzer et al. (1995).

Hypotheses and Findings Regarding Coping

In this section, we explicate why we hypothesized that mothers of adults with mental illness would use different coping strategies than mothers of adults with mental retardation. According to Lazarus and Folkman (1984), cognitive appraisal and coping are two components in the stress process. An individual assesses or appraises the possibility of mastering or altering the stressful situation (Folkman, 1984), and copes accordingly. Emotion-focused coping strategies (cognitive and behavioral efforts to reduce or manage emotional distress) are most likely to be used in situations in which there are high levels of uncertainty and when the individual perceives few possibilities for effective change. In contrast, problem-focused coping strategies (cognitive and behavioral problem-solving strategies aimed at altering or managing the stressor) are most effective in situations in which the individual feels a sense of personal efficacy and perceives the possibility for making positive change. Hence, the degree of predictability and control over the caregiving context may influence how mothers cope.

There are three reasons why the caregiving context of mothers of adults with mental illness is more unpredictable and less under their control than the caregiving context of mothers of adults with mental retardation, and hence would lead to the use of different types of coping strategies. First, mothers of adults with mental illness face more behavior problems in their son or daughter than mothers of adults with mental retardation. Second, the lack of adequately funded community-based services for persons with serious mental illness also contributes to parental feelings that they are unable to change the caregiving situation. Lastly, the stigma of mental illness may also fuel a mother's sense of powerlessness and social isolation, which may further reduce coping efficacy. On the basis of these differences in the caregiving context, we hypothesized that mothers of adults with mental illness would report greater use of emotion-focused coping strategies, and mothers of adults with mental retardation would report greater use of problem-focused coping strategies.

Table 13.2 Analysis of Covariance of Use of Coping Strategies by Mothers of Adults With Mental Retardation and Mothers of Adults With Mental Illness

Coping Strategy	Mothers of Adults with Mental Retardation[a]	Mothers of Adults with Mental Illness[a]	F
Problem-focused coping			
Active coping	11.57	11.75	0.35
Planning	12.18	12.22	0.02
Positive reinterpretation and growth	12.62	12.58	0.01
Emotion-focused coping			
Focus on and venting emotions	8.60	9.65	11.07***
Denial	5.59	6.13	4.70*
Behavioral disengagement	6.50	7.11	5.96**
Mental disengagement	7.53	8.74	22.04***

[a] Means are adjusted for the gender of the adult with disabilities.

* $p < .05$. ** $p < .01$. *** $p < .001$.

We found mixed support for our predictions. (See Table 13.2.) Contrary to our hypothesis, there were no differences in the extent to which the two groups of caregiving mothers used the problem-focused coping strategies of active coping, planning, or positive reinterpretation and growth. However, we found support for the expected differences with respect to emotion-focused coping. Mothers of adults with mental illness were significantly more likely than mothers of adults with mental retardation to use each of the emotion-focused coping strategies. Note that all of these comparisons controlled for the possible influence of the gender of the adult with disabilities, as this variable differentiated the two diagnostic groups.

However, differences in the use of various types of coping strategies can provide us with only a partial understanding of how mothers of adults with different types of disabilities respond to their caregiving challenge. In particular, it is unwarranted to assume that such differences in coping use translate into differences in the effects of coping. In order to determine the effectiveness of coping, it is necessary to examine its association with measures of psychological well-being.

Controversy exists in the literature regarding the nature of effects of emotion-focused coping. On the one hand, Folkman and Lazarus (1980) posit that greater use of emotion-focused coping in situations that are characterized by uncertainty should be beneficial by helping people manage emotions and reduce distress. However, past research has indicated that the opposite may occur in the caregiving context, as caregivers who use emotion-focused coping strategies have higher levels of depression and distress (Haley et al., 1987; Li, Seltzer, & Greenberg, in press).

We addressed the question of how the use of emotion-focused coping is related to depressive symptoms via a series of multiple regression analyses. (See Table 13.3.) Separate analyses were conducted for mothers of adults with mental illness and mothers of adults with mental retardation. For all of the analyses, the dependent variable was depressive symptoms. A separate regression model was estimated for each of the four emotion-focused coping strategies. Each model included three sets of independent variables: the control variables (maternal age, level of education, family income, marital status, health status, and the gender of the adult with disabilities), the sources of stress (caregiving demands, behavior problems), and one of the coping strategies. Finally, in preliminary analyses, we tested the interaction effects of each of the two sources of stress by each of the coping strategies in order to assess whether coping buffered the effects of stress, and such interactions were included only when significant.

We found that for both mothers of adults with mental illness and mothers of adults with mental retardation, those who relied on emotion-focused coping had significantly higher levels of depressive symptoms. There was no evidence of moderating (i.e., buffering) effects for emotion-focused coping depending on levels of stress. Rather, the use of these coping strategies had direct and negative effects on depressive symptoms. Although emotion-focused coping strategies may serve to create emotional distance between the stressful situation and the person affected by the situation, such strategies do not alter the boundaries or nature of the stressful situation.

Next we turned to the use of problem-focused coping strategies. The findings of past research on caregivers for the elderly show mixed effects of the use of this type of coping. Some studies reported no effect of problem-focused coping (Pruchno & Kleban, 1993; Pruchno & Resch, 1989), whereas others reported that problem-focused coping was associated with better mental health outcomes (Haley et al., 1987; Pratt et al., 1985). Bandura's (1986) theory may clarify the controversy. He suggested that coping strategies will have stress-buffering effects only when an individ-

Table 13.3 Effects of Emotion-Focused Coping on Depressive Symptoms in Mothers of Adults With Disabilities

A. Mothers of Adults with Mental Illness

Independent Variables	Focus on and Venting Emotions	Denial	Behavioral Disengagement	Mental Disengagement
Maternal age	.02	.03	−.02	.02
Level of education	−.17	−.11	−.12	−.21
Family income	−.06	−.01	−.03	.02
Marital status	.12	.09	.12	.10
Maternal health	−.20	−.19	−.20	−.16
Gender of adult	.07	.07	.09	.08
Caregiving demands	.27**	.22*	.22*	.24*
Behavior problems	.04	.05	.02	.03
Coping[a]	**.23***	**.27***	**.33***	**.27***
R^2	.23	.25	.28	.25

B. Mothers of Adults with Mental Retardation

Independent Variables	Focus on and Venting Emotions	Denial	Behavioral Disengagement	Mental Disengagement
Maternal age	.06	.01	−.01	.02
Level of education	−.01	.03	.03	.04
Family income	−.10	−.04	−.06	−.10
Marital status	−.06	−.04	−.06	.00
Maternal health	−.22***	−.26***	−.25***	−.18***
Gender of adult	.07	.10*	.06	.07
Caregiving demands	.05	.04	.05	.07
Behavior problems	.05	.11*	.09	.05
Coping[a]	**.31***	**.27***	**.28***	**.41***
R^2	.23	.22	.22	.30

Note: The coefficients shown are standardized regression coefficients.
[a] Each coping strategy was entered into only one regression model.
* $p < .05$; ** $p < .01$; *** $p < .001$.

ual holds the expectation that a certain course of action has a high likelihood of leading to the desired outcome. Therefore, for mothers of adults with mental illness, we hypothesize that problem-focused coping will not be effective in reducing the negative effects of stress, but for mothers of adults with mental retardation, we expect that problem-focused coping will effectively buffer the stresses of caregiving.

Our findings were supportive of these expectations. (See Table 13.4.) We conducted three additional regression analyses for mothers of adults with mental illness and three for mothers of adults with mental retardation, modeled after those described above, but this time including problem-focused coping variables. In support of our hypotheses, for mothers of adults with mental illness, none of the three problem-focused coping strategies had a significant effect on level of depressive symptoms. (See Table 13.4A) For mothers of adults with mental retardation, in contrast, the use of active coping was associated with significantly lower levels of depressive symptoms. (See Table 13.4B) The use of planning and positive reinterpretation and growth had stress-buffering effects. In other words, when mothers faced high levels of caregiving demands, the use of the coping strategies of planning and positive reinterpretation and growth reduced the negative effects of this source of stress. Hence, their level of depressive symptoms was no higher than those mothers whose son or daughter did not have high levels of caregiving demands.

We believe that the reason why problem-focused coping strategies did not buffer the effect of stress for mothers of adults with mental illness is that these mothers are confronted on a daily basis with a caregiving context over which they can expert only limited control, due both to the stigmatizing and unpredictable nature of the behavior problems of their son or daughter and to the reluctance of mental health professionals to involve families as allies in the treatment process. Conversely, mothers of adults with mental retardation can rely on the relative stability of their child's functioning and the lower frequency of behavior problems, and therefore they can exert considerably greater influence and authority over the daily life of their adult child. Professionals also have been more responsive to the needs of these families, and by embracing them as collaborators in the treatment process, they validate their role as a primary support to the adult with mental retardation.

Additional insight in interpreting these findings comes from the work of Taylor (1983) who proposed a theory of cognitive adaptation in the face of stressful events. Among the factors that account for recovery from stressful events, two stand out as particularly important: a search for meaning in the experience, and an attempt to regain mastery over the event. In support of this perspective, our findings indicated that the use of positive reinterpretation and growth, which is a search for meaning, had a buffering effect for mothers of adults with mental retardation. Further, active coping, which is a way of asserting mastery, was negatively associated with depressive symptoms for these mothers. Although both mothers of

Table 13.4 Effects of Problem-Focused Coping on Depressive Symptoms in Mothers of Adults with Disabilities

A. Mothers of Adults with Mental Illness

Independent Variables	Active Coping	Planning	Positive Reinterpretation and Growth
Maternal age	−.02	−.02	−.02
Level of education	−.18	−.19	−.18
Family income	−.06	−.06	−.06
Marital status	.11	.11	.11
Maternal health	−.19	−.20	−.20
Gender of adult	.08	.08	.08
Caregiving demands	.23*	.24*	.23*
Behavior problems	.10	.10	.10
Coping[a]	**−.04**	**.03**	**−.02**
R^2	.19	.19	.19

B. Mothers of Adults with Mental Retardation

Independent Variables	Active Coping	Planning	Positive Reinterpretation and Growth
Maternal age	.00	.00	.01
Level of education	.01	.00	−.01
Family income	−.09	−.08	−.08
Marital status	−.08	−.09	−.09
Maternal health	−.27***	−.29***	−.26***
Gender of adult	.06	.07	.07
Caregiving demands	.03	.04	.04
Behavior problems	.11*	.12*	.11*
Coping[a]	**−.12***	**−.10***	**−.17***
Coping x caregiving demands		**−.14****	**−.17****
R^2	.16	.18	.20

Note: The coefficients shown are standardized regression coefficients.
[a] Each coping strategy was entered into only one regression model.
* $p <.05$; ** $p <.01$; *** $p <.001$.

adults with mental illness and mothers of adults with mental retardation used these strategies with equal frequency, the effect of using these coping strategies was different in the two caregiving contexts. Although mothers of adults with mental illness may search for meaning and may attempt to assert mastery over their caregiving role, these coping strategies were ineffective, possibly because of their lack of control over the caregiving context. Hence, the equivalent use of these coping strategies in different caregiving contexts did not translate into the same mental health outcomes.

In conclusion, we found support for our expectation that the caregiving context differentiates coping effectiveness for mothers of adults with mental retardation as compared with mothers of adults with mental illness. The unpredictability of the caregiving context for mothers of adults with mental illness erodes their sense of self-efficacy and mastery. These effects are exacerbated by social and institutional structures that stigmatize families of persons with mental illness and that have in the past tended to blame rather than support them in their caregiving efforts. In contrast, mothers of adults with mental retardation experience a greater degree of control over their caregiving context and are likely to be rewarded when they use problem-focused coping strategies by reducing their level of distress. Hence, both the nature of the immediate caregiving context as well as the larger social structural context in which caregiving occurs determine whether the use of particular coping strategies will have beneficial, harmful, or no effects on psychological well-being.

THE CAREGIVING CONTEXT AS A FUNCTION OF KINSHIP RELATIONSHIP

Overview of Wife and Daughter Caregivers

In our third study, we are examining how the kinship relationship between the person providing the care and the person receiving it defines the context of caregiving. Specifically, we contrast wives who are caring for their elderly husband with adult daughters who are caring for their elderly parent. We look to the kinship relationship as a defining feature of the caregiving context because we hypothesize that it lends meaning to the objective tasks that comprise the caregiving role.

Wife and daughter caregivers experience a caregiving challenge marked by both similarities and differences. The similarities are evident with respect to the characteristics of the two groups of care recipients. In our study, both husband and parent care recipients are elderly (mean age was 75.8 for husband recipients and 84.2 for parent recipients). There was no difference between husband and parent care recipients in the prevalence of the types of medical problems that caused their need for care, with approximately 17% of both groups having dementia, 10% reporting heart disease, and 10% having had a stroke. Fewer than 10% of the others in either group reported any single diagnosis. It is also noteworthy that the objective stresses of caregiving are not different for wives and daughters, as the two types of care recipients do not differ in severity of functional limitations or behavior problems. Thus, our samples of wives who care for their elderly husband and daughters who care for their elderly parent have highly similar caregiving challenges with respect to the age, types of health problems, functional limitations, and behavior problems manifested by the family member to whom care was provided.

In other respects, however, these two groups of caregivers are highly distinct. First, wives and daughters are members of different generations and are at different stages of life, which result in divergent positions in the social structure. The wives in our sample are considerably older (mean ages for wives and daughters were 70.9 and 57.5, respectively), less likely to be employed (24.3% of the wives and 54.3% of the daughters were employed), less likely to be high school graduates (72.0% of the wives and 94.0% of the daughters had at least a high school education), and are in poorer health (33.3% of the wives vs. 19.7% of the daughters in fair or poor health). These demographic profiles index cohort differences that may influence the caregiving role, such as socioeconomic status and access to resources. Because of their more limited education and rates of employment, the social class of a wife in our study may be more dependent on her husband's status than is the case in later generations. When the husband becomes ill, wives in this cohort may be more negatively affected socially and financially than wives in younger cohorts, which may impact on their ability to withstand the stresses of caregiving.

Second, wives and daughters differ in their prior expectations of the relationship with the care recipient. For wives, caregiving is an extension of prior exchange of support and assistance in the marital relationship. In contrast, the flow of support exchanged between daughter and parent undergoes a number of shifts at various points of the life course, starting with total dependency during the daughter's early childhood and becoming more egalitarian in adulthood. Therefore, the onset of caregiving for a parent represents a reversal of prior roles, as well as a departure from the adult-to-adult relationship which was more or less devoid of care given by either party.

Third, as noted earlier, there are different normative expectations for wives than for adult children in the caregiving role. When a husband becomes ill, social norms are that the wife is the expected source of help and assistance for him. In contrast, when an aging parent becomes ill, the determination of which child will assume the role of caregiver is more ambiguous. Although the caregiving role falls more heavily on daughters than sons (Hooyman & Gonyea, 1995), there is evidence that the extent of past transfers of financial support from the parent to the child is predictive of which child will assume the caregiving role subsequently (Henretta, Hill, Li, Soldo, & Wolf, 1997). Thus, the wife-daughter contrast is one of clear versus ambiguous societal expectations regarding who will become the caregiver.

Fourth, the salience of the caregiving role is different for wives than for daughters. Past research suggests that the wife role is more salient than the role of adult daughter (Richards, Bengtson, & Miller, 1989; Rossi & Rossi, 1990). In addition to the obvious differences between the spousal and parent-child relationships, spouses generally co-reside, and are at a stage of life when the caregiver has few competing family and work demands. In contrast, when the caregiver is an adult child and the care recipient is her aged parent, they typically live apart, and the caregiving role often competes with multiple family and work roles. These differences may help to explain why wife and daughter caregivers may differ in role saliency.

As in our prior analysis of the effect of the disability of the care recipient, the context of caregiving is important because it may affect how caregiving is experienced. In the present example, although the objective stresses of caregiving are similar for wife and daughter caregivers, the divergence in the two caregiving contexts may result in differences in how factors such as social support affect whether caregiving stress takes a toll on the psychological well-being of the caregiver.

Social Support and Caregiving

The stress of caregiving for elderly family members has been well-documented in the literature, with higher rates of depressive symptoms observed among caregivers than their non-caregiving age peers (Aneshensel et al., 1995; Lawton et al., 1991). Yet, as we have noted, there is great heterogeneity in the mental health of caregivers. Pearlin et al.'s (1981) stress process model is useful in accounting for the reasons why caregivers who face similar challenges have different levels of psychological well-being. According to the stress process model, personal and social resources can determine the extent to which stress takes a toll. Among these resources is social support.

Caregivers who have access to the support of others have a lower level of depressive symptoms than those without social support (Fengler & Goodrich, 1979; Fiore, Becker, & Coppel, 1983; George & Gwyther, 1986; Gilhooly, 1984; Haley et al., 1987; Zarit et al., 1980). However, there is little in the caregiving literature that clarifies the specific mechanisms by which social support reduces depression. The general literature on social support (i.e., the literature not restricted to caregivers) is more informative in this regard, and clarifies the conditions under which support either buffers the effect of stress or directly boosts psychological well-being. The buffering effects model posits that the beneficial effect of social support derives primarily from its protective properties in the presence of high levels of stress (e.g., Gerin, Milner, Chawla, & Pickering, 1995; Kessler & Essex, 1982; Kessler & McLeod, 1985). Past research has shown that a buffering effect is most likely to be observed in conjunction with functional indicators of social support, such as receiving emotional support (Cohen & Wills, 1985). The direct effects model posits that social support enhances well-being irrespective of stress level (Fryman, 1981; Lin, 1986; Seeman, Berkman, Blazer, & Rowe, 1994; Williams, Ware, & Donald, 1981). Past research has shown that the direct effect is most likely to be observed in conjunction with structural indicators of social support, such as having a large social support network or participating in social activities (Murrell, Norris, & Chipley, 1992). Hence, the type of support (functional or structural) will determine the mechanism by which social support has its effect (buffering or direct).

However, we hypothesize that whether social support has a direct or a buffering effect in any given situation is dependent in part on the caregiving context. To investigate this idea, we focus on the fit between the context in which caregiving stress is experienced and the type of support received. Specifically, we hypothesize that wives and daughters in the caregiving role benefit from different types of social support.

Hypotheses Regarding Social Support Effects in Two Caregiving Contexts

As in our prior analysis of caregiving for adults with mental retardation and mental illness, we conceptualized the stress of caregiving to include the care recipient's limitations in activities of daily living (both personal and instrumental) and behavior problems, because when the care recipient is more functionally dependent and exhibits more problem behaviors, the demands of caregiving are greater and the caregiving role is more difficult (Aneshensel et al., 1995).

We investigated two dimensions of social support received by caregivers—social participation and emotional support. Social participation refers to the frequency with which an individual participates in social activities. This is a structural support measure which has been shown in past research to have a direct effect on psychological well-being. Emotional support refers to the receipt of reassurance and respect from members of an individual's personal network and having someone in whom to confide (Antonucci & Akiyama, 1987). This is a functional support measure for which buffering effects have been suggested in past research. As noted earlier, our measure of psychological well-being was level of depressive symptoms.

We hypothesized that social participation would not be related to the level of depressive symptoms in wives caring for their aging husbands because participating in social activities might compete with a wife's role as a caregiver. To participate in social activities, a wife may have to leave her husband at home, whereas previously they participated together in these social occasions. We posit that the beneficial effect of social participation reported in past research may not be found for wife caregivers because the wife's worry about her husband when she is not with him may counterbalance potential positive effects of social participation, as does the reminder that she is increasingly alone in social situations (Pearlin, Turner, & Semple, 1989).

In contrast, we hypothesized that social participation will have a direct positive effect on psychological well-being for daughter caregivers, as suggested by previous research (Haley et al., 1987; Lin, 1986). Participation in social activities may provide a break from the demands of caring for a parent and may offer a vehicle for maintaining ongoing social relationships and roles. Further, as daughters tend not to socialize with their aging parents in the same way that wives socialize with their husbands, we do not expect that the increasing infirmity of an aging parent will have the same disruptive effect on a daughter's social life as does the infirmity of a husband on a wife's social life.

We hypothesized that emotional support would buffer the effects of caregiving stress for both wives and daughters and that the buffering effects of emotional support would be particularly evident in moderating the effects of behavior problems on well-being. The behavior problems faced by family caregivers of older persons are often intermittent and unpredictable, similar to those faced by families of persons with mental illness. In their theory of optimal matching, Cutrona and Russell (1990) suggest that, in comparison with instrumental support, emotional support more optimally fits the needs of individuals facing stressors over which they perceive little control.

Although we predicted that emotional support would have a buffering effect for both daughters and wives, we expected a stronger effect for wives. We base this hypothesis on the greater salience of the wife role, which is central to a woman's self-concept and identity, particularly during the later years of the life course (Rossi & Rossi, 1990). Past research has shown that emotional support has a greater impact on stresses emerging from highly salient roles than those linked with less central roles (Krause, 1994; Krause & Borawski-Clark, 1994). Anticipating the loss of the role of wife may challenge a woman's sense of purpose and meaning of life (Skaff & Pearlin, 1992). Therefore, wife caregivers may be particularly in need of reassurance and support from others to reinforce feelings of self-worth. Moreover, when a husband becomes ill or disabled, his wife experiences a loss of emotional support from him. Pearlin et al. (1989) described the loss of love, affection, and reciprocity of exchange with the spouse as one of the most painful losses and powerful sources of strain experienced by spousal caregivers. The emotional support provided by a wife's social support network can make her feel loved and cared for in the context of this loss.

For daughter caregivers, the buffering effect of emotional support was expected to be weaker than for wives. This is because the daughter role is less central to a woman's self-concept at this stage of life than other roles (Richards et al., 1989). Moreover, adult daughters tend to be less reliant on their aging parents to fulfill their emotional needs than are wives on their husbands, and thus we expect less of an impact on the loss of emotional support from the care recipient on daughters than on wives.

To summarize, for wives caring for their aging husband, emotional support was hypothesized to have a strong buffering effect on stress, but social participation was not expected to have any effect on their psychological well-being. For daughters caring for their aging parent, emotional support was hypothesized to buffer the effect of stress on depressive symptoms, but to a lesser extent than for wives. However, social participation was hypothesized to have a direct negative effect on depressive symptoms for daughter caregivers.

Methods Used to Investigate the Influence of Kinship
Relationship on the Caregiving Context

We recruited a probability sample of caregivers in Wisconsin. Our sample was a subset of a larger probability sample drawn by random digit dialing techniques for the State of Wisconsin Bureau on Aging in 1991. The larger sample consisted of 2250 persons age 60 or older and 500 persons younger than age 60 who provided care to someone age 60 or older. To ensure a sufficiently large pool of caregivers, we supplemented this base with an additional thousand households also contacted through random digit dialing procedures.

We telephoned all of these persons in 1993 and screened them to determine their current caregiving status. If a wife or a daughter provided assistance to a husband or a parent, due to his or her aging or illness or disability, with at least one of the following tasks, she was included in our study: housework, preparing meals, finances, yard work, shopping, taking medications, getting around inside the house, eating, dressing, bathing, using the toilet, and getting in and out of bed. Of the wives and daughters who met study criteria, 73.8% agreed to participate. Only caregivers of care recipients who lived in community-based settings (non-institutionalized) were included in this analysis ($n = 103$ for wife caregivers and $n = 149$ for daughter caregivers).

During home visits, each caregiver was interviewed and completed a set of self-administered standardized questionnaires. As in our earlier study of coping in aging mothers of adults with mental retardation and mental illness, the dependent variable used in this analysis was depressive symptoms, which was measured by the CES-D (Radloff, 1977). Daughter caregivers had significantly lower levels of depressive symptoms than wife caregivers (a mean of 9.31 versus 11.90 on the CES-D). These levels of depressive symptoms were roughly comparable to those characteristic of their age peers in the general population (Gatz & Hurwicz, 1990).

We had two measures of caregiving stress, which were conceptually similar to those used in our prior analysis of coping, although different instruments were used to operationalize these concepts. Caregiving stress was indicated by behavior problems and by limitations in functional abilities. We assessed functional abilities with respect to 14 activities of daily living (e.g., dressing, medication management, meal preparation). Behavior problems were measured by a 14-item scale (Pearlin, Mullan, Semple, & Skaff, 1990). Sample items include how often the care recipient hides belongings and forgets about them, dresses the wrong way, and swears or uses foul language.

The two dimensions of social support we examined in this study were social participation and emotional support. Social participation was measured by the frequency of social activities engaged in by the caregiver. Using a modified version of a measure developed for the National Survey of Families and Households (Sweet & Bumpass, 1987), respondents rated the frequency of participating in five types of social activities: spending social time with relatives, spending social time with people with whom the respondent works, spending social time with friends and neighbors, attending a social event at church or synagogue, and participating in a group recreational activity. Daughters had a significantly higher level of social participation than wives. Emotional support was measured by variables derived from the convoy model developed by Antonucci and Akiyama (1987). Respondents were first asked to list up to ten persons with whom they exchanged support. Then they indicated whether each person provided them with the following four types of emotional support: someone in whom they could confide, a source of reassurance when feeling uncertain, someone to talk with when upset, nervous or depressed, and someone to show them respect. A total score of emotional support was obtained by summing the availability of these four types of support from all members in the network. Although the difference in emotional support between wives and daughters was not statistically significant, the level for daughters was higher than that for wives.

We addressed the question of how social support was related to depressive symptoms in wife and daughter caregivers via a series of multiple regression analyses. We analyzed the wife and daughter caregiver samples separately because of their distinct demographic profiles and their different positions in the life course. For all of these analyses, the dependent variable was depressive symptoms. Each model consisted of three sets of variables: characteristics of the caregiver (included for control purposes), sources of stress (functional limitations and behavior problems), and one measure of social support. The analysis of each type of social support was conducted in a separate model. We first tested the main effect of social participation. Next, in order to test the buffering effect of emotional support, we created interaction terms for each of the types of stress (functional limitations by emotional support, behavior problem by emotional support). Only significant interactions were included in the final models. Additional details about the methods used in this analysis can be found in Li et al. (1997).

Different Effects of Social Support for Wife and Daughter Caregivers

Overall, we found that different aspects of social support affected the psychological well-being of wife and daughter caregivers in different ways. Specifically, for wife caregivers, social participation did not have an effect on depressive symptoms, which was consistent with our hypothesis. (See Table 13.5.) We speculate that the potential benefits of social participation were counterbalanced for wife caregivers because participating in social activities posed role conflicts for them, in many cases taking them away from their husband to whom they now must provide care, but who in the past may have joined them as a marital partner in these social activities.

In contrast, for daughter caregivers, social participation was found to be significantly related to psychological well-being. The more a daughter caregiver participated in social activities, the less likely she was to have feelings of depression, regardless of the level of caregiving stress. Social participation gives these daughters a break from the demands of caregiving and allows them to continue ongoing social relationships.

A different picture emerged from our analysis of the effects of emotional support. As shown in Table 13.6, we found that emotional support buffered the stresses emanating from the behavior problems of the care recipient for both wives and daughters. For wives, the significant interaction of behavior problems by emotional support indicates that when the husband had a higher level of behavior problems, wives who received more emotional support from their friends and family members had lower levels of depressive symptoms than wives who had less emotional support. But under the low stress condition (i.e., when the husband had fewer behavior problems), emotional support was not significantly related to wives' depressive symptoms. Our interpretation is that when a husband develops behavioral problems, he may no longer be a source of emotional support to his wife. In this situation, emotional support from others may compensate at least to some extent for the loss of the husband's emotional support and for the stress of the husband's behavior problems.

For daughter caregivers, emotional support also was found to buffer the effect of stress of the behavior problems of their parent. (See Table 13.6.) We interpret this finding in the context of role reversal. When the daughter caregiver has to regulate parental behavior problems, she increasingly assumes a parent-like role. This reversal of roles may be disturbing for the adult daughter, but emotional support from family and friends may buffer the stress.

Table 13.5 Effects of Social Participation on Depressive Symptoms for Wife and Daughter Caregivers

Independent Variables	Wife Caregivers	Daughter Caregivers
Age	−.14	−.29***
Education	−.04	−.07
Employment	−.02	−.07
Duration of caregiving	−.05	.12
Health	−.45***	−.20**
Functional limitations of care recipient	−.04	−.06
Behavior problems of care recipient	.20*	.42***
Social participation	**−.14**	**−.18***
R^2	.31	.37

Note: The coefficients shown are standardized regression coefficients.
* $p <.05$; ** $p <.01$; *** $p <.001$.

Table 13.6 Effects of Emotional Support on Depressive Symptoms for Wife and Daughter Caregivers

Independent Variables	Wife Caregivers	Daughter Caregivers
Age	−.12	−.30***
Education	.04	−.06
Employment	−.03	−.09
Duration of caregiving	−.06	.14‡
Health	−.41***	−.22**
Functional limitations of care recipient	.02	−.01
Behavior problems of care recipient	.34***	.35***
Emotional support	**−.23***	**−.05**
Behavior problems × emotional support	**−.24****	**−.14***
R^2	.39	.37

Note: The coefficients shown are standardized regression coefficients.
‡ $p <.06$; * $p <.05$; ** $p < .01$; *** $p <.001$

As we predicted, the buffering effect of emotional support was stronger for wives than for daughters. Although not portrayed in the table, we found that emotional support accounted for a greater percentage of the variance in depressive symptoms of wives than of daughters (5.0% versus 1.8%, respectively). Hence, our prediction that emotional support would be more strongly related to wives' psychological well-being than daughters' received some affirmation.

We believe that the different pattern of effects of social support was a result of differences in the context of caregiving, in particular differences due to the type of kinship relationship between caregiver and care recipient. Stronger stress-buffering effects were found for wives, for whom the caregiving role was conceptualized as more salient than for daughters. However, only daughters benefitted from social participation, which was directly related to their psychological well-being. For wives, however, the positive benefits of social participation may have been offset by the stress associated with being away from her husband while she participates in social activities.

New Research Directions and Implications for Theories of the Stress Process

A central aim of our program of research on caregiving has been to investigate whether the effectiveness of social and psychological resources in reducing distress varies systematically across different caregiving contexts. Our cross-sectional data indicate that the social context of caregiving, indeed, matters. In our comparative study of mothers of adults with disabilities, we found that the use of problem-focused coping buffered the effects of stress only for mothers of adults with mental retardation. In other research not reported in this chapter, we found additional differences between the two groups in how the stress process operated. For example, mothers of adults with mental illness were found to be more vulnerable to the positive and negative aspects of their social support networks than mothers of adults with mental retardation (Greenberg et al., 1997). Also, we found that the factors that predicted the end of co-residence between parents and adult child differed for the two caregiving situations; adults with mental illness were likely to move away from the parental home when there was stress in the family, whereas adults with mental retardation were likely to move away when the mother's caregiving capacity declined (Seltzer et al., 1997). Thus, there is ample evidence of differences in the effects of coping and social support processes in these two groups.

Similarly, in our comparative study of wife and daughter caregivers, we found that social participation reduced depression among daughters, but not wives. Also, emotional support more strongly buffered the effects of stress associated with the care recipient's behavior problems for wives than for daughters. In other research not reported in this chapter, we found that wife and daughter caregivers also differed in their subjective reactions to the transitions of caregiving and in how the temporal dimensions of caregiving affected their psychological well-being (Seltzer & Li, 1996). Hence, there is considerable evidence that the type of kinship relationship conditions the nature of the caregiving experience for these two groups.

We recognize that the research we have conducted thus far on the interplay between the caregiving context and stress and coping processes represents only a beginning effort to understand these complex relationships. The caregiving context is shaped not only by the nature of the adult's disability and kinship relationship of the caregiver to the care recipient, but also by the timing of the onset of caregiving in the individual's life course (Pearlin & Skaff, 1996) and characteristics of the larger social structure in which the caregiving role is enacted (Pearlin, 1989). We offer several directions for future research that take a broader view of the caregiving context and that investigate how the larger social context interacts with individual well-being.

One promising area of research which thus far has received little attention in the caregiving literature, but which we have discussed earlier in this chapter, is the investigation of how social services condition the use and effects of individual coping efforts. The coping efforts of caregivers are enacted in the context of service systems which may be either supportive of such efforts or which may create additional obstacles for the caregiver to overcome. Earlier in this chapter, we noted that families of persons with mental retardation interact with a larger system that tends to be more responsive to and supportive of their caregiving efforts than to those of families of persons with mental illness. Little research has been conducted that has directly measured or analyzed how the rippling effects of these service system differences influence individual coping efforts. It is possible that parents of adults with mental illness would develop more effective coping strategies and a greater sense of confidence and efficacy as caregivers if they were to be included as collaborators or allies in the treatment process. One direction for future research, therefore, is to investigate the mechanisms by which the orientation of the service system toward family involvement conditions the effectiveness of parental coping efforts in reducing caregiving stress.

Second, the stigma of mental illness has long been recognized as having a pervasive negative effect. Stigma, like racism and sexism, is a powerful yet frequently denied societal condition that is beyond the individual's power to change. Surprisingly, little research has examined the impact of stigma on the well-being of families of persons with serious mental illness (Greenberg, Greenley, McKee, Brown, & Griffin-Francell, 1993; Lefley, 1985). We speculate that stigma encourages the use of emotion-focused coping strategies, as most individuals experience stigma as beyond their control. Research is needed to examine this hypothesis as well as other mechanisms or processes by which social stigma may influence individual psychological well-being.

Future research on social stigma should be mindful that objective indicators of social stigma (indexed by surveys of community attitudes toward mental illness and mental retardation) may be distinct from the subjective perception of families of the extent of social acceptance or stigma. Objective and subjective indicators of the social context of caregiving may be quite divergent, not only because of differences in the salience of issues of mental illness and mental retardation to the general community versus parent caregivers, but also because of the internalized stigma that may affect parental perceptions of the external context. It would also be fruitful to explore cohort differences in this regard, as younger generations of parents of adults with mental illness have experienced a service system that is less likely to blame them for their child's difficulties than the generation we have studied. Similarly, the extent of social acceptance of mental retardation has increased, and younger generations of parents have come to expect legal protections and mandated services not even dreamed of by older cohorts. Hence, internalized stigma may be less of an issue for future generations of parent caregivers.

Another direction for future research is investigating life-course variation in the effects of different social and psychological resources, such as social support. During the past decade, researchers have theorized that for social support to be effective, there must be a good fit between the types of problems confronting individuals and the type of social supports provided (Cutrona & Russell, 1990; Pearlin & Skaff, 1996). However, there has been mixed support for this hypothesis. A life-course perspective sensitizes us to the fact that similar problems may require different types of support depending on one's location in the life course. As described in this chapter, we found that although adult daughters and wives faced similar caregiving stressors, certain types of support (i.e., social participation) reduced caregiving stress for daughters, but did not have a similar effect for wives. Social participation may have a more profound effect on the well-being of daughter than wife caregivers because of differences in the social expectations and norms associated with their different stages in the life course. Whereas after a person has reached old age, the social norms and expectations regarding social participation are more ambiguous and individualistic, in middle age, social participation is clearly normative and intimately linked to many family, work, and community roles that are important sources of self-worth and esteem. These differences in societal expectations tied to different stages of the life course are found in various life course theories of human development (e.g., Buhler, 1968; Erikson, 1950; Neugarten, Moore, & Lowe, 1965; Settersen & Hagestad, 1996a, 1996b). This would suggest that theories of "optimal matching" between types of stressors and types of support could be elaborated by taking into account the individual's location in the life course.

Lastly, future research could address how the life-course trajectories of parental caregivers diverge from those of parents of unaffected children. There are normative expectations regarding when adults make life-course transitions, such as completing schooling, getting a job, etc. (Settersen & Hagestad, 1996a, 1996b). Particularly in the case of mental retardation, which occurs relatively early in the parents' adulthood, there may a fundamental alteration in the subsequent shape of the life course. Having a child with a disability may disrupt parental education, alter employment patterns, and affect decisions about future childbearing. A different profile may be characteristic of parents of persons who have mental illness, due to the later onset of this disability in the family life course. The disruptions of mental illness may be less prominent in the realm of parental achievements and attainments and more evident in their interpersonal relationships and changed expectations for the future. Research is needed to determine the extent of these disruptions and their impact on parental psychological well-being.

To conclude, by studying the well-being of caregivers through a comparative lens, we have brought the context in which this role is carried out into the foreground. The contrast between caregivers who face similar challenges in different contexts highlights our basic premise that the behaviors comprising the caregiving role take on unique meaning because of the larger social context, and thus have unique effects. The dynamic interplay between the social context and the stress process shapes the course of individual development among women who are family caregivers.

REFERENCES

Aneshensel, C. S., Pearlin, L. I., Mullan, J. T., Zarit, S. H., & Whitlach, C. F. (1995). *Profiles in caregiving: The unexpected career.* New York: Academic Press.

Antonucci, T. C., & Akiyama, H. (1987). Social networks in adult life and a preliminary examination of the convoy model. *Journal of Gerontology, 42,* 519–527.

Bandura, A. (1986). *Social foundations of thought and action: A social cognitive theory.* Englewood Cliffs, NJ: Prentice-Hall.

Braddock, D., Hemp, R., Bachelder, L., & Fujiura, G. (1995). *The state of the states in developmental disabilities.* Washington, DC: American Association on Mental Retardation.

Brody, E. M. (1985). Parent care as a normative family stress. *The Gerontololgist, 25,* 19–29.

Bruininks, R. H., Hill, B. K., Weatherman, R. F., & Woodcock, R. W. (1986). *Inventory for client and agency planning (ICAP).* Allen, TX: DLM Teaching Resources.

Buhler, C. (1968). The course of human life as a psychological problem. *Human Development, 11,* 184–200.

Cantor, M. H. (1983). Strain among caregivers. *The Gerontologist, 23,* 597–604.

Carver, C. S., Scheier, M. F., & Weintraub, J. K. (1989). Assessing coping strategies: A theoretically based approach. *Journal of Personality and Social Psychology, 56,* 267–283.

Cattanach, L., & Tebes, J. (1991). The nature of elder impairment and its impact on family caregivers' health and psychosocial functioning. *The Gerontologist, 31,* 246–255.

Clipp, E. C., & George, L. K. (1993). Dementia and cancer: A comparison of spouse caregivers. *The Gerontologist, 33,* 534–541.

Cohen, S., & Wills, T. A. (1985). Stress, social support, and the buffering hypothesis. *Psychological Bulletin, 98,* 310–357.

Cutrona, E. C., & Russell, D. W. (1990). Type of social support and specific stress: Toward a theory of optimal matching. In B. R. Sarason, I.G. Sarason, & G. R. Pierce (Eds.), *Social support: An interactional view* (pp. 319–366). New York: Wiley.

Dura, J. R., Haywood-Niler, E., & Kiecolt-Glaser, J. K. (1990). Spousal caregivers of persons with Alzheimer's and Parkinson's disease dementia: A preliminary comparison. *The Gerontologist, 30,* 332–336.

Dura, J., Stukenberg, K., & Kiecolt-Glaser, J. K. (1990). Chronic stress and depressive disorders in older adults. *Journal of Abnormal Psychology, 99,* 284–290.

Erikson, E. H. (1950). *Childhood and society.* New York: Norton.

Eyman, R. K., & Widaman, K. F. (1987). Life-span development of institutionalized and community-based mentally retarded persons, revisited. *American Journal of Mental Deficiency, 91,* 559–569.

Fengler, A. P., & Goodrich, N. (1979). Wives of elderly disabled men: The hidden patients. *The Gerontologist, 19,* 175–183.

Fiore, J., Becker, J., & Coppel, D. B. (1983). Social network interactions: A buffer or a stress. *American Journal of Community Psychology, 11,* 423–439.

Folkman, S. (1984). Personal control and stress and coping processes: A theoretical analysis. *Journal of Personality and Social Psychology, 46,* 839–852.

Folkman, S., & Lazarus, R. S. (1980). An analysis of coping in a middle-aged community sample. *Journal of Health and Social Behavior, 21,* 219–239.

Francell, C. G., Conn, V. S., & Gray, D. P. (1988). Families' perceptions of burden of care from chronic mentally ill relatives. *Hospital and Community Psychiatry, 39,* 1296–1300.

Fryman, M. I. (1981). Social support, life events and psychiatric symptoms: A study of direct, conditional and interaction effects. *Social Psychiatry, 16,* 69–78.

Gatz, M., & Hurwicz, M. (1990). Are old people more depressed? Cross-sectional data on Center for Epidemiological Studies Depression Scale factors. *Psychology and Aging, 5,* 284–290.

George, L. K. (1989). Stress, social support, and depression over the life-course. In K. S. Markides & C. L. Cooper (Eds.), *Aging, stress and health* (pp. 241–267). New York: Wiley.

George, L. K. (1993). Sociological perspectives on life transitions. *Annual Review of Sociology, 19,* 353–373.

George, L. K., & Gwyther, L. P. (1986). Caregiver well-being: A multidimensional examination of family caregivers of demented adults. *The Gerontologist, 26,* 253–259.

Gerin, W., Milner, D., Chawla, S., & Pickering, T. G. (1995). Social support as a moderator of cardiovascular reactivity in women: A test of the direct effects and buffering hypotheses. *Psychosomatic Medicine, 57,* 16–22.

Gilhooly, M. L. M. (1984). The impact of caregiving on caregivers: Factors associated with the psychological well-being of people supporting a dementia relative in the community. *British Journal of Medical Psychology, 57,* 35–44.

Greenberg, J. S. (1995). The other side of caring: Adult children with mental illness as support to their mothers in later life. *Social Work, 40,* 414–423.

Greenberg, J. S., Greenley, J. R., McKee, D., Brown, R., & Griffin-Francell, C. (1993). Mothers caring for an adult child with schizophrenia. *Family Relations, 42,* 205–211.

Greenberg, J. S., Seltzer, M. M., & Greenley, J. R. (1993). Aging parents of adults with disabilities: The gratifications and frustrations of later-life caregiving. *The Gerontologist, 33,* 542–550.

Greenberg, J. S., Seltzer, M. M., Krauss, M. W., & Kim, H. (1997). The differential effects of social support on the psychological well-being of aging mothers of adults with mental illness or mental retardation. *Family Relations, 46,* 383–394.

Haley, W. E., Levine, E. G., Brown, S. L., & Bartolucci, A. A. (1987). Stress, appraisal, coping, and social support as predictors of adaptational outcome among dementia caregivers. *Psychology and Aging, 2,* 323–330.

Harper, S., & Lund, D. A. (1990). Wives, husbands, and daughters caring for institutionalized dementia and noninstitutionalized dementia patients: Toward a model for caregiving burden. *International Journal of Aging and Human Development, 30,* 241–262.

Hatfield, A. (1988). Issues in the psycho-education for families of the mentally ill. *International Journal of Mental Health, 1,* 48–64.

Henretta, J. C., Hill, M. S., Li., W., Soldo, B., & Wolf, A. (1997). Selection of children to provide care: The effect of earlier parental transfers. *Journal of Gerontology: Psychological and Social Sciences, 52B,* 110–119.

Holden, D., & Lewine, R. R. J. (1982). How families evaluate professionals, resources, and the effects of illness. *Schizophrenia Bulletin, 8,* 626–633.

Holroyd, J., & McArthur, D. (1976). Mental retardation and stress in the parents: A contrast between Down syndrome and childhood autism. *American Journal of Mental Deficiency, 80,* 431–436.

Hooyman, N. R., & Gonyea, J. (1995). *Feminist perspectives on family care: Policies for gender justice.* Thousand Oaks, CA: Sage.

Karlin, N. & Bell, P. A. (1992). Self-efficacy, affect, and seeking support between caregivers of dementia and non-dementia patients. *Journal of Women and Aging, 4,* 59–77.

Kessler, R. C., & Essex, M. (1982). Marital status and depression: The role of coping resources. *Social Forces, 61,* 484–507.

Kessler, R. C., & McLeod, J. D. (1985). Social support and mental health in community samples. In S. Cohen & S. L. Syme (Eds.), *Social support and health* (pp. 219–240). New York: Academic Press.

Kiecolt-Glaser, J. K., Dura, J. R., Speicher, C. E., Trask, J., & Glaser, R. (1991). Spousal caregivers of dementia victims: Longitudinal changes in immunity and health. *Psychosomatic Medicine, 53,* 345–362.

Kramer, B. J. (1997). Gain in the caregiving experience: Where are we? What next? *The Gerontologist, 37,* 218–232.

Krause, N. (1994). Stressors in salient social roles and well-being in later life. *Journal of Gerontology: Psychological Sciences, 49,* P137–148.

Krause, N., & Borawski-Clark, E. (1994). Clarifying the functions of social support in later life. *Research on Aging, 16,* 251–279.

Lawton, M. P., Moss, M., Kleban, M. H., Glisksman, A., & Rovine, M. (1991). A two-factor model of caregiving appraisal and psychological well-being. *Journal of Gerontology: Psychological Sciences, 46,* P181–189.

Lazarus, R. S., & Folkman, S. (1984). *Stress, appraisal, and coping.* New York: Springer Publishing Co.

Lefley, H. P. (1987). Impact of mental illness in families of mental health professionals. *The Journal of Nervous and Mental Disorder, 175,* 613–619.

Li, L. W., Seltzer, M. M., & Greenberg, J. S. (1997). Social support and depressive symptoms: Differential patterns in wife and daughter caregivers. *Journal of Gerontology: Social Sciences, 52B,* S200–S211.

Li, L. W., Seltzer, M. M., & Greenberg, J. S. (in press). Changes in depressive symptoms among daughter caregivers: An 18-month longitudinal study. *Psychology and Aging.*

Lin, N. (1986). Modeling the effects of social support. In N. Lin, A. Dean, & W. Ensel (Eds.), *Social support, life events, and depression* (pp. 173–212). New York: Academic Press.

Mattlin, J. A., Wethington, E., & Kessler, R. C. (1990). Situational determinants of coping and coping effectiveness. *Journal of Health and Social Behavior, 31*, 103–122.

Murrell, S. A., Norris, F. H., & Chipley, Q. T. (1992). Functional versus structural social support, desirable events, and positive affect in older adults. *Psychology and Aging, 6*, 562–570.

Neugarten, B. L., Moore, J. W., & Lowe, J. C. (1965). Age norms, age constraints, and adult socialization. *American Journal of Sociology, 70*, 710–717.

Pearlin, L. I. (1989). The sociological study of stress. *Journal of Health and Social Behavior, 30*, 241–256.

Pearlin, L. I., Lieberman, M., Menaghan, E., & Mullan, J. T. (1981). The stress process. *Journal of Health and Social Behavior, 22*, 337–356.

Pearlin, L. I., Mullan, J. T., Semple, S. J., & Skaff, M. M. (1990). Caregiving and the stress process: A overview of concepts and their measures. *The Gerontologist, 30*, 583–595.

Pearlin, L. I., & Skaff, M. M. (1996). Stress and the life course: A paradigmatic alliance. *The Gerontologist, 36*, 239–247.

Pearlin, L. I., Turner, H., & Semple, S. (1989). Coping and the mediation of caregiver stress. In E. Light & B. Lebowitz (Eds.), *Alzheimer's disease treatment, and family stress: Directions for research.* Rockville, MD: US Department of Health and Human Services.

Pratt, C., Schmall, V., Wright, S., & Cleveland, M. (1985). Burden and coping strategies of caregivers to Alzheimer's patients. *Family Relations, 34*, 27–33.

Pruchno, R. A., & Kleban, M. H. (1993). Caring for an institutionalized parent: The role of coping strategies. *Psychology and Aging, 8*, 18–25.

Pruchno, R. A., Patrick, J. H., & Burant, C. J. (1996). Mental health of aging women with children who are chronically disabled: Examination of a two-factor model. *Journal of Gerontology: Social Sciences, 51B*, S284–296.

Pruchno, R. A., Peters, N. D., & Burant, C. J. (1995). Mental health of co-resident family caregivers: Examination of a two-factor model. *Journal of Gerontology: Psychological Sciences, 50B*, P247–256.

Pruchno, R. A., & Resch, N. L. (1989). Mental health of caregiving spouses: Coping as mediator, moderator, or main effect? *Psychology and Aging, 4*, 454–463.

Quayhagen, M. P., & Quayhagen, M. (1988). Alzheimer's stress: Coping with the caregiving role. *The Gerontologist, 28*, 391–396.

Rabins, P. V., Fitting, M. D., Eastman, J., & Fetting, J. (1990). The emotional impact of caring for the chronically ill. *Psychosomatics, 31*, 331–336.

Radloff, L. (1977). The CES-D scale: A self-report depression scale for research in the general population. *Applied Psychological Measurement, 1*, 385–401.

Reibschleger, J. L. (1991). Families of chronically mentally ill: Siblings speak to social workers. *Health and Social Work, 16*, 94–103.

Richards, L. N., Bengtson, V. L., & Miller, R. B. (1989). The generation in the middle: Perceptions of changes in adults' intergenerational relationships. In K. Kreppner & R. M. Lerner (Eds.), *Family systems and life-span development* (pp. 341–366). Hillsdale, NJ: Erlbaum.

Rossi, A. S., & Rossi, P. H. (1990). *Of human bonding: Parent-child relations across the life course*. New York: Aldine de Gruyter.

Rossi, P. H., Wright, J. D., Fisher, G. A., & Willis, G. (1987). The urban homeless: Estimating composition and size. *Science, 235*, 1336–1341.

Ryff, C. D. (1987). The place of personality and social structure research in social psychology. *Journal of Personality and Social Psychology, 53*, 1192–1202.

Seeman, T. E., Berkman, L. F., Blazer, D., & Rowe, J. (1994). Social ties and support and neuroendocrine function: The MacArthur studies of successful aging. *Annals of Behavioral Medicine, 16*, 95–106.

Seltzer, M. M., Greenberg, J. S., & Krauss, M. W. (1995). A comparison of coping strategies of aging mothers of adults with mental illness or mental retardation. *Psychology and Aging, 10*, 64–75.

Seltzer, M. M., Greenberg, J. S., Krauss, M. W., & Hong, J. (1997). Predictors and outcomes of the end of co-resident caregiving in aging families of adults with mental retardation or mental illness. *Family Relations, 46*, 13–22.

Seltzer, M. M., & Krauss, M. W. (1994). Aging parents with co-resident adult children: The impact of lifelong caregiving. In M. M. Seltzer, M. W. Krauss, & M. P. Janicki (Eds.), *Life course perspectives on adulthood and old age* (pp. 3–28). Washington, DC: American Association on Mental Retardation.

Seltzer, M. M., Krauss, M. W., & Tsunematsu, N. (1993). Adults with Down syndrome and their aging mothers: Diagnostic group differences. *American Journal on Mental Retardation, 97*, 464–508.

Seltzer, M. M., & Li, L. W. (1996). The transitions of caregiving: Subjective and objective definitions. *The Gerontologist, 36*, 614–626.

Settersen, R. A., & Hagestad, G. O. (1996a). What's the latest? Cultural age deadlines for family transitions. *The Gerontologist, 36*, 178–188.

Settersen, R. A., & Hagestad, G. O. (1996b). What's the latest? II. Cultural age deadlines for educational and work transitions. *The Gerontologist, 36*, 602–613.

Sistler, A. (1989). Adaptive coping of older caregiving spouses. *Social Work, 34*, 415–420.

Skaff, M. M., & Pearlin, L. Z. (1992). Caregiving: Role engulfment and the loss of self. *The Gerontologist, 32*, 656–664.

Stoller, E., & Pugliesi, K. (1989). Other roles of caregivers: Competing responsibilities or supportive resources? *Journal of Gerontology: Social Sciences, 44*, S231–238.

Sweet, J. A., & Bumpass, L. (1987). *American families and households.* New York: Russell Sage Foundation.

Taylor, S. E. (1983). Adjustment to threatening events: A theory of cognitive adaptation. *American Psychologist, 38,* 1161–1173.

Thoits, P. A. (1995). Stress, coping, and social support processes: Where are we? What next? *Journal of Health and Social Behavior,* Extra Issue, 53–79.

Turnbull, H. R., Turnbull, A. P., Bronicki, C. J., Summers, J. A., & Roeder-Gordon, C. (1989). *Disability and family: A guide to decisions for adulthood.* Baltimore, MD: Paul H. Brookes.

Williams, A., Ware, J. E., & Donald, C. A. (1981). A model of mental health, life events, and social supports applicable to general population. *Journal of Health and Social Behavior, 22,* 324–336.

Zarit, S. H., Reever, K. E., & Bach-Peterson, J. (1980). Relatives of the impaired elderly: Correlates of feelings of burden. *The Gerontologist, 20,* 649–655.

CHAPTER 14

Linking Social Structure and Self-Concept: Variations in Sense of Mastery

Marilyn McKean Skaff

Nearly two decades ago, Rosenberg and Pearlin (1978) wrote, "If social science is to go beyond the level of description, it is imperative to understand how a demographic variable enters the individual's life, is converted into interpersonal experiences, is processed by a particular cognitive structure, and reflects the individual's relationship to his environment." (p. 72). Environmental forces find many expressions in people's lives, but none is more clear nor more powerful than in the shaping of the ways people think about themselves, their self-concepts (George, 1990; Marshall, 1995). A particularly important component of the environments in which people live their lives entails those social structures having hierarchically ordered statuses, such as economic and occupational classes, gender, and ethnicity. These kinds of structures, where access to opportunities, privilege, and respect are unequally distributed, have a pivotal part in molding self-concept (Ryff, 1989).

It is no mystery that this is so. These systems of inequality influence the people with whom we interact and the conditions under which interactions occur and, of paramount importance, they influence the quality of the roles we occupy in major social institutions—notably family and occupational roles. In larger measure, the location of people within the ubiquitous social structures unavoidably exerts an impact on how people come to unders both their outer worlds and their inner selves (George, 1993). Social structure structures experience, and the structure of experience, in turn, underlies our concepts of self (Marmot, Ryff, Bumpass, Shipley, & Marks, 1997).

In emphasizing the omnipresence of social structures in people's lives and their importance to the formation of self-concepts, I do not wish to imply either a mechanical or unidirectional process. On the contrary, people occupying similar statuses may come to entertain dissimilar conceptions of themselves. Indeed, it is an enduring research challenge to explain such variability. Some of the explanation, undoubtedly, rests with the fact that our research typically falls short of observing all of people's relevant statuses, relationships, and roles. Another likely explanation is that people's lives are undergoing constant changes as their statuses shift and as the accumulation and mix of experiences undergo alterations. Such changes mean that self-concept itself is a dynamic construct, malleable across the life course; it is a process rather than a static entity (Marshall, 1996; Skinner, 1995). A dynamic view of the relationship between social structure and self-concept also requires an acknowledgment of the potential for the impact of individuals on social structure (e.g., the women's movement).

A significant part of individuals' identity consists of those roles and statuses indicative of their location on the tapestry of social structure. More subtle, perhaps, are the traits, behaviors, and beliefs that develop as part of the individuals' self-concepts by virtue of experiences that are at least partially organized by structural locations. Roles and statuses stand as vital intermediate links in everyday life between social structure and individual self-concept (George, 1990, 1993).

Of course, a life-span perspective is required to gauge fully the effects of social structure on self-concept: individuals' views of themselves are the result of an accumulation of experiences over a life time, experiences that to some degree are organized by those individuals' location within social structures and systems of inequality. However, if self-concept is seen as malleable throughout the life span, a process rather than a static product, we should be able to identify conditions in the current lives of people that explain some of the variation in self-concept.

This chapter attempts to establish such a link within the context of one specific role: that of family caregiver to a relative with Alzheimer's Disease. The examination of experience within this specific informal role combines role and stress theories (Pearlin, Lieberman, Menaghan, & Mullan, 1981; Pearlin, Mullan, Semple, & Skaff, 1991). There is abundant evidence that the caregiver role is one that contains all the elements of the stress process. Further, because of the inexorable progression of Alzheimer's disease, it is likely to provide a challenge to the mastery of caregivers, regardless of their location in the social structure. Within the caregiving role, we seek to explain at least a part of the relationship between one aspect of self-concept, sense of mastery, and social status, represented by household income, through conditions within the role of caregiver. To do so, we are empirically linking three conceptual levels: the macro/social-structural level (income), the meso level (the caregiving role), and the micro level (individual sense of mastery).

The basic question being asked is how income level comes to affect caregivers' beliefs about how much general control they have over what happens in their lives. Income is being used here as one representation of status within social structure. Admittedly, income alone is far from perfect as an indicator of one's location within the status hierarchy. However, economic resources do represent far more than just dollars—in a way, serving as a surrogate for other socially recognized indicators of status such as education, prestige, and lifestyle. It is not viewed as an individual characteristic, but rather as one imperfect indicator of the larger social forces at work, providing structure for the experiences of those who share similar locations (Marshall, 1994). Sense of mastery or control is what Mirowsky and Ross (1984) refer to as a "socially transmitted, and thus socially structured, conception of reality." (p. 2). In people's daily experience lie messages regarding the real and assumed control that they can exert over the important facets of their lives. Economic realities do affect opportunities and resources, which in turn become internalized as attitudes toward the self (Ryff, 1989).

As mentioned above, when we search for linkages between income and mastery within the caregiving role, an important part of the unexplained variance in the relationship between income and mastery will reside in the history of individual lives. Another source might be found in those domains in the participants' lives that we are not able to examine, including other roles and relationships beyond the caregiving role. However, our task involves establishing whether at least some of the relationship between income and mastery can be explained by conditions within the caregiver role. To do so, we must first ascertain whether caregivers' sense of mastery does vary by income level. Second, we must identify those conditions within the caregiving role that vary by SES. Finally, we examine whether these economic variations in conditions of caregiving help explain some of the relationship between SES and sense of mastery. Before addressing these questions empirically, we shall consider the conceptual underpinnings of the proposed model.

THE THEORETICAL MODEL

Figure 14.1 presents the basic theoretical model to be tested. This model suggests that the level of family income will have an influence on daily experience within the caregiving role, and that those conditions, in turn, will have an effect on the caregiver's sense of control. It is also assumed that there will be a direct path leading from income to mastery, based on previous life experience and other roles outside caregiving. The goal, therefore, is to understand how much of the total relationship between income and mastery is explained indirectly through the conditions of caregiving. As illustrated in the model, the links to be examined involve three conceptual areas: SES, chronic role strain, and mastery. First, I shall consider the evidence for a relationship between SES (represented here by income) and sense of mastery. Second, I examine the literature on social structure and stress. Finally, I discuss the literature on the relationship between conditions within a chronic stressful role and sense of mastery.

SOCIAL ORIGINS OF SENSE OF MASTERY

Defining Mastery

A sense of control or mastery has been referred to by a myriad of names. As it is used here, mastery refers to the general degree to which people feel they can control the forces that affect their own lives (Pearlin, 1983)—one way in which individuals view themselves in relation to the world. Feelings of control may vary by specific life domains; for example, the

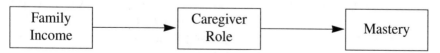

Figure 14.1 Theoretical model: Caregiver role as a mediator in the relationship between income and mastery.

level of mastery may vary from one of an individual's multiple roles to another. As used here, mastery refers to global feelings of control, much as self-esteem is used to refer to global positive self-evaluations (Rosenberg, 1979). However it may be labeled or operationalized, feelings of control have been found repeatedly to be related to psychological well-being (Pearlin et al., 1981; Turner & Noh, 1988). Although sense of control or mastery has often been treated as a resource or as moderating variable in stress research, in the model to be tested here, it is treated as an outcome. As such, it is the malleability of mastery as an aspect of self-concept in which we are interested.

Linking Social Structure and Mastery

In order to establish the connections between status within a stratified order, the experiences and quality of caregiving, and mastery, it is first necessary to observe whether people's sense of mastery varies with social status. Whereas the evidence is mixed for a relationship between mastery and ethnicity (Miller, Campbell, Farran, Kaufman, & Davis, 1995; Mirowsky & Ross, 1984; Skaff, 1995), age (Brandtstadter & Rothermund, 1994; Lachman, 1986; Pitcher & Hong, 1986) and gender (Ross & Mirowsky, 1989; Thoits, 1987), in general, evidence has been pretty consistent that those with higher income and education report a greater sense of control over their lives (Downey & Moen, 1987; Mirowsky & Ross, 1984; Pearlin & Radabaugh, 1976; Ross & Mirowsky, 1992). In fact, personal control has been identified as an explanation of the relationship that has been found between social class and psychological distress (Turner & Noh, 1983).

Although there has been little empirical work establishing the mechanisms linking social structure and mastery, Ross and Mirowsky (1989) have described the conditions that link social class to a sense of powerlessness, the inverse of mastery. These relevant conditions among lower class persons include a) an inability to achieve one's ends; b) inadequate resources and opportunities; c) restricted alternatives; and d) the likelihood that the jobs occupied will provide limited autonomy. Specifically, the sense of not being able to control one's life reflects a realistic perception for those who lack financial resources. However, although these powerful lessons about individual control occur early and can be persistent, it can also be asserted that experiences appearing at later points in the life course can alter perceptions of control. For example, in a study specifically examining the relationship between income and sense of control in a sample of women heading households, Downey and Moen (1987) found that sense of personal efficacy rose over time in relation to increases in income. In our earlier work with the same sample of caregivers used in the present analysis, the malleability of mastery was demonstrated in response to caregiving experiences. Thus, it was found that sense of mastery declined over a 3-year period in those who continued to care for their relative during that time, it remained level in those who placed their relative in a care facility, and increased in those whose Alzheimer's disease relative had died (Skaff, Pearlin, & Mullan, 1996).

Social Roles as Intermediate Links
Between SES and Mastery

Our next task is to consider the mechanisms that might link economic status and sense of mastery. If social roles are the linking mechanisms between macro/social-structural factors and the individual, then we should be able to identify structurally organized conditions within those roles that help explain individual differences (George, 1990; Marmot et al., 1997; Marshall, 1990). Life-course theorists tend to link macro and micro levels through work and the family. From a developmental perspective, it is in interacting with other family members that a child first learns what is controllable. Of course, these lessons may be influenced by ethnic and cultural characteristics of the family and gender, as well as economic factors, but it is the family's access to resources via income that has a major influence on the context in which the child develops (Bronfenbrenner, 1986). The mechanisms through which these lessons of personal control are transmitted may include parenting styles (Baumrind, 1977), maternal responsiveness (Skinner, 1995), and more generally communication of family belief systems about control and a readiness to put these beliefs to test (Gecas, 1989). A child who grows up in an authoritarian family learns at an early age that control lies in the hands of powerful others. Likewise, a family whose relationship to the social power structure is one of dependence on external powerful others (employers, government, etc.) for its welfare transmits beliefs about powerlessness to its offspring. The type and extent of education the child receives will undoubtedly be influenced by the family's location in the social structure and may further reinforce the child's beliefs about the efficacy of his/her own efforts (Skinner, 1995).

If we were to believe that ideas of personal mastery, once formed, were stable, no further discussion would be necessary. An important underpinning of the current discussion, therefore, is our belief that sense of mastery is malleable; that is, it is responsive to the current and changing conditions of peoples' lives. It is easy to believe that the experiences of control or lack of such on the job and within the family—experiences likely to be organized at least partially parallel to the income structure—will have an important impact on the adult's feelings about personal control.

It be must noted that we are interested in more than role occupancy; the focus here, rather, is on the quality of the experiences within the role. Because institutional social roles usually represent arenas of considerable importance to people, chronic strain within these roles is likely to have a powerful influence on well-being, including views of self. Pearlin and associates (1981) found that sense of mastery was susceptible to diminishment as a result of enduring or chronic strain within major roles such as work, parenting, and marriage. They attributed this to the steady reminder that one lacks the ability to change the enduring, difficult conditions within roles of central importance.

SES and Stress

There is evidence that stress is not evenly distributed, but rather varies as a result of location on the social system (for an excellent review, see Aneshensel, 1992). There are generally two perspectives on the relationship between SES and stress (Kessler, 1979). One perspective attributes SES differences in stress to differential exposure, whereas the other emphasizes differential vulnerability. Pearlin and Lieberman (1979) found that those with low SES were exposed to the most severe role strains. However, Kessler, Price, and Wortman (1985) found that it was not differential exposure that was responsible for SES differences in distress, but rather that stressful experience had more adverse effects on those of low SES, primarily due to differential access to resources. It is not the purpose of this chapter to debate the relative strengths of these two perspectives; they are certainly not mutually exclusive. However, they do suggest some of the potential sources of SES differences in the experience of stress. Although it is unlikely that SES is related to the assumption of the caregiving role (something we are unable to test with our data), there may be greater strains experienced within the caregiving role by those with fewer resources. "Vulnerability" to stress includes differential access to such resources as social support and coping. Kiecolt (1994) suggests that social structure may influence beliefs people hold about the options and strategies that are available to them. Brown and Harris (1978) found that lower-class respondents in their study were more vulnerable due to their access to fewer confidants.

Stress and Mastery

The final link in our model is that between stressful life experience and sense of mastery. The literature on social stress provides fertile ground for an examination of how social structure might be linked to sense of mastery. Unfortunately, far too often in stress research, demographic variables are "controlled for" without considering how they might be implicated in the relationships being investigated.

There is evidence that chronic stress can indeed erode one's sense of control (Kiecolt, 1994; Pearlin et al., 1981; Pitcher & Hong, 1986; Rodin, 1986; Skaff et al., 1996). Pearlin (1989) suggests that mastery is affected by chronic strain because such strain serves as a constant reminder of people's impotence. The process of living with chronic stress can implicate the self in several ways: through unfavorable reflected appraisals, through self-perceptions of incompetence, or through unfavorable social comparisons (Kiecolt, 1994).

Caregiving as a Mediating Context
Between SES and Mastery

In this chapter, we focus on the qualities of experience within one particular role—one that has been called an unexpected "informal role" to distinguish it from institutional roles for which there is prior socialization (Pearlin & Aneshensel, 1994). It is within this informal role that we have a strategic opportunity to examine the relationship between social class and mastery under conditions of chronic stress—stress that resides within a structured set of relationships.

There are several points in the caregiving career where income may make a difference. Although Alzheimer's disease (AD) appears to be an equal-opportunity disease, striking at all levels of the economic structure, its consequences for families are not equal. Thus, there is a possibility that economic considerations influence the individuals selected to assume the role of caregiver. Further, it is reasonable to believe that once the role of caregiver has been assumed, the experiences within that role may vary with the caregiver's location on that structure. For example, economic level may influence a) the stressors the caregivers face; b) the social support they receive; c) the way they cognitively frame their conditions as caregivers; and d) the degree to which they feel burdened or overwhelmed by caregiving.

In many ways, AD caregivers have been placed in a situation guaranteed to reduce self-perceptions of control. There is nothing that can be done to halt the inexorable progression of the disease. Little can be done to alter cognitive decline, to delay increasing dependence, or to fend off the onset of problem behaviors. This is not to say that people cannot or do not cope in a myriad of creative ways with the objective and subjective conditions of caring for a relative with AD. However, AD caregiving stands as an opportunity to observe how the sense of mastery of people at different locations in the social structure is affected by a situation highly predictive of stressors resistant to amelioration.

Although it is tempting to assume that life as a caregiver should be easier for those with greater economic resources, one could also argue the reverse: the uncontrollable aspects of the caregiving relationship are more familiar to those with fewer such resources and therefore less detrimental to their sense of mastery (Miller et al., 1995). It is possible that those who are accustomed to intractable life problems and who have lower expectations of control might posses coping mechanisms—what Heckhausen & Schulz (1995) and others have called "secondary control"—that would allow them to redefine the stressors to be less damaging to their sense of personal control.

When we attempt to explain the links between SES and sense of mastery, we shall consider four areas: the conditions of caregiving, i.e., the primary objective stressors confronted by the caregivers as they care for their relative; the subjective assessment of the amount of hardship experienced by the caregiver; the social resources available to them, both emotional and instrumental; and the ways in which the caregivers cope with the stress of caregiving. That is, it will be possible to determine if economic status affects the sense of mastery both directly and indirectly through the chronic stressors to which they are exposed and the psychosocial resources to which they have access.

THE STUDY

The data that were used to test the model come from the first wave of a longitudinal study of stress and coping in a sample of 555 spouses and adult children caring for a family member with Alzheimer's disease or a related dementing disorder. The caregivers were recruited from a list of persons who had contacted local chapters of the Alzheimer's Association in the San Francisco Bay Area and Los Angeles County. We attempted to contact everyone on those lists who self-identified as primary caregiver (either spouse or adult child) to a noninstitutionalized person with Alzheimer's or a related disorder. Of the 1,740 persons contacted by telephone, over 1000 did not meet our inclusion criteria. A total of 164 persons refused to participate. No information is known about the eligibility of most of those who refused or those persons we were unable to contact; therefore an accurate response rate is difficult to calculate. Although this sample may not be representative of all caregivers everywhere, the distribution of characteristics is broad enough to allow us to examine their relationship with other attributes of the caregivers. (For more information about the study see Aneshensel, Pearlin, Mullan, Zarit, & Whitlatch, 1995.)

The data were collected in structured interviews conducted in the caregivers' homes. The characteristics of the sample are presented in Table 14.1. The participants are relatively well-educated, on average having slightly more than one year of college. The caregivers ranged in age from 27 to 88, with a mean age of 61.9 years (spouse caregivers: 70 years; adult children, 51 years). The average family income in this sample was slightly over $34,000 (SD = $22,000).

Variables in the Model

Mastery was measured by the 7-item Pearlin mastery scale (Pearlin & Schooler, 1978), a scale that is widely used and found to be both reliable and valid as a measure of global control. Income is represented by the annual household income in thousands of dollars, recoded for the regression analyses to midpoints of categories of income.

As mentioned earlier, the first task is to ascertain whether sense of mastery in this sample of Alzheimer's caregivers is related to structural variables. Although we are primarily interested in the relationship between family income and mastery, Table 14.2 presents correlations between mastery and a variety of demographic variables. Mastery is significantly related to income ($r = .21, p < .001$). It is also positively related to education, although the relationship is not as strong as that between income and mastery. There is a significant negative relationship between age of the caregiver and sense of mastery ($r = -.13, p < .01$). Mastery is not related to either race (comparing Whites with others) or to gender.

The second step in the analysis is to determine the relationship between conditions of caregiving and both income and mastery. In order for variables representing caregiving conditions to be included in the analytic model, it is required that they be related to both income and mastery, since it is only through the presence of both relationships that the indirect effects of income can be established (Table 14.3).

Table 14.1 Sample Characteristics of Alzheimer's Caregivers

Variable	Spousal Caregivers ($n = 326$)	Adult Child Caregivers ($n = 229$)
Gender		
Female	58%	84%
Male	42	16
Race		
White	87	80
Black	7	15
Asian	2	3
Hispanic	4	2
Age		
< 44	1	27
45–54	5	39
55–64	17	28
65–74	45	6
75–88	32	—
Education		
< High school	18	6
High school	29	25
Some college	22	32
College graduate	14	18
College +	17	19

Stressors

First, the question asked is whether the stressors faced by the caregivers varied with the level of family income. Thus, we might expect to find that people of different economic statuses are differently sensitive to similar conditions.

The primary stressors resulting from the care of the AD patient include the symptoms of cognitive decline displayed by the patient, Cognitive Difficulty; the ADL help given by the caregiver to the patient; and the Problem Behaviors with which the caregiver must contend (see appendix for scale items and alphas). These comprise what we have called the objective primary stressors (Pearlin et al., 1990). Although the actual cognitive and physical condition of the patient is not likely to be directly affected by economic level, the amount of care that is provided, and, therefore, the

Table 14.2 Correlations Between Mastery and Demographic Variables

	Mastery	Income	Education	Gender	Age	Race
Mastery	1.00					
Income	.21***	1.00				
Education	.15***	.43***	1.00			
Gender	.07	.07	.06	1.00		
Age	−.13**	−.20***	−.16***	.31***	1.00	
Race	−.08	.17***	.15***	.01	.12**	1.00

* *p* < .05 ** *p* < .01 *** *p* < .001

perception of the level of these stressors might be affected by financial standing.

As Table 14.3 illustrates, income is not related to cognitive difficulty—no amount of income can affect the inexorable course of cognitive decline. However, the higher the family income, the fewer the ADLs for which caregivers provide assistance, and the fewer problem behaviors they report. Because mastery is not significantly related to any of the primary stressors, none of the objective primary stressors was included in the final model.

Psychosocial Resources

Although the availability of adequate financial resources is expected to be related directly to mastery, we would expect some of that relationship to be indirect through psychosocial resources available to the caregiver. These resources include both social support and the ways in which the

Table 14.3 Correlations Between SES, Mastery, and Caregiver Conditions

	Mastery	Income
Primary Stressors		
Cognitive Difficulty	.06	−.06
ADLs	−.05	−.16***
Problem Behaviors	−.08	−.13**
Overload	−.27***	−.16***
Psychosocial Resources		
Instrumental Support	.09*	.12**
Emotional Support	.32***	.15***
Cognitive Reframing	−.10*	−.20***

* *p* < .05 ** *p* < .01 *** *p* <.001

caregiver copes with the stress of caregiving. There are two indicators of the amount of social support caregivers received. First, instrumental support represents the amount of help from both formal and informal sources that the caregiver received with patient care and household chores. The scores range from 0 to 4, representing the presence or absence of each type of help. The second measure, Emotional Support, refers to the amount of perceived support the caregiver receives from friends and family (see appendix).

In Table 14.3 we see that instrumental support is positively correlated with both mastery and income. That is, those who have higher family income receive more help with the chores they face as caregivers, and the more help they receive, the higher is their sense of mastery. Likewise, those with higher incomes also feel more supported emotionally, and emotional support is related to higher mastery.

In addition to social support, another resource that we expect to be related to both SES and mastery is the style of coping that is used by the caregivers in dealing with the stressors (Pearlin & Schooler, 1978). One domain of cognitive coping is negatively related to both SES and to mastery: the use of Cognitive Reframing. That is, those with lower incomes are more likely to use methods of coping with caregiving that include trying to make some sense of the illness, telling themselves that this is something to expect as people get older, and praying for strength to keep going on.

Overload

In the model proposed, it is postulated that the effects of income on mastery will be partially mediated through the influence of financial resources on the caregiver's subjective level of stress or burden, as well as on psychosocial resources. An important measure of the subjective stress experienced by the caregivers is the sense of Overload, an assessment by the caregiver that they have too much to do, they are exhausted when they go to bed, and have no time for themselves. Overload is negatively related to both income and to mastery.

Path Analysis: Linking Income to Mastery Through the Caregiver Role

We are viewing the conditions within the caregiving role as mediators in the relationship between income and sense of mastery. This model was tested using a two-stage path analysis in order to examine both the direct effect of income on mastery, as well as its indirect effects through conditions within the caregiving role (See Figure 14.2). (In doing so, we are ignoring the correlations among the caregiving variables.) Because the relationship between caregiver and care recipient (spouse vs. adult child) is related to both income and mastery and has been found to have important and pervasive effects on caregiving experiences (Aneshensel et al., 1995), it will be controlled in the analyses.

In the first step, each of the psychosocial resource variables was regressed on income, controlling for relationship. Then, mastery was regressed on all preceding variables in the model. The path coefficients presented in Figure 14.2 are the standardized regression coefficients (unstandardized coefficients in parentheses).

It is not in the effect of each individual path that we are most interested, as much as in the total effect. However, there are a few points of interest that bear mentioning. One rather surprising finding is that although income is slightly related ($p < .09$) to the amount of instrumental help the caregiver receives, this is not significantly related to mastery. Perhaps when a caregiver needs to turn to others for help with daily tasks, their own sense of mastery is not enhanced. (This could also be an artifact of combining both formal and informal help.)

An important portion of the effect of income on mastery appears to operate through its effect on both overload and emotional support. Greater financial resources are related to both lower levels of subjective stress and higher levels of emotional support, both of which are strongly related to sense of mastery. Income is negatively related to the tendency on the part of the caregiver to use cognitive reframing, a means of coping with the stressors of caregiving, however, this coping mechanism is subsequently only slightly related to mastery.

Overall, the effect of each of these paths is relatively weak, but their combined effect is more impressive. Thus, we see that the analytic model supports the theoretical model, helping to explain part of the relationship between income and mastery through conditions within the caregiver role.

Another way to compare the direct and indirect relationship between income and mastery is illustrated in Table 14.4. In a two-step regression analysis, examining the relationship between income and mastery, with and without the caregiving variables, the beta for income in the first step (representing the correlation between income and mastery with relationship controlled) is .18 ($p < .001$). When the caregiving role variables are included in the regression analysis, the relationship between income and mastery is .10. Thus, nearly half of the relationship between the two is indirect through income's effect on the lives of caregivers.

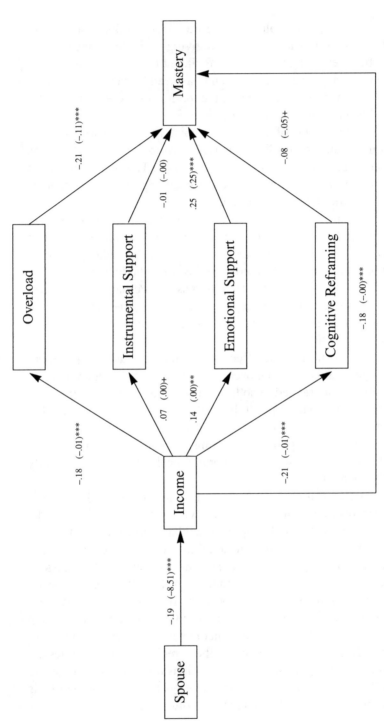

Figure 14.2 Analytic model: Path analysis of the direct and indirect effects of income on mastery, mediated by caregiver role.

+ *p* <.10; * *p* <.05; ** *p* <.01; *** *p* <.001

Standardized regression coefficients (unstandardized in parentheses)

Table 14.4 Regression Analyses: Mastery Regressed on a) Income Alone and b) on all Variables in the Model (Controlling for Relationship)

	Model a	Model b
Spouse	−.16***	−.16***
Income	.18***	.10*
Overload		−.21***
Instrumental Support		−.01
Emotional Support		.25
Cognitive Reframing		−.08+
R^2	.04***	.19***

$+ p < .10; * p < .05; ** p < .01 *** p < .001$
Table presents standardized regression coefficients.

WHAT DOES ALL THIS MEAN? SOME DANGLING QUESTIONS AND FUTURE DIRECTIONS FOR RESEARCH

Returning to the quote with which we began, Rosenberg and Pearlin (1978) suggested that we need to understand how demographic variables are translated into individual experience with the environment. In this chapter, we have examined how one demographic variable, income, is translated into the way individuals view of one aspect of their relationship to the environment: their sense of mastery. Two potential links in this translation that Rosenberg and Pearlin identified are interpersonal experiences and cognitive structures. Using a stress process model, we have taken one step in this examination by looking at how income affects psychosocial resources (social support and cognitive coping), as well as the perception of stress in the context of the caregiving role, and how those factors help explain the relationship between income and sense of mastery.

This is but a beginning in an attempt to understand how social status comes to have an impact on people's sense of self. It has been demonstrated that part of that relationship is channeled indirectly through psychosocial resources, more specifically, the degree of emotional support people perceive, and to a lesser degree, the use of cognitive reframing to cope with the stressors inherent in caregiving. An important link between income and mastery is the effect that financial resources have on a subjective sense of caregiver burden, their level of stress within an informal role. To the extent that caregivers with fewer financial resources feel an imbalance between the burdens of caregiving and the amount of time and energy they have available, their sense of mastery is threatened.

In the lives of caregivers, income cannot prevent or control the cognitive decline of the person with Alzheimer's disease; however, it does provide choices, alternatives, security. Those with more money were less likely to be involved in the daily care of their relative and less likely to report the difficult, problematic behaviors that can be very distressing for caregivers, although these primary stressors were not related to mastery. If we think of the stressors inherent in lower-income families, it is likely that the challenges of caregiving are only a part of the constellation of stressors they face each day. The other resources that appear to go along with financial resources may help explain why objective conditions of caregiving are less likely to have a direct impact on caregivers' sense of mastery.

There is little in the literature to guide interpretation of the effect of income on the caregiver's perception of social support. Brown and Harris (1978) found that lower-class respondents had fewer confidants, which led to greater vulnerability to depression. It is possible that those caregivers with low incomes have less time to cultivate supportive relationships; that the people they might turn to have problems of their own that might preempt their providing support.

There is some disagreement about social class differences in coping. Pearlin and Schooler (1978) found that those with low income and education were less likely to use efficacious coping mechanisms. Although we have viewed mastery as an outcome in these analyses, it is quite likely that the relation between coping and mastery is a reciprocal one. Ross and Mirowsky (1989) found that problem-focused coping (usually treated as a more effective approach to coping than emotion-focused or cognitive coping) was more likely to be found among those with higher mastery.

Inherent in the stress process model is the implication of the self (Pearlin et al., 1981; Pearlin et al., 1990). One relatively unexplored area is the individual variation in the degree to which stress arouses self-examination. Folkman's (1984) work on appraisal suggests a point in the process at which individuals might vary on their assessment of the threats involved in a stressful situation. Another potential avenue lies in the work on the mechanisms with which we evaluate where we are: reflected appraisals, self-perceptions, and social comparisons (Rosenberg & Pearlin, 1978). We might ask whether there are differences between people at various locations on the social structure in the nature and use of these mechanisms. How might SES affect the people to whom we look for appraisals of our performance, the standards against which we judge ourselves, or those to whom we compare ourselves? What we see when we observe our self is far from an objective picture. It is influenced partially by mechanisms in place that determine the information we use to make such observations. This information includes where we stand in comparison to what we should be, what others think of us, and where we are in relation to others in similar circumstances.

Previous analyses with the same data set revealed that respondents with lower income are more likely to report that they have gained personally (e.g., grown as a person and become more self-confident) as a result of their caregiving experience (Skaff & Pearlin, 1992). This way of positively framing the experience in some aspects resembles our measure of coping by cognitive reframing. The tendency to use emotion-focused coping and a positive evaluation of the impact of stressful conditions on one's self may represent a lifetime of confronting problems that do not have easy solutions. Those who truly have a history of limited control over their lives and fates may be less likely to see difficult circumstances as a reflection of their own inadequacy, yet it appears that sense of mastery is not increased by such cognitive redefining.

In this chapter, mastery is treated in a relatively unorthodox manner in that it is viewed as an outcome, a malleable self-view. This is in contrast to its typical role as a stable characteristic that moderates the effects of stress on well-being. One important area that is not addressed here, and needs to be, is the relationship between global mastery and domain specific control. One might ask whether it is possible to feel control in a specific area of life (e.g., caregiving), but feel little mastery in relation to the world in general, and whether these differences might covary with location within social structure.

We have a long way to go before we understand what people really mean when they report feelings of control (see Moss & Perkinson, 1995) and the specific experiences that underlie a global sense of control. A challenge that lies before us is to understand such self-views in the context of the realities of people's daily lives. It is when stressful life circumstances direct our attention to ourselves, i.e., change the way we define and evaluate our worth, including our level of control over ourselves and our environment, that those circumstances have the potential to affect our well-being.

Can we say anything about "vulnerability?" Cautiously, at best. If we define vulnerability as having fewer resources, then it would appear that our caregivers with lower income are indeed more vulnerable. The psychosocial resources that are related to income do appear to have an impact on their sense of mastery—in itself, an important resource. Our results suggest that the burdens of caregiving have a stronger impact on perception of stress among those with fewer financial resources. When caregiving is added to already challenging life circumstances, it is not surprising that such respondents would report having more to do than they can handle, or being exhausted when they go to bed at night. However, vulnerability implies a deficit that lies within the individual, rather than with the inequalities within a structured system. If people perceive less emotional support from those around them and feel more burdened by their caregiving perhaps "realistic" is a more equitable label than "vulnerable." The same could be said for their assessment of their control over their lives.

The results presented here do lend some support to other work that found differential access to resources helped explain SES differences in distress (Kessler et al., 1985). However, it was not possible to test adequately the exposure hypotheses: whether income was related to becoming a caregiver. Future work might examine whether Alzheimer's is indeed an equal-opportunity disease, and whether assumption of caregiving is related to financial resources.

CAVEATS

There are some important caveats that bear mentioning in regard to these analyses. First, a path model has been tested, implying a direction of causation. It is acknowledged that the relationships examined are quite likely to be reciprocal. Further, income is but one representation of social class. It is, however, one that is frequently used in research—usually as a "control;" therefore, it behooves us to understand how it actually affects the independent as well as the dependent variables that we study. There are other important social-structural variables that have not been included and that undoubtedly have an important impact on mastery and possibly on the relationship between income and mastery. In controlling for relationship between the caregiver and care recipient, we have at least partially "controlled for" age. However, it is quite possible that the relationships we observed may differ depending partly on the age of the caregiver.

For example, in analyses not presented here, it was found that whereas income is more strongly related to mastery than education for younger caregivers, the opposite was true for older caregivers. Similarly, Rosenberg and Pearlin (1978) found social structure to have different effects at different ages.

Another important variable that needs to be considered is race. Previous work has indicated that African American caregivers report higher mastery and that they differ on the predictors of that mastery (Skaff, 1995). Finally, although gender was not related to mastery or income, it is quite possible that the paths linking income and mastery are different for women and men. Likewise, there may be important differences between resources of spouses and adult children that need further clarification.

Although we have been able to account for 19% of the variance in mastery, there is a great deal that is left unexplained by the model presented here. In that unexplained variance lies a lifetime of socialization and accumulated experience of just how much control people actually have. As Ross and Mirowsky (1989) phrase it, "The sense of not controlling one's life reflects awareness of objective conditions" (p. 207).

CONCLUSION

The evidence presented here provides support for the suggestion that, if we are to understand how social structure affects well-being, it is indeed imperative that we begin to look at people's everyday lives (Pearlin, 1989; Ryff, 1989). The question yet to be answered is what the mechanisms are to explain these links we have observed. Unfortunately, these data do not allow that level of analysis, but do give us some sense of where to direct our future inquiries. The bridge between social structure and individual self-concept appears to be built, at least partially, upon the psychosocial resources with which people confront stressors in their lives. Income does appear to have an impact on self-concept—in this case, on sense of control. The challenge remains to understand the sources of these feelings within the context of daily experiences and the mechanisms by which they are converted into global attitudes about the self.

Appendix

Cognitive Difficulty (alpha = .86)

Now, I/d like to ask you some questions about your (relative's) memory and difficulty (he/she) may have doing some things. How difficult is it for your (relative) to:

A. Remember recent events
B. Know what day of the week it is
C. Remember (his/her) name
D. Remember words
E. Understand simple instructions
F. Find (his/her) way around the house
G. Speak sentences
H. Recognize people that (he/she) knows

Response categories: (4) Can't do at all; (3) Very difficult; (2) Fairly difficult; (1) Just a little difficult; (0) Not at all difficult.

Problem Behaviors (alpha = .79)

In the past week, on how many days did you personally have to deal with the following behavior of your (relative)? On how many days did (he/she):

A. Keep you up at night
B. Repeat questions/stories
C. Try to dress the wrong way
D. Have a bowel or bladder "accident"
E. Hide belongings and forget about them
F. Cry easily
G. Act depressed or downhearted
H. Cling to you or follow you around
I. Become restless or agitated
J. Become irritable or angry
K. Swear or use foul language
L. Become suspicious, or believe someone is going to harm (him/her)
M. Threaten people
N. Show sexual behavior or interests at wrong time/place

Response categories: (4) 5/more days; (3) 3–4 days; (2) 1–2 days; (1) No days.

Overload (alpha = .78)

Here are some statements about your energy level and the time it takes to do the things you have to do. How much does each statement describe you?

A. You are exhausted when you go to bed at night
B. You have more things to do than you can handle
C. You don't have time just for yourself

Response categories: (4) completely; (3) Quite a bit; (2) Somewhat; (1) Not at all.

Emotional Support (alpha = .87)

Let's turn now to the help and support you get from your friends and relatives. Thinking about your friends and family, other than your (relative), please indicate the extent to which you agree or disagree with the following statements.

A. There is really no one who understands what you are going through (reversed)
B. The people close to you let you know that they care about you
C. You have a friend or relative in whose opinions you have confidence
D. You have someone who you feel you can trust
E. You have people around you who help you to keep your spirits up
F. There are people in your life who make you feel good about yourself
G. You have at least one friend or relative you can really confide in
H. You have at least one friend or relative you want to be with when you are feeling down or discouraged

Response categories: (4) Strongly agree; (3) Agree; (2) Disagree; (1) Strongly disagree.

Cognitive Reframing (alpha = .49)

Here are ways that some people think about caregiving and about their relative with memory problems. How often do you think in these ways? How often do you:

A. Try to make sense of the illness
B. Pray for strength to keep going
C. Remind yourself that this is something to expect as people get older

Response categories: (4) Very often; (3) Fairly often; (2) Once in a while; (1) Never.

REFERENCES

Aneshensel, C. S. (1992). Social stress: Theory and research. *Annual Review of Sociology, 18*, 15–38.

Aneshensel, C. S., Pearlin, L. I., Mullan, J. T., Zarit, S. H., & Whitlatch, C. J. (1995). *Profiles in caregiving: The unexpected career*. San Diego, CA: Academic Press.

Baumrind, D. (1977). *Socialization determinants of personal agency*. Paper presented at the Biennial Meeting of the Society for Research in Child Development, New Orleans.

Brandtstadter, J. & Rothermund, K. (1994). Self-percepts of control in middle and later adulthood: Buffering losses by rescaling goals. *Psychology and Aging, 9*(2), 265–273.

Bronfenbrenner, U. (1986). Ecology of the family as a context for human development: Research perspectives. *Developmental Psychology, 22*(6), 723–742.

Brown, G., & Harris, T. (1978). *Social origins of depression: A study of psychiatric disorder in women*. London: Tavistock.

Downey, G., & Moen, P. (1987). Personal efficacy, income, and family traditions: A longitudinal study of women heading households. *Journal of Health and Social Behavior, 28*, 320–333.

Folkman, S. (1984). Personal control and stress and coping processes: A theoretical analysis. *Journal of Personality and Social Psychology, 46*, 839–852.

Gecas, V. (1989). The social psychology of self-efficacy. *Annual Review of Sociology, 15*, 291–316.

George, L. K. (1990). Social structure, social processes, and social-psychological states. In R. H. Binstock & L. K. George (Eds.), *Handbook of aging and the social sciences (3rd ed.)* (pp. 186–204). New York: Academic Press.

George, L. K. (1993). Sociological perspectives on life transitions. *Annual Review of Sociology, 19*, 351–371.

Heckhausen, J., & Schultz, R. (1995). A life-span theory of control. *Psychological Review, 102*(2), 284–304.

Kessler, R. C. (1979). Stress, social status, and psychological distress. *Journal of Health and Social Behavior, 20*, 259–272.

Kessler, R. C., Price, R. H., & Wortman, C. B. (1985). Social factors in psychopathology: Stress, social support, and coping processes. *Annual Review of Psychology, 36*, 531–572.

Kiecolt, K. J. (1994). Stress and the decision to change oneself. *Social Psychology Quarterly, 57*(1), 49–63.

Lachman, M. E. (1986). Personal control in later life: Stability, change, and cognitive correlates. In M. M. Baltes & P. B. Baltes (Eds.), *The psychology of control and aging* (pp. 207–236). Hillsdale, NJ: Erlbaum.

Marmot, M., Ryff, C. D., Bumpass, L. L., Shipley, M., & Marks, N. F. (1997). Social inequalities in health: Next questions and converging evidence. *Social Science and Medicine, 44*(6), 901–910.

Marshall, V. W. (1993). The micro-macro link in the sociology of aging. In C. Hummel and C. J. D'Epinay (Eds.), *Images of aging in Western societies* (pp. 337–371). Geneva: Centre for Interdisciplinary Gerontology, University of Geneva.

Marshall, V. W. (1994). Sociology, psychology, and the theoretical legacy of the Kansas City Studies. *The Gerontologist, 34*(6), 768–774.

Marshall, V. W. (1996). The state of theory in aging and the social sciences. In R. H. Binstock, L. K. George, V. W. Marshall, G. C. Myers, & J. H. Schulz (Eds.), *Handbook of aging and the social sciences* (pp. 12–30). San Diego, CA: Academic Press.

Miller, B., Campbell, R. T., Farran, C. J., Kaufman, J. E., & Davis, L. (1995). Race, control, mastery, and caregiver distress. *Journal of Gerontology: Social Sciences, 50B*(6), 5374–5382.

Mirowsky, J. & Ross, C. E. (1984). Mexican culture and its emotional contradictions. *Journal of Health and Social Behavior, 25,* 2–13.

Moss, M., & Perkinson, M. (1995, November). *The Ms-tery of mastery: The meaning of mastery for care-giving middle-aged women.* Paper presented in a symposium at the Annual Meeting of The Gerontological Society of America, Los Angeles.

Pearlin, L. I. (1983). Role strains and personal stress. In H. B. Kaplan (Ed.), *Psychosocial stress: Trends in theory and research* (pp. 3–32). New York: Academic Press.

Pearlin, L. I. (1989) The sociological study of stress. *Journal of Health and Social Behavior, 30,* 240–256.

Pearlin, L. I., & Aneshensel, C.A. (1994). Caregiving: The unexpected career. *Social Justice Research, 7,* 373–390.

Pearlin, L. I., & Lieberman, M. A. (1979). Social sources of emotional distress. *Research in Community and Mental Health, 1,* 217–248.

Pearlin, L. I., Lieberman, M. A., Menaghan, E. G., & Mullan, J. T. (1981). The stress process. *Journal of Health and Social Behavior, 22,* 337–356.

Pearlin, L. I., Mullan, J. T., Semple, S. J., & Skaff, M. M. (1990). Caregiving and the stress process: An overview of concepts and their measures. *The Gerontologist, 30*(5), 583–594.

Pearlin, L. I., & Radabaugh, C. W. (1976). Economic strains and the coping functions of alcohol. *American Journal of Sociology, 82,* 652–663.

Pearlin, L. I., & Schooler, C. (1978). The structure of coping. *Journal of Health and Social Behavior, 19,* 2–21.

Pitcher, B. L., & Hong, S. Y. (1986). Older men's perceptions of personal control: The effect of health status. *Sociological Perspectives, 29*(3), 397–419.

Rodin, J. (1986). Aging and health: Effects of the sense of control. *Science, 233,* 1271–1276.

Rosenberg, M. (1979). *Conceiving the self.* New York: Basic Books.

Rosenberg, M., & Pearlin, L. I. (1978). Social class and self-esteem among children and adults. *American Journal of Sociology, 84*(1), 53–77.

Ross, C. E., & Mirowsky, J. (1989). Explaining the social patterns of depression: Control and problem solving—or support and talking? *Journal of Health and Social Behavior, 30,* 206–219.

Ross, C. E., & Mirowsky, J. (1992). Households, employment, and the sense of control. *Social Psychology Quarterly, 55*(3), 217–235.

Ryff, C. D. (1989). Happiness is everything, or is it? Explorations on the meaning of psychological well-being. *Journal of Personality and Social Behavior, 57*(6), 1069–1081.

Skaff, M. M. (1995, November). *Religion in the stress process: Coping with caregiving.* Paper presented in a symposium at the Annual Meeting of The Gerontological Society of America, Los Angeles.

Skaff, M. M., & Pearlin, L. I. (1992). Caregiving: Role engulfment and the loss of self. *The Gerontologist, 32*(5), 656–664.

Skaff, M. M., Pearlin, L. I., & Mullan, J. T. (1996). Transitions in the caregiving career: Effects on sense of mastery. *The Gerontologist, 11*(2), 247–257.

Skinner, E. A. (1995). *Perceived control, motivation, and coping.* Thousand Oaks, CA: Sage.

Thoits, P. A. (1987). Gender and marital status differences in control and distress: Common stress versus unique stress explanations. *Journal of Health and Social Behavior, 28,* 7–22.

Turner, R. J., & Noh, S. (1983). Class and psychological vulnerability among women: The significance of social support and personal control. *Journal of Health and Social Behavior, 24,* 2–15.

Turner, J. J., & Noh, S. (1988). Physical disability and depression: A longitudinal analysis. *Journal of Health and Social Behavior, 29,* 23–37.

CHAPTER 15

Intersections of Society, Family, and Self Among Hispanics in Middle and Later Life

Sonia Miner &
Julian Montoro-Rodriguez

INTRODUCTION AND BACKGROUND

The sense of self (e.g., well-being, life satisfaction, self-esteem, and belief system) is grounded in several factors associated with the larger society primarily involving economic, physical health, and social conditions. For Hispanics, issues of acculturation, discriminatory barriers, family support patterns, and norms of familism often compound more commonly experienced societal factors to shape the sense of self in later life. This phenomenon can be linked to the sociocultural grounding of self, which refers to the societal and cultural influence on the perception of self (Markus, 1989; Ryff, Lee, & Na, 1996).

This chapter focuses on the link between the society, culture, family, and the sense of self among middle-aged and elderly Hispanic persons in the United States. This population was chosen because of the varied macro (society), meso (family) and micro (individual) experiences of Hispanic persons which are influenced by place of birth, language, values, ethnicity, immigration, and residence patterns. Specifically, we are interested in the influences of socioeconomic status, health, acculturation (English language proficiency, foreign birth, length of time in the U.S., enclave residence, etc.), ethnic origin, norms of familism, and family structure on the sense of self and well-being (psychosocial indicators of happiness, depression, and self esteem) among middle- and later-life Hispanics living in the United States.

Recent social science research has focused on contrasts between cultures and the distinctions between individualistic, collectivistic, independent, and interdependent constructions of the self in society. Recognition of this psychological fundamental is thought to have an influence on the most basic aspects of human experience, including emotions, beliefs and behavior (Ryff et al., 1996). Those with an individualistic frame of reference would be expected to derive well-being from a more personal perspective (i.e., health, socioeconomic status, education level, gender). On the other hand, those with a collectivistic or interdependent construction of the self would be expected to derive their well-being from beliefs about the supportive responsibilities of the group (i.e., family). There is some evidence to suggest that the countries from which Hispanics immigrate have a more collectivistic attitude with regard to family support norms and the definition of self, when compared to the attitudes of U.S. native-born persons. We attempt to determine the differences in self and well-being between Hispanics who are more closely tied to their ethnic origin (e.g., first-generation immigrants, speak Spanish regularly, reside in Spanish enclaves, and have been residents of U.S. for a short duration) and those who have become acculturated to the more individualistic Anglo attitudes in the U.S.

WELL-BEING AND THE SELF

Ryff et al. (1996) provide a universal definition of well-being, "Well-being is above all a human construction. It is an attempt to define the contours of a healthy, positive life. To understand essential features of wellness is thus to grasp core values that shape the human experience and embody human hopes (p. 19)." Here, when we refer to well-being, we are defining this concept using psychological indicators of happiness, mental health, and sense of self. We operationalize psychosocial well-being to include three measures; global happiness, depression level, and self-esteem (or mastery). Other studies of non-Hispanic populations have examined more complex conceptualizations of well-being, including positive relations with others, autonomy, environmental mastery, purpose in life, and personal growth (Ryff et al., 1996). While our research is limited in its ability to tap into all of these levels of well-being, we provide an examination of what we believe are the most basic dimensions of the self.

CONCEPTS AND RESEARCH ON HISPANIC WELL-BEING IN LATER LIFE

Societal Barriers to Well-Being

The concept of psychological adjustment refers to one's subjective impression of his or her overall happiness, life satisfaction, and well-being. We argue that micro-level psychological adjustment is affected by macro societal variables (acculturation level, cultural familistic beliefs, ethnicity) and meso factors (family structure and contact). Societal variables include income, education level, wealth, and other variables that, in turn, have an impact on the sense of self. In addition, we consider subjective health and functional needs limitations to be indicators of access to societal resources (George, 1995), since these characteristics are often influenced by the societal availability of health care (or lack thereof).

Easterlin (1973) and others found a strong direct correlation between socioeconomic status and life satisfaction. Research indicates an inverse relationship between social class and psychological distress (i.e., lower education level is associated with higher depressive symptom scores) (Krause, 1991). Many Hispanic persons, with the possible exception of some older Cuban immigrants, experience barriers to high socioeconomic status (Bean & Tienda, 1987). Another affect of lower income occupations and low socioeconomic status may include a lack of health insurance benefits, which can in turn negatively affect health status (George, 1995). Studies on general and Hispanic populations find that level of functional need and health status has a consistent direct effect on well-being, life satisfaction, and depression (Larson, 1978; Markides, Costley, & Rodriguez, 1981). For all groups in U.S. society, independence and good physical health are important predictors of the sense of self. Research on older Hispanics has indicated that depression is related to issues of health, functional disability, and dependency, with those dependent and in poor health being the most depressed (Markides & Martin, 1990). Other factors affecting depression include discriminatory barriers to resources (including income and education), family structure, living arrangements (Markides & Martin, 1990), and gender (Mendes de Leon & Markides, 1988). We will consider family structure and living arrangement effects on well-being later in this chapter.

Much of the literature on mental well-being of Hispanics in later life compares these ethnic groups to Anglos in the U.S. Our research focuses only on Hispanics and the differences within that group, but it is useful to apply these comparative studies to a description of the differences among acculturated and nonacculturated Hispanics. In other words, there are Hispanics that are more traditional (e.g., retaining the cultural beliefs and language of origin) and those who are more acculturated (similar to Anglos). With this in mind, we can apply the available literature to the linkage between the social structure (society) and the self. For instance, Antures, Gordon, Gaitz, & Scott (1974) describe the social stress model as one where the group that is perceived as a minority group will suffer from higher psychological distress because they "absorb the added stresses caused by racial bigotry and discrimination" (p. 362). That societal stress is expected to be more detrimental to nonacculturated versus acculturated Hispanics in an Anglo-dominated culture such as the United States.

Acculturation, Culture, and the Self

In addition to sociodemographic and health factors, certain acculturation and cultural influences can be important macro-level predictors of well-being. For example, being a minority group member in a society may be likely to add stress in the form of racism, bigotry, language differences, lack of access to services, etc., which then affect an individual's sense of mastery and self-concept. The potential exists for minority individuals to decrease the societal stress by conforming to the norms and behaviors of that society (i.e., by speaking the dominant language, etc.). In contrast, another argument states that by adopting the values/language/beliefs of the dominant culture, Hispanics may lose some of their sense of self through an oppression of their culture of origin. We suggest that it is a combination of societal barriers and individual adaptations (through acculturation) that influence the sense of self among older Hispanics who reside in the United States.

To study the level of acculturation of Hispanics in middle and later life, researchers have considered measures such as the predominant language spoken (Cuellar, Harris, & Jasso, 1980; Taylor, Hurley, & Riley, 1986), place of birth, time of contact with the new culture (Markides, Rudkin, Angel, & Espino, 1995), and generation level (Griffith, 1983). Other research has proposed the development of scales using questions pertaining to self-classification and preferences for language, movies, television, radio, foods, and music (Cuellar, Arnold, & Maldonado, 1995; Marin, Sabogal, Marin, Otero-Sabogal, & Perez-Stable, 1987).

Markides et al. (1995) use a definition of acculturation which is measured by time in the U.S. and find that it is linked to well-being among middle- and later-life Hispanic persons. The term "acculturation" is used in their study to refer to a process of change experienced by members of a minority (i.e., Hispanic immigrants in the United States) towards the adoption of the majority group's culture (i.e., Anglo-American). This process of adaptation is frequently viewed as stressful by the minority group (Berry, 1980). The process of acculturation, however, is not a unidirectional phenomenon, since the two groups are mutually influenced by one another (Negy & Woods, 1992). Acculturation my be a selective phenomenon, with an individual adopting new values, beliefs, and customs while simultaneously retaining traditional values, beliefs, attitudes, and behaviors (Keefe & Padilla, 1987).

Some of the classic studies on Hispanic acculturation have focused on the residential and occupational environments of immigrants (Portes & Bach, 1985; Sanders & Nee, 1987). Specifically, these researchers argue that immigration into an ethnic enclave economy can either help (Portes and Bach, 1985) or hinder (Sanders & Nee, 1987) economic success and acculturation into mainstream society. Proponents of the enclave economy theory argue that a large Hispanic population in the community serves to buffer the effects of discrimination and barriers to success in American society. This perspective argues that members of ethnic minority groups can gradually work their way into the dominant culture by living and working with those who speak their language and understand their cultural practices, values, and beliefs (Portes & Bach, 1987). It could be assumed by this graduated approach that immigrants and their descendents who live in ethnic enclaves have a higher degree of well-being than those who are immersed into the dominant culture without this advantage. While the literature in this area is focused mostly on explaining economic assimilation of immigrants, we believe that it is useful to use the same framework to illustrate the process of linking macro-societal structure to micro or individual well-being through the process of acculturation. Those living in Hispanic enclave communities with neighbors and businesses owned by Spanish-speaking persons may find it easier to adjust to American society. The social stress model described above can be applied to this perspective by suggesting that a Hispanic enclave environment could serve to decrease the effects of the discrimination of the larger society. When adjustment and acculturation is less stressful, we can assume that well-being will be relatively high. Therefore, the size of the population of Spanish-speaking persons will serve as a link or moderator between the macro societal and micro individual level outcomes (e.g., well-being).

The empirical evidence available on Hispanic acculturation and its relationship to well-being is inconclusive (for a review see Kaplan & Marks, 1990; Negy & Woods, 1992). The research in this area tends to involve persons of all ages in multigenerational households, rather than focusing on Hispanics in middle and later life. Some of these studies have found that Hispanics in the U.S. who identify more with the traditional Hispanic culture are better psychologically adjusted than those who identify more with Anglo-American culture (Ramirez, 1969), especially when the acculturated individuals have family members who identify strongly with the culture of origin (Szapocznik & Truss, 1978). In contrast, other research has suggested that biculturality (identifying with both Anglo and traditional Hispanic culture) is highly associated with subjective well-being among Hispanics (Lang, Munoz, Bernal & Sorensen, 1982). However, Lang et al. (1982) suggested that greater satisfaction with life was expressed by those who were bicultured, but oriented more toward Hispanic than Anglo culture. It may be that acculturation helps the adaptation process of the individual to the societal demands, but that those who remain collectivistic in their cultural and family orientation have the highest levels of well-being.

Acculturation, measured by length of time in the U.S., was studied by Markides et al. (1995) who found recent migrants to be less depressed than native-born and long-term residents. This supports the "healthy migrant" viewpoint that only the strongest, healthiest individuals will immigrate from another country and settle in a foreign environment (Markides et al., 1995). This selectivity argument must be acknowledged when comparing the well-being of foreign born to native-born Hispanics. It may appear as if those who are less acculturated have a higher level of life satisfaction and well-being, but there is a process which selects only the hearty individuals for foreign immigration. The subsequent generations (more acculturated) in the new country will not have this benefit, and will appear less healthy, either physically or mentally, when compared to the migrants (less acculturated).

Other research disputes the above findings to suggest that those who are less acculturated or assimilated will be less successful in a dominant society and will experience unhappiness, especially as their children become more assimilated into the society (Gordon, 1964; Markides, Liang, & Jackson, 1990). The less acculturated may hold greater norms of familism and be disappointed when their expectations go unmet (Markides & Martin, 1990). Many of the relationships that we have discussed here have brought in the element of family belief systems and expectations. We will focus the next section on the meso level, which involves family structure and beliefs, as these factors span between society, culture, and the sense of self.

In sum, the literature is not clearly understood with regard to the effects of acculturation on the sense of self among older Hispanics. Some of the previous research has suggested that acculuturation provides a bridge between the society and the individual which results in a positive sense of well-being. In contrast, others argue that the self and life satisfaction are related to retaining one's sense of Hispanic culture and family beliefs while living in the dominant Anglo society.

Cultural Familism and the Self

The description of well-being introduced earlier can be expanded to include a component of family beliefs as a predictor of positive outlook and the sense of self. Familism as a cultural belief system refers to feelings of loyalty, reciprocity and solidarity towards members of the family (Triandis, Marin, Betancourt, Lisansky, & Chang, 1982). Familism has been proposed as one of the most important culture-specific values of Hispanics, which includes a strong identification and attachment of individuals to their nuclear and extended families. The family is viewed as the single most important institution for Hispanics as well as an extension of the self (Marin, 1993; Sabogal, Marin, Otero-Sabogal, Marin, & Perez-Stable, 1987). Here, we define the concept of familistic attitude measured by values and beliefs surrounding intergenerational support patterns. Specifically, familistic attitudes are those beliefs that parents and adult children should provide basic necessities (housing, finances, support, etc.) for one another if, for some reason, they cannot provide for themselves. Identifying familism as a concept in this research can help to distinguish those who have a collective versus an individualistic definition of the self. This serves as a key element to linking the macro cultural sphere to the individual level (micro) sense of self and well-being.

Family Structure, Support, and Interaction

Family support and interaction is considered one of the self-system mechanisms which increase an individual's subjective impression of life satisfaction. Social isolation among elderly persons is associated with higher depression, when compared to those who report active engagement in supportive social networks (Krause, 1991). Researchers have pointed to the effects of acculturation on depression among Hispanics which are mediated by the system of support, interaction, and norms of obligation to members of the family. Hispanic families are perceived as protecting their members against physical and emotional stress. The importance of that familial reliance can help to explain what some have called "the relatively trouble-free adaptation" of Hispanic immigrants (Cohen, 1979; Grebler, Moore, & Guzman, 1970). On the other hand, we have seen that family systems can also serve as a source of distress if: (1) one feels too dependent on their family, (2) if members of the family have different familistic expectations (Markides & Martin, 1990) and/or (3) if members are progressing at varying rates of acculturation (Markides et al., 1990; Szapocznik & Truss, 1978).

The perspective described in this chapter, which includes an examination of the effects of macro (societal) and meso (family) structure variables to describe Hispanic psychological adjustment after midlife, has only been utilized to a limited degree in the literature. This chapter attempts to pull these areas together to provide a more comprehensive approach to linking the societal, family, and individual spheres of social life for older Hispanics.

CONCEPTUAL FRAMEWORK

The self is ultimately linked to the society, but in the case of Hispanics in later life, this process is compounded by the degree to which one retains values of other societies (cultural beliefs of immigrants or decendants of immigrants), barriers to well-being that are associated with ethnicity, the degree to which they conform to American society (acculturation), and the effects of family structure and support. We illustrate this idea in Figure 15.1 below.

The macro structure is represented in this model by the sociodemographic and the culture/accculturation components. The sociodemographic components include income level, wealth, education, gender, age, urban residence, and health variables. Culture includes ethnic origin and cultural familistic beliefs. Acculturation refers to the length of time in the U.S., foreign vs. native birth, Spanish language utilization, and enclave residence. Hispanics in the United States can be either native- or foreign-born. The primary sources of Hispanic immigration are Mexico, Puerto Rico, Cuba,

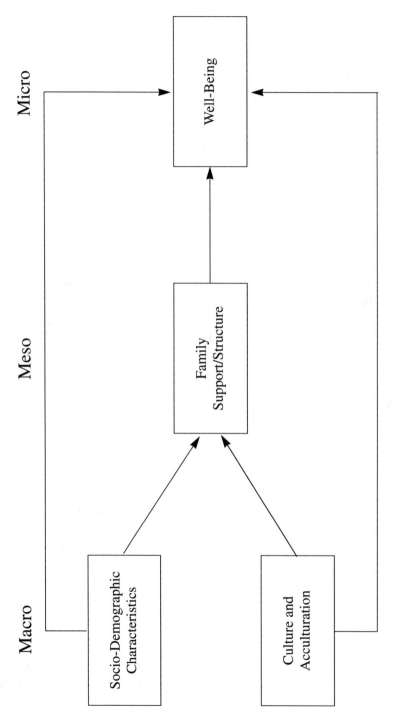

Figure 15.1 Macro and meso predictors of well-being among middle- and later-life Hispanics.

and Latin America. Foreign birth and the amount of time residing in the United States are important predictors of whether an individual has adopted the cultural beliefs and behavior of the dominant society (acculturation). In addition, whether the individual speaks English is another indicator of acculturation.

Enclave residence is included in the culture/acculturation sphere because it is assumed that those who live among others who are similar to themselves will have smoother transitions into the dominant culture and therefore higher levels of psychological well-being. The enclave may serve as a buffer to the negative effects of discrimination from the larger American society.

The meso structure is represented in the model by living arrangement and family structure variables. According to our model, these characteristics combine with the macro structure to influence well-being of Hispanic persons in middle and later life. However, family structure and support are also hypothesized to be affected by macro-structure variables. [Several researchers have noted that acculturation and family beliefs are linked to support functioning, and contact in Hispanic families (Lubben & Becerra, 1987; Wallace et al., 1994), with those who are more acculturated and less familistic showing lower levels of informal support.] Ultimately, we are interested in the effects of acculturation and cultural beliefs on level of family contact and support and finally the sense of self.

Other examples of effects of macro structure on families include that of ethnic discrimination, which often causes barriers to income that then go on to cause older Hispanics to live together in an extended family household rather than to live independently in separate nuclear family units. Being in such close proximity to family can either positively or negatively affect well-being, depending on whether the older person has retained ethnic values of familism, or, on the other hand, has adopted the more Anglo value of individuality.

We are interested in the effects of sociodemographic characteristics, structural barriers, culture, acculturation, enclave residence and familistic beliefs on the level of family contact and support which would ultimately affect the sense of self. However, we note that these macro and meso components of the model also directly affect well-being. For example, income level is directly related to global happiness (Easterlin, 1973; Ryff, 1995) and English language proficiency may have a direct effect on a person's self esteem. To illustrate these effects, we have indicated in the model where these macro and meso characteristics are directly linked to the sense of self (well-being).

Markides and Martin (1990) point out that the relationship between acculturation, family relationships, and well-being is quite complex. We hope to increase our understanding of these processes by empirically testing the following questions: Does acculturation weaken the norms of familism among Hispanics? What is the effect of this process on actual family structure, interaction, and support in middle and later life? Are happiness, depression, and self-esteem related to structural factors, culture, adaptations, family beliefs, and behaviors for older Hispanics living in the U.S.? Which sphere of social life has the greatest impact on satisfaction and well-being, the macro societal or the meso family level? What factors serve as links between the society, family and the self?

DATA AND METHODS

In order to ground our model in empirical research, we are using the National Survey of Families and Households (NSFH1) to analyze the responses of the Hispanic population aged 50 and over ($n = 226$) with regard to issues of society, family, and self. While the sample size is not ideal, it does provide us with an exploratory examination of our research questions. The majority of the respondents in this study are women (60%). About 10% of the respondents had been in the U.S. less than 20 years, which indicates that many respondents were either born in this country or were young migrants. Thirty-one percent of the respondents spoke Spanish ($n = 71$) at the interview, 53% were foreign-born ($n = 121$) and 62% ($n = 141$) were of Mexican ethnicity.

Dependent Variables

The main dependent variables in this research are measures of well-being (happiness, depression, and self-esteem). In addition, we will treat some other variables as dependent in the initial analyses, such as: norms of familism, support from adult children, and social contact with relatives. However, these measures will also serve as independent predictors of well-being and self esteem, as shown in Figure 15.1. Emotional well-being is measured by a global happiness item ("Overall, how would you say you are feeling these days?" 1 = very happy, 7 = very unhappy), as well as a 12-item depression scale (irritability, poor appetite, blues, trouble with concentration, depression, fatigue, fear, insomnia, withdrawal, loneliness, sadness, and lethargy). Reliability for the depression scale is excellent (alpha = .93). Self-esteem is measured by a four-item measure of agreement with the following questions: "I have always felt pretty sure my life would work out the way I wanted it to," "I feel that I'm a person of worth, at least on an equal plane with others," "On the whole, I am satisfied with myself," and "I am able to do things as well as other people." The reliability for this measure is less desirable, but still in the acceptable range (alpha = .60).

Norms of familism are measured by a five-item scale which measures the agreement with statements about whether respondents feel that older people should provide housing, economic support, and help with college expenses to adult children in need, and whether adult children should provide care, housing, and money to needy parents. This scale has acceptable reliability (alpha = .70). Actual support received is measured by responses to a series of five questions that ask whether a respondent has received regular support provided from adult children in: advice and listening to problems, news about mutual relatives and friends, help with household tasks and transportation, financial assistance, and companionship. Those with no children are coded as having 0 types of support from children. Social contact involves frequency of spending a social evening with relatives, coded 0 = never, 4 = several times per week.

Independent Variables

According to our model, the independent predictors of well-being include macro structural, cultural, and meso family variables. The sociodemographic macro-level variables include socioeconomic status, which includes a measure of family income, education (both measured continuously) and a dichotomous measure of homeownership (wealth). Demographic variables include age, gender (1 = female), residence patterns (urban = 1, other = 0), and health status, which is measured by level of functional disability (limited ability to care for personal needs, move around the house, work for pay, perform day-to-day household tasks, climb a flight of stairs, and walk six blocks).

Other macro level indicators include the degree of acculturation, which is measured by foreign birth, number of years in U.S., and whether the respondent speaks Spanish or English in the interview, and ethnicity, coded with the use of three dichotomous variables representing Mexican, Puerto Rican and "other".[1] Acculturation has been measured in several different ways with varying levels of detail. Some studies have simply used the time of residence in the U.S. (Markides et al., 1995), while others have developed elaborate scales of behavioral acculturation levels (Burnam, Telles, Karno, Hough, & Escobar, 1987; Cuellar et al., 1995; Szapocznik, Scopetta, Kurtines, & Aranalde, 1978) including several measures of language spoken in different settings, the language of the media preferred, food, dance, etc. We use three measures of acculturation in this analysis: foreign birth, time in the U.S. measured continuously (those born in the U.S. are coded with their age in years), and whether or not Spanish language is spoken at the time of the interview. Further information about the level of acculturation and the acculturation process is obtained by examining the contextual measure of the percentage of Spanish origin individuals in the county of residence. This will provide us with an idea of whether living in an ethnic enclave buffers the negative effects of being in a minority group in an Anglo-dominated society. We realize the limitations of these measures, but we feel that they do provide some information about the acculturation level of the individual. The familistic attitude scale (see above in dependent variables section) is used as an independent predictor of well-being in most of our analyses.

Our model suggests that family or meso-level variables serve to link macro and micro spheres. Meso-level variables include number of children, close proximity to nearest child (1 = nearest child lives within 25 miles), and living arrangements. Living alone was coded as a dummy variable (1 = live alone). Due to the small sample size, we were concerned about adding too many variables to the model. However, future research could examine other family structure variables such as household size, quality of relationships with family members, etc. In the analysis predicting well-being, we do include measures of the level of social interaction and support between respondents and their kin (see above in the dependent variable section).

The methods used in these analyses predicting familism, family contact/support, and well-being involved OLS regression techniques. For the measures of well-being, the independent variables were added in steps in order to show the relative influence of (1) sociodemographic variables and structural barriers (i.e., age, gender, urban residence, income, education, and functional limitations), (2) cultural values, acculturation, and enclave status (i.e., familism, Spanish language, time in U.S., ethnicity, foreign birth, and percent Spanish speaking in county), and (3) family structure, living arrangements, and available support/contact from kin.

---

1. In the analyses, Mexican ethnicity is the reference category.

RESULTS

Table 15.1 reports the global happiness, depression and self esteem scale means for selected variables for Hispanics age 50 and over. Men are happier and less depressed than women. There is a positive relationship between age and sense of self. Those who are older appear to have a higher self-esteem than the younger respondents. Health and functional needs were very important positive predictors of happiness and depression. Those in poor health with functional disabilities have lower levels of perceived emotional well-being (less happy and more depressed) and poor self-esteem.

Ethnic variations appear, with the Cuban/other group feeling the happiest and Puerto Ricans reporting the highest level of depression. Respondents who spoke Spanish at the interview reported higher levels of self-esteem when compared to those who spoke English. This provides some insight into the question regarding whether acculturation affects the sense of well-being, and gives support to the suggestion that those who suppress their culture and language may suffer in their sense of self. However, it should also be noted that this group reports the highest level of depression, when compared to English speakers. Other acculturation variables are important as well. Those who spent the shortest amount of time in the U.S. have a higher self-esteem, when compared to those who have been here longer. Those who live in low-concentration Hispanic communities were happier than those in counties with more Hispanics. This may reflect a pattern that may disappear once income and education are controlled. Higher levels of cultural familism is related to better self-esteem.

Interestingly, the group with no children had the highest level of self-esteem, when compared to respondents with children. Perhaps Hispanics with children feel lower self-esteem, especially if their children are more acculturated. People who visit with relatives report higher levels of happiness and lower depression levels than their more isolated counterparts. Similar to some of the literature, dependence on support from children is related to greater levels of depression. We now turn to the multivariate results which control for the independent variables in our model.

Table 15.2 reports the results of the analyses predicting familism, support from children and visiting with relatives. Acculturation variables did not predict support or visiting behaviors, but the time living in the U.S. was a significant predictor of familism. Those who have been in the U.S. fewer years are more familistic than those who have been here a long time (or since birth). This may reflect a pattern, where those who have been in the U.S. for less time are more dependent on their family ties than those

Table 15.1 Means for Happiness, Depression and Self-Esteem Scales by Selected Variables

		Happiness	Depression	Self-Esteem
Sociodemographic Variables				
Gender	Men	5.46	3.64	3.40
	Women	5.28	5.13	3.20
Age	50–59	5.22	4.45	3.27
	60–69	5.49	4.73	3.20
	70+	5.48	4.55	3.48
Residence	Urban	5.35	4.57	3.25
	Non-Urban	5.35	4.45	3.56
Family Income	0–9,999	5.22	4.35	3.40
	10–19,999	5.42	3.84	3.24
	20–29,999	5.66	5.04	3.13
	30–39,999	5.72	6.10	2.90
	40,000+	5.33	4.74	3.25
Education	0–11	5.33	4.97	3.28
	H.S.	5.50	3.55	3.06
	Coll.+	5.25	3.45	3.59
Needs	0	5.54	3.35	3.90
	1	5.38	4.71	3.40
	2+	4.89	7.79	2.93
Hispanic Culture And Acculturation				
Ethnic	Mexican	5.39	4.36	3.29
	Puerto Rican	4.92	5.51	3.13
	Cuban/Other	5.69	4.37	3.38
Spanish Speaker	Yes	5.39	4.84	3.59
	No	5.34	4.42	3.14
Foreign Birth	Yes	5.40	4.37	3.30
	No	5.30	4.78	3.25
Time in U.S.	0–19yr	5.13	4.73	3.78
	20–39	5.47	3.69	3.22
	40+	5.33	4.91	3.25
% Spanish in County	0–4%	5.79	4.55	3.25
	5–10%	4.75	6.14	3.66
	11–20%	5.21	5.04	3.07
	20%+	5.41	4.41	3.31

continued

Table 15.1 *(continued)*

		Happiness	Depression	Self-Esteem
Familism	0	5.55	4.36	2.72
	1	5.00	6.72	2.58
	2+	5.31	4.43	3.37
Available Family/				
Support & Interaction				
Children	0	5.17	4.04	3.63
	1	4.92	4.32	3.33
	2	5.80	4.12	3.20
	3+	5.37	4.83	3.22
Living with others		5.40	4.62	3.77
Arrangement alone		5.23	4.40	3.03
Visit kin	Never	4.79	5.92	2.95
	5/year	5.20	4.35	3.53
	1/month	5.21	5.16	3.20
	weekly+	5.82	3.68	3.18
Supp. Child	0	5.34	3.96	3.41
	1	5.57	3.64	3.25
	2+	5.34	5.03	3.21

who have been here longer or were native to the U.S. Puerto Ricans report more familistic beliefs than do Mexicans (the reference category). Those categorized as "other" Hispanics (Latin American or Cuban) reported getting less support from their children than did the Mexican origin ethnic group. Living close to (within 25 miles) of core relatives had a positive effect on feelings of familism, support and visiting. Those who have more children, urban dwellers, and females have greater chances of receiving support from a child. Interestingly, neither familism nor enclave residence have a significant effect on support received or visiting behaviors. It is true that those with less time in the U.S. (less acculturated) have greater norms of familism; however, other acculturation measures do not significantly predict the dependent variables described in Table 15.2.

The model predicting support from children had the highest degree of explained variance ($R^2 = .284$) of the three. The model predicting the frequency of visiting relatives was not particularly informative. The only significant predictor of this phenomenon was proximity to core kin, with those who have nearby relatives visiting more frequently.

Table 15.2 Coefficients (and Standard Error) of Regression Analyses Predicting Familism, Support From Children and Frequency of Visiting Relatives

Independent Variables	Familism	Support	Visiting
Gender	−.134	1.248***	−.257
	(.227)	(.264)	(.187)
Age	.013	.033	−.010
	(.018)	(.021)	(.015)
Urban	.143	1.118*	.155
	(.422)	(.492)	(.373)
Family Inc.	−.010	.017	−.004
	(.009)	(.011)	(.008)
Education	−.006	.011	−.018
	(.030)	(.035)	(.025)
Own home	.490*	−.103	.220
	(.242)	(.286)	(.201)
Needs	.058	−.030	−.097
	(.064)	(.075)	(.058)
Puerto Rican	.778*	−.091	.008
	(.357)	(.421)	(.303)
Other Hispanic	.256	−.885*	.073
	(.354)	(.413)	(.304)
Spanish Lang.	.231	−.554	.082
	(.326)	(.380)	(.269)
Foreign Birth	−.432	.332	−.361
	(.373)	(.436)	(.315)
Time here	−.025*	−.001	−.005
	(.010)	(.012)	(.009)
Familism	——	−.098	−.055
		(.088)	(.061)
County % Hispanic	.008	−.005	−.006
	(.005)	(.006)	(.004)
Live Alone	−.215	−.360	.333
	(.298)	(.348)	(.246)
Children	−.011	.151***	−.001
	(.039)	(.046)	(.033)
Core relatives	.927**	1.769***	.971***
within 25 miles	(.327)	(.389)	(.278)
Intercept	2.692**	−2.988*	2.501**
	(1.136)	(1.344)	(.968)
Adjusted R^2	.102	.284	.050
N	192	192	184

*p <= .05, **p <= .01, ***p <= .001

Tables 15.3, 15.4 and 15.5 report the findings of the OLS regression analyses predicting the happiness, depression, and self-esteem of Hispanics in middle and later life. In all three tables, independent variables are added in steps to show the effects of structural barriers, acculturation, and family structure/behaviors.

Table 15.3 predicts happiness among Hispanics. Similar to the findings of research on well-being for the general population, functional needs are an important predictor of happiness. Those with fewer reported health limitations reported greater happiness. Those who report high levels of familistic beliefs are more likely to feel happy. This may reflect a general optimistic attitude that includes a supportive feeling toward family. One finding in this table that seemed perplexing was the seemingly contrary effects of relative visits and relative proximity. Those with core family living within 25 miles report lower happiness scores, but those who have more visits with relatives are more happy. This may reflect the fact that some nearby relatives (perhaps even co-residing family members) may be serving as a source of strain, rather than having all positive effects. Another possibility is that nearby relatives have a negative effect on levels of happiness by not visiting enough or not meeting the social expectations of the middle-aged or elderly person. Visiting relatives may be a more welcome kin interaction and increase the happiness of Hispanic individuals in middle and later life. Adding family structure and behavior variables to the analysis is responsible for adding to the variance explained in the model ($R^2 = .10$). Interestingly, none of the true acculturation variables had any significant effect on happiness among middle-aged and elderly Hispanics in this sample, and they did not serve to increase the explained variance in the model. However, familistic beliefs, which are associated with time in the U.S., served as a strong predictor of happiness.

Table 15.4 illustrates the findings for the model predicting depression. Once again, the acculturation variables have relatively little predictive influence, but familistic attitude does have a significant effect. The pattern associated with family beliefs here suggests that those who have high levels of obligation toward family members are less depressed and those who do not have strong support beliefs have a greater problem with depression. Functional needs are significantly related to well-being. Similar to the pattern of well-being and happiness (reported in Table 15.3), those with more functional limitations are more depressed. These results confirm earlier research, which finds disabilities to be negatively related to psychological health in the general elderly population. There are some significant findings associated with the family structure measures. Similar to the results

Table 15.3 Coefficients (and Standard Error) for Regression Analyses Predicting Happiness for Respondents Age 50+ With the Predictor Variables Added in Steps

	Step 1	Step 2	Step 3
Gender	−.052	−.024	.068
	(.241)	(.259)	(.273)
Age	.005	−.010	−.006
	(.014)	(.020)	(.021)
Urban	−.142	−.093	−.287
	(.465)	(.526)	(.562)
Family Income	.007	.004	.005
	(.009)	(.010)	(.011)
Education	−.032	−.037	−.055
	(.032)	(.036)	(.036)
Own home	.353	.203	.075
	(.249)	(.292)	(.285)
Needs	−.141*	−.160*	−.168*
	(.065)	(.078)	(.080)
Puerto Rican[a]		−.675	−.632
		(.430)	(.432)
Other Hisp.[a]		.295	.425
		(.424)	(.439)
Spanish Language		.058	.009
		(.388)	(.382)
Foreign Birth		.427	.395
		(.442)	(.444)
Time here		.008	.010
		(.013)	(.012)
Familism		.133	.198*
		(.090)	(.090)
County % Hisp.		−.002	.002
		(.006)	(.006)
Live Alone			−.273
			(.341)
Children			−.049
			(.047)
Core relatives within 25 mi.			−1.117**
			(.420)
Visit relatives			.459***
			(.109)
Support from Children			.100
			(.074)
Intercept	5.273***	5.443***	5.198***
	(1.113)	(1.329)	(1.415)
Adjusted R^2	.005	.005	.100
N	195	178	172

*$p <= .05$, **$p <= .01$, ***$p <= .001$.
[a] Reference category is Mexican ethnicity.

Table 15.4 Coefficients (and Standard Error) for Regression Analyses Predicting Depression Scale for Respondents Age 50+ With the Predictor Variables Added in Steps

	Step 1	Step 2	Step 3
Gender	1.390*	1.244	1.113
	(.627)	(.671)	(.706)
Age	–.016	–.010	–.017
	(.036)	(.050)	(.053)
Urban	.508	.812	1.920
	(1.295)	(1.380)	(1.562)
Family Income	.014	.014	–.006
	(.024)	(.027)	(.028)
Education	–.113	–.146	–.074
	(.081)	(.090)	(.091)
Own home	–.169	.315	.251
	(.634)	(.734)	(.734)
Needs	.913***	.965***	1.006***
	(.169)	(.197)	(.205)
Puerto Rican[a]		.894	.762
		(1.071)	(1.081)
Other Hisp.[a]		.195	–.079
		(1.021)	(1.071)
Spanish Language		.345	.374
		(.952)	(.955)
Foreign Birth		–.642	–.769
		(1.085)	(1.100)
Time here		–.012	–.033
		(.032)	(.032)
Familism		–.418*	–.511*
		(.215)	(.218)
County % Hisp.		–.016	–.026
		(.016)	(.016)
Live alone			–.331
			(.893)
Children			.175
			(.121)
Core relatives within 25 mi.			1.622**
			(1.103)
Visit relatives			–.712**
			(.282)
Support from children			.093
			(.189)
Intercept	3.530	5.610	3.582
	(2.921)	(3.291)	(3.664)
Adjusted R^2	.172	.170	.221
N	186	171	165

*p <= .05, **p <= .01, ***p <= .001.
[a] Reference category is Mexican ethnicity.

for happiness reported in table 15.3, the family structure variables have a strange result. Living within 25 miles of a core relative (parent, child or sibling) is associated with higher depression, but frequent visits with relatives are associated with lower depression levels reported. It is possible that nearby family members are a drain on a person's sense of self and well-being in some instances. For example, perhaps close proximity to children or parents create stresses for caregiving to those generations, which do not allow for as many benefits as they do costs. Having "family neighbors" is not enough to have a positive effect on well-being, but to have relatives who visit does appear to increase well-being. Family structure variables are modest contributors to the model predicting depression, as the addition of the family variables in step 3 increased the proportion of the variance explained (from R^2 .17 to .22).

Table 15.5 reports the model predicting the self-esteem of middle-aged and elderly Hispanic persons. This model shows a drastic increase in the explained variance once familism and acculturation variables are added (R^2 = .025 to .167), with only a slight increase after the family structure and behavior variables were added (R^2 = .171) to the model. Examination of the correlations (not shown here) revealed that the familism variable was responsible for this vast increase in the amount of variance explained by the model. Familism and self-esteem were correlated at the .57 level, which is moderately high, but not enough for concern about multicollinearity. Close examination of these two measures finds no problems associated with overlapping meaning. Those respondents with a high degree of familism also have greater feelings of self-esteem. In addition to familism, Spanish language spoken at the interview is positively related to self-esteem. It is possible that the translation into Spanish had a slightly different meaning for the self-esteem variable. However, it is also possible that adopting the (often) second language of English has the effect of oppression of one's native culture and therefore a decline in the way one feels about one's self. Learning a second language may also make one feel less proficient at the art of communication, causing a decreased sense of mastery. This finding was a relatively consistent effect, even as we adjusted the specifications and variables in the model.

Functional needs and living alone are negatively related to self-esteem. Functional limitations have been shown to be a major predictor of well-being, whether it is measured as happiness, depression, or self-esteem.

It is worth noting that the contextual measure of the percent of Spanish persons in the county of residence does not have a significant effect on the sense of self measured by happiness, depression, or self-esteem. This

Table 15.5 Coefficients (and Standard Error) for Regression Analyses Predicting Self-Esteem for Respondents Age 50+ With the Predictor Variables Added in Steps

	Step 1	Step 2	Step 3
Gender	−.209	−.212	−.165
	(.146)	(.139)	(.154)
Age	.003	.015	.015
	(.008)	(.011)	(.012)
Urban	−.317	−.467	−.464
	(.254)	(.255)	(.285)
Family Income	−.008	−.001	−.006
	(.005)	(.005)	(.006)
Education	.014	.030	.025
	(.018)	(.018)	(.019)
Own home	.278	.131	.107
	(.148)	(.151)	(.155)
Needs	−.076	−.080*	−.102*
	(.042)	(.040)	(.046)
Puerto Rican[a]		−.007	−.073
		(.226)	(.236)
Other Hisp.[a]		.204	.112
		(.220)	(.238)
Spanish Language		.598**	.478*
		(.198)	(.207)
Foreign Birth		−.270	−.107
		(.239)	(.252)
Time here		−.003	.001
		(.006)	(.007)
Familism		.197***	.189***
		(.045)	(.047)
County % Hisp.		−.001	.000
		(.003)	(.003)
Live Alone			−.430*
			(.188)
Children			−.039
			(.026)
Core relatives within 25 mi.			−.143
			(.230)
Visit relatives			−.004
			(.059)
Support from Children			.003
			(.041)
Intercept	3.442***	2.088**	2.527***
	(.655)	(.679)	(.783)
Adjusted R²	025	.167	.171
N	184	182	174

*p <= .05, **p <= .01, ***p <= .001.
[a] Reference category is Mexican ethnicity.

variable was added to the analysis to determine whether residence in an enclave type of setting would have an effect on well-being (see Portes & Bach, 1985). Ethnic enclaves have received a large amount of attention in the literature (especially the issue of economic well-being) but did not predict the sense of self as it was defined here. These and other findings have shown that the sense of self among later-life Hispanics is better predicted by functional health, familistic attitudes, and family structure than by macro variables such as income, education, urban residence, and enclave residence. Occasionally the ethnic and acculturation variables predicted the well-being outcomes, but it is not a consistent pattern in the results.

DISCUSSION AND CONCLUSIONS

This research focused on the linking of the society, family, and self among middle-aged and elderly Hispanic persons. The relationship between structural barriers, culture, acculturation, family availability, behaviors, and beliefs on the individual's well-being were defined, conceptualized, and examined empirically. These factors were broken down into macro, meso and micro spheres so that we could more easily trace the process of linkage between these areas. We begin our discussion of this research by examining the findings as they indicate individualistic vs. collectivistic attitudes and beliefs among Hispanics in later life. We then turn to the macro (societal and cultural) and then the meso level (family structure and behavior) factors associated with well-being.

Cultural Perspective: Familistic Attitudes and Behaviors

Our earlier discussion described the difference between an individualistic versus collectivistic cultural perspective of the relationship between the self and the society (see Ryff et. al., 1996). Hispanics are thought to have a more collectivistic perception of the role of family in the individual's well-being. We found evidence of this collectivistic philosophy through the examination of familistic attitudes and beliefs. Specifically, those older Hispanics who hold intergenerational support norms of obligation are more likely to experience high levels of well-being. The self in the collective perspective is associated with the perceived supportive responsibilities of the group (i.e., family).

There was a relationship between the macro socioeconomic predictor of wealth (measured by home ownership) and collectivistic beliefs. Those who own their homes are more likely to report familistic attitudes and support beliefs. However, it is not clear whether this relationship is simply an artifact of the way that familism is measured in the data set used. Most of the intergenerational support beliefs measured here are related to the issue of economic support (i.e., college expenses, let parent/child live in household if they were having difficulties, provide financial assistance to parent/child). Future research could examine more in-depth measures of intergenerational obligation, such as emotional support beliefs (expectations of love, personal caregiving tasks and responsibilities, etc.).

There were some interethnic variations in the degree of collectivisitic attitude and behaviors exhibited. Puerto Ricans were more collectivistic as a group than their other ethnic counterparts, due to their higher familistic attitude scores. This belief did not translate into more actual support between Puerto Ricans and their kin compared to the other groups, but there was less actual support provided by children to the respondents in the "other Hispanic" category. Further research using larger samples of each Hispanic ethnic group is needed to get a better idea of the interethnic variations among older Hispanics in the U.S.

Acculturation is related to collectivistic beliefs among later-life Hispanic persons. More collectivistic attitude was found among those who were less acculturated (lived fewer years in the United States). However, acculturation variables were not successful predictors of actual support behavior, which was best explained by family structure variables. We did expect those with lower acculturation levels to be more familistic, which conforms to the notion that as Hispanics become acculturated into the dominant society, their attitudes begin to resemble the more individualistic attitudes that have been attributed to Anglos. However, since this study did not actually compare Hispanics to the Anglo population, we can not be sure that Anglos actually exhibit a more individualistic perspective. This would be a potential direction of future research. We were not able to examine this relationship between Hispanics and Anglos, due to our interest in the issue of acculturation, which is only comparable among other Hispanics, as this issue is moot among most native-born Anglos who have little ethnic identification outside of the U.S.

Macro Sphere Influence on Well-Being

Our model specified societal and cultural influences on individual well-being. We found that socioeconomic status, gender, and age were not significant predictors of well-being. Easterlin's argument that well-being is almost completely explained by economic status was not supported here. It appears as if the Hispanic population does not weigh socioeconomic characteristics heavily in their perception of the sense of self, when compared to the general populations represented in Easterlin's research. It is also possible that there is less variability in the income and wealth distribution in the Hispanic population studied here, therefore the impact of the gap between the rich and the poor is not as evident. Future research using larger samples of Hispanics (i.e., NHANES III) might be more successful in the examination of the effects of socioeconomic conditions as they shape the sense of self among Hispanics after midlife.

Although we found no association between socioeconomic status and well-being, we did find that functional disability status (health) was consistently related to happiness, depression, and self-esteem. This relationship between health and well-being among Hispanics is similar to that found in the general population. Ultimately, our research reported that the macro level is associated with the micro outcome because health status is highly associated with access to social and economic resources in society (George, 1995). Barriers to health care in U.S. society, which are related to the attainment of socioeconomic resources, may play an important role in the definition of the sense of self for older Hispanics. Obviously, those persons who are not insured have fewer opportunities for preventative care and tend to postpone treatment until their health problems become more acute.

The perception of self is entertwined with the experience of independence, interdependence, and dependency. Similar to the results of Markides' research, we found that those who report dependence on others have more psychological problems and a lower overall well-being (Markides & Martin, 1990). We did not find that there was a significant effect of receiving support from children on well-being, but we did find that reporting the need for help with tasks and movement (functional disability) was negatively related to well-being. This finding is probably due to the way that support from children is measured in this data set. Many of the items involve receipt of expressive support, and only one item relates to the receipt of instrumental assistance. Further research in this area would do well to examine who typically assists frail Hispanics and how this need for assistance shapes their sense of self and well-being.

In our conceptual model, discrimination is represented in the societal sphere. We suggest, for example, that discrimination against Hispanics in the dominant Anglo society has an effect on the levels of socioeconomic and health resources attained. Markides et al., (1980) describe the "social stress model" which argues that the harsh treatment experienced by a minority group in a dominant society is more detrimental to the well-being of nonacculturated persons than to their more acculturated counterparts. Acculturation, according to this model, serves as a buffer to the harsh treatment of the group perceived by the host society as "foreigners." Residence in a Spanish neighborhood or enclave would be expected to buffer the effects of the negative experiences in the dominant Anglo society, because nonacculturated persons could readily communicate and understand the world around them.

Our research found little support for the social stress model when describing the well-being of Hispanics after midlife. In other words, when we tested for the effects of acculturation, most often, we found no significant effects of acculturation on well-being. In the few instances, where relationships were noted, they tended to be in the opposite direction of that anticipated by the social stress model. For example, Spanish-language speakers reported having a higher sense of self-esteem. Further, the persons living in high Spanish concentration areas were not significantly more likely to report high levels of well-being.

There tends to be a conflict in the literature with regard to whether acculturation is a cost or benefit to one's sense of self. We find some evidence to suggest that a costly relationship exists. Specifically, those who have been in the U.S. longer report a lower level of familism, and familistic attitude is highly associated with well-being. A person who has high levels of familistic attitude tends to be happier, less depressed, and possess a better self-esteem, when compared to their counterparts with lower levels of family obligation beliefs. Again, the results that show lower self-esteem among English speakers would confirm this suspicion. However, it should also be noted that the other variables that measured acculturation, such as foreign birth and percentage Spanish speaking in the county, were not significant predictors of well-being.

One area that we were not able to test was the issue of biculturality. Previous researchers report that there are benefits associated with understanding both Hispanic and Anglo culture. They also argue that those who can maintain a bicultured perspective, while being slightly more oriented toward Hispanic culture are most satisfied with their life and sense of self (Lang et al., 1982: Ramirez, 1969). Further research would benefit from determining the role of the family in the relationship between cultural perspective and well-being. This suggests the possibility of interaction effects between these spheres as they are related to the sense of self. We now turn to a discussion of the meso sphere and the relationship to the self.

Meso Sphere and Well-Being

Families most likely play a role as a mediating system of support which ultimately is associated with the sense of self for Hispanics. It is possible that the family can serve as a source of positive feelings, distress, or both. Our research on Hispanic well-being found some curious results with regard to proximity to family and visiting behavior. In some instances, close proximity to "core" family members (parents, children or siblings) was associated with a poor sense of well-being. However, in contrast, those who visited regularly with relatives reported the highest level of well-being. For this reason, we find it difficult to provide a precise explanation for the effect of family variables on the sense of self. A larger data set with more precise measures of family structure (e.g., household size, quality of relationships, etc.) is necessary to examine this issue more closely. Further analysis of these linkages would include interactions between family and functional limitations (dependence level), differing levels of familism (family and individual levels), expectations of family, and whether family members are progressing at different levels of acculturation.

REFERENCES

Antures, G., Gordon, C., Gaitz, C. M., & Scott, J. (1974). Ethnicity Socio-economic Status and the Etiology of Psychological Distress. *Sociology & Social Research, 58*, 361–368.

Bean, F., & Tienda, M. (1987). *The Hispanic population in the United States in the 1980s*. New York: Russell Sage Foundation.

Berry, J. W. (1980). Acculturation as varieties of adaptation. In A. M. Padilla (Ed.), *Acculturation: Theory, models and some new findings*. Boulder, CO: Westview.

Burnam, M. A., Telles, C. A., Karno, M., Hough, R. L., & Escobar, J. (1987). Measurement of acculturation in a community population of Mexican Americans. *Hispanic Journal of Behavioral Sciences, 9*, 105–130.

Cohen, R. (1979). *Culture, disease and stress among Latino immigrants*. Washington, DC: Smithsonian Institution.

Cuellar, I., Arnold, B., & Maldanado, R. (1995). Acculturation Rating Scale for Mexican Americans-II: A revision of the original ARSMA Scale. *Hispanic Journal of Behavioral Sciences, 17*, 275–304.

Cuellar, I., Harris, L. C., & Jasso, R. (1980). An Acculturation Scale for Mexican-

Americans: Normal and clinical populations. *Hispanic Journal of Behavioral Sciences, 2,* 199–217.

Easterlin, R. A. (1973). Does money buy happiness? *The Public Interest, 3,* 3–10.

George, L. (1995). Social factors and illness. In R. Binstock & L. George (Eds.), *Handbook of aging and social sciences* (4th ed., pp. 229–252). New York; Academic Press.

Gordon, M. (1964). *Assimilation in American life: The role of race, religion and national origins.* New York: Oxford University Press.

Grebler, I., Moore, J. W., & Guzman, R. C. (1970). *The Mexican American people.* New York: Free Press.

Griffith, J. (1983). Relationship between acculturation and psychological impairment in adult Mexican Americans. *Hispanic Journal of Behavioral Sciences, 5,* 431–459.

Kaplan, M. S., & Marks, G. (1990). Adverse effects of acculturation: Psychological distress among Mexican American young adults. *Social Science and Medicine, 31,* 1313–1319.

Keefe, S. F., & Padilla, A. M. (1987). *Chicano ethnicity.* Albuquerque, NM: University of New Mexico Press.

Krause, N. (1991). Stress and isolation from close ties in later life. *Journal of Gerontology: Social Sciences, 46,* S183–S194.

Lang, J. G., Munoz, R. F., Bernal, G., & Sorensen, J. L. (1982). Quality of life and psychological well-being in a bicultural Latino community. *Hispanic Journal of Behavioral Sciences, 4,* 433–450.

Larson, R. (1978). Thirty years of research on subjective well-being of older Americans. *Journal of Gerontology, 33,* 109–125.

Lubben, J. E., & Becerra, R. M. (1987). Social support among Black, Mexican and Chinese elderly. In D. E. Gelfand & C. M. Berresi (Eds.), *Ethnic dimensions of aging* (pp. 130–144). New York, Springer Publishing Co.

Marin, G. (1993). Influence of acculturation on familism and self-identification among Hispanics. In M. E. Bernal, & G. P. Knight (Eds.), *Ethnic identity.* Albany, NY: State University of New York Press.

Marin, G., Sabogal, F., Marin, B. V., Otero-Sabogal, R., & Perez-Stable, E. J. (1987). Development of a short acculturation scale for Hispanics. *Hispanic Journal of Behavioral Sciences, 9,* 183–202.

Markides, K. S., Costley, D. S., & Rodriguez, L. (1981). Perceptions of intergenerational relations and psychological well-being among elderly Mexican Americans: A causal model. *International Jounal of Aging and Human Development, 13,* 43–52.

Markides, K. S., Liang, J., & Jackson, J. S. (1990). Race, ethnicity and aging: Conceptual and methodological issues. In R. Binstock & L. George (Eds.), *Handbook of aging and social sciences* (3rd ed., pp. 112–129). New York: Academic Press.

Markides, K. S., & Martin, H. W. (1990). *Older Mexican Americans: Selected findings from two San Antonio studies.* Tomas Rivera Center Publication.

Markides, K. S., Martin, H. W., & Sizemore, M. (1980). Psychological distress among elderly Mexican Americans and Anglos. *Ethnicity, 7*, 298–309.

Markides, K. S., Rudkin, L., Angel, R. & Espino, D. V. (1995). Health status of Hispanic elderly in the United States. Washington, DC: National Academy of Sciences Publication.

Markus, H. (1989). *Culture and the self.* Unpublished manuscript, University of Michigan.

Mendes De Leon, C. F., & Markides, K. S. (1988). Depressive symptoms among Mexican Americans: A three generations study. *American Journal of Epidemiology, 127*, 150–160.

Negy, C. & Woods, D. J. (1992). The importance of acculturation in understanding research with Hispanic-Americans. *Hispanic Journal of Behavioral Sciences, 14*, 244–247.

Portes, A., & Bach, R. L. (1985). *Latin journey.* Berkeley, CA: University of California Press.

Ramirez, M. (1969). Identification with Mexican American values and psychological adjustment in Mexican American adolescents. *International Journal of Social Psychiatry, 15*, 151–156.

Rogers, L. P., & Markides, K. S. (1989). Well-being in the postparental stage in Mexican-American women. *Research on Aging, 11*, (4):508–516.

Ryff, C. D. (1995). *Mechanisms of self-evaluation: Linking social structure to well-being.* Presentation at the June 1995 Summer Institute on Aging on Society and Self, Madison, WI.

Ryff, C. D., Lee, Y., & Na, K. (1996). Through the lens of culture: Psychological well-being at midlife. Unpublished manuscript.

Sabogal, F., Marin, G., Otero-Sabogal, R., Marin, B. V., & Perez-Stable, L. (1987). Hispanic familism and acculturation: What changes and what doesn't? *Hispanic Journal of Behavioral Sciences, 9*, 397–412.

Sanders, J., & Nee, V. (1987). Limits of ethnic solidarity in the enclave economy. *American Sociological Review, 52*, 745–773.

Szapocznik, J., Scopetta, M. A., Kurtines, W., & Aranalde, M. (1978). Theory and measurement of acculturation. *Interamerican Journal of Psychology, 12*, 113–130.

Szapocznik, J., & Truss, C. (1978). Intergenerational sources of role conflict in Cuban mothers. In M. Montiel (Ed.), *Families: Critical issues for policy and programs in human services.* Washington, DC: National Coalition of Hispanic Mental Health and Human Services Organizations.

Taylor, V. I., Hurley, E. C., & Riley, M. T. (1986). The influence of acculturation upon the adjustment of preschool Mexican-American children of single parent families. *Family Therapy, 13*, 246–256.

Triandis, H. C., Marin, G., Betancourt, H., Lisansky, J., & Chang, B. (1982). Dimensions of familism among Hispanics and mainstream navy recruits. Dept of Psychology, University of Illinois.

U.S. Bureau of the Census. (1993). *Hispanic Americans Today*. (Current Population Reports, P23–183). Washington, DC: U.S. Government Printing Office.

Wallace, S. P., Campbell, K., & Lew-Ting, C. (1994). Structural barriers to the use of formal in-home services by elderly Latinos. *Journal of Gerontology, Social Sciences, 49*, S253–S263.

CHAPTER 16

The Social Psychology of Values: Effects of Individual Development, Social Change, and Family Transmission Over the Life Span

Robert E. L. Roberts & Vern L. Bengtson

W hat accounts for the things we value in adulthood? Do the moral and ethical standards we claim in mid- and later life merely echo orientations we learned as children and adolescents? Or are values continually formed and transformed throughout life, reflecting the progression of developmental processes and the twists and turns of our biographical experiences? And just how do our value orientations relate to the larger sociocultural milieu? To what extent does social change promote change in individual value orientations, and vice versa?

Our aim in this chapter is to explore linkages among adult development, social change, and human values. The specific focus is to identify individual and social-structural factors accounting for lifetime stability and

Support for this research was provided by grants from the Spencer Foundation and the National Institute on Aging (R37 AG07977). The authors wish to thank Mary Anthony for invaluable research assistance and Linda Hall for expert technical assistance.

change in two values—individualism and materialism. Our choice of these values reflects an interest in understanding social trends in value orientations in the United States over the past half century. We note that many observers, from de Tocqueville to Christopher Lasch, have portrayed the American character as imbued with a particular reverence for individual autonomy and material attainments. Indeed, several studies confirm these observations, and suggest that late 20th-century America is becoming even more individualist and materialistic over time (Bellah, Madsen, Sullivan, Swidler, & Tipton, 1985; Putnam, 1996).[1] Our research explores the complex interplay between developmental and socio-historical processes underlying this cultural change.

Though secular trends in value orientations are relatively easy to document, drawing conclusions about the reasons for these shifts and forecasting future trends is very difficult. The primary hurdle is that not much is known about the malleability of value orientations across the adult lifespan. In particular, it remains unclear whether value orientations are "fixed" dimensions of one's personality in adulthood or remain pliable in response to aging processes, ongoing socialization in primary relationships, and changing social conditions.

Perhaps the clearest statement of the "fixed" position was articulated by Mannheim (1922/1952) who argued that value orientations were formed primarily in late adolescence/early adulthood as each new generation made "fresh contact" with the sociopolitical conditions of the day. These values were then carried forward throughout adulthood, shaping one's overall outlook in broad strokes until death. From this perspective, secular trends reflect the replacement of older cohorts (through mortality) with younger ones whose values reflect the distinctive sociohistorical conditions they experienced as adolescents (Alwin, 1990; Putnam, 1996). If America is becoming more individualistic, then it is because older, more collectivistic cohorts are being replaced by their more individualist heirs.

The alternative approach is to view value orientations as more pliant over the adult life course. Proponents of this approach argue that individuals' orientations remain susceptible to a confluence of influential forces reflecting age-based changes in physical and mental functioning, ongoing and new interpersonal relationships, and dramatic changes in the social milieu (Converse, 1987; Roberts & Bengtson, 1996). Thus, while one may enter

---

1. Although some researchers argue that there has been a shift toward "post-materialist" values: a complex of liberal humanist beliefs thought to underlie movements such as environmentalism, feminism, and libertarianism (Abrahamson & Ingelhart, 1987, 1995).

adulthood with well-formed value orientations, these outlooks may be altered in response to changes in health or functional status, relational experiences at home and work, and profound sociohistorical events and processes.

As one might guess, there is evidence to support both positions. Several well-known studies document dramatic long-term effects of early social conditions on lifetime values and other orientations (Alwin, Cohen, & Newcomb, 1991; Elder, 1974; Jennings, 1987; Marwell, Aiken, & Demerath, 1987). Yet other studies find either no connection between adolescent social experiences and later values (Converse, 1964, 1987) or effects limited to smaller subpopulations and/or very specific attitudes (Alwin, 1990; Schuman & Rieger, 1992; Schuman & Scott, 1989; Sears, 1983). Still other studies have found evidence that family members do exert influence on one another's values throughout adulthood (Acock & Bengtson, 1978; Bengtson, 1975; McBroom, Reed, Burns, Hargraves, Trankel, 1987; but cf. Jennings & Niemi, 1968; Connell, 1972).

Our goal in this chapter is provide the basis for a deeper understanding of secular trends in values by assessing the extent to which individual development, intergenerational influences, and sociohistorical change affect value orientations over a lifetime. By exploring these intersections of self and society in aging, we engage many of the theoretical issues raised in earlier chapters of this volume. Our central concern is with documenting the multiplicity and complexity of influences that flow between the developing individual and the many social contexts she or he inhabits. Our analysis is organized around three specific questions:

(1) How stable are individuals' endorsements of individualism and materialism over the adult life-span?
(2) What are the distinct contributions of life-span/aging processes, social-structural location, and historical change to individual changes in these value orientations?
(3) To what extent does stability and change in these values reflect intergenerational socialization processes in adulthood?

Prior to engaging the data, we discuss the classic obstacles that have plagued researchers who have attempted to draw conclusions about the diverse and interrelated effects of individual aging, interpersonal relationships, and macrosocial change on value orientations. We then propose a novel analytic strategy that we apply to a unique set of longitudinal data to distinguish these often indistinguishable influences on social psychological development.

PROBLEMS OF TIME AND SOCIAL STRUCTURE IN THE SOCIAL PSYCHOLOGY OF HUMAN VALUES

Human development is commonly viewed as the product of a complex interplay of mutually influential organismic and socio-environmental processes (Tudge, Gray, & Hogan, 1997). Numerous theories aim to specify the rich connections that link the developing person to his or her *oik* (e.g., Bronfenbrenner, 1979; House & Mortimer, 1990; Mannheim, 1922/1952; Tudge et al., 1997). However, empirical validation of these theoretical models has been limited by recalcitrant problems of research design and interpretation that make it difficult to distinguish organismic from environmental influences.[2] Particularly troublesome is the fact that individuals and their environments are continuously changing, leading to a "chicken and egg" problem of determining which factor(s) are temporally and causally prior to developmental change. Further complicating the issue is the fact that individuals are embedded within multiple overlapping socioenvironmental contexts that link their immediate experiences to events unfolding, in varying rhythms, across increasingly larger levels of social organization. In this section, we discuss how these temporal and structural complexities of human experience bear upon the social psychological study of values.

Temporal Complexity

Social psychological processes in human development are notoriously difficult to study because of the multiplicity of "clocks" that time individual and social aging. As Alwin et al. (1991) note, the primary challenge for developmental research is to untangle the unique and joint effects of complex forces that operate along two somewhat asynchronous timelines: biographical and historical. This challenge is even more daunting considering that each timeline encompasses a multidimensional array of developmental influences. For example, biographical time encompasses: (1) biological/maturational change, (2) shifting dynamics of key interpersonal relationships, and (3) transitions across key roles and statuses that characterize the life course (George & Gold, 1991; Hagestad & Neugarten, 1985). Historical time presents an equally complex metric insofar as it

---

2. Although some theorists (notably those promoting an ecological view) eschew the search for distinct influences, arguing instead that organism and environment be conceptualized as a holistic unity (e.g., Bronfenbrenner, 1979).

subsumes cyclical shifts in the political, economic, and cultural climates, as well as changes elicited by dramatic macrosocial events (e.g., the Great Depression, World War II).

Structural Complexity

Temporal complexity in developmental research is compounded by an equally thorny set of issues related to the subject's exposure to mutually influential and continually changing micro- and macro-social contexts. One can get a sense of this structural complexity by considering the problem of accounting for developmental influences on any social psychological attribute (e.g., beliefs, attitudes, values) of any individual at any given time. At the very least, formative influences operating at three levels of analysis must be considered. First, at the most general level, are macrosocial influences such as large-scale events, cultural practices, and/or political-economic configurations that distinguish the thoughts, feelings, and behaviors common to one population from those of another. Second, an intermediate level of influence consists of the ideographic social contexts that define each person's unique social biography. At this level, relationships and interactions with family members, friends, and others combine with local socioeconomic conditions to shape further each individual's distinctive outlooks and behaviors. Third, and most specific, are influences that reflect each individual's unique biopsychological development, especially with regard to the timing and magnitude of developmental changes one experiences. We use "structural complexity" as a shorthand for the notion that change or inertia at any of these three analytic levels has simultaneous and lingering implications for what unfolds at each of the others. This interdependence of individual and social contexts creates a complex field of potential direct and indirect factors that shape social psychological phenomena such as identities, attitudes, and values over time.

Temporal and Structural Effects on Value Orientations

Never are the temporal and structural complexities of interpretation more evident than when addressing the life-span development of value orientations. This is because values reflect perfectly the paradox of the social self. On the one hand, value orientations appear to be central dimensions of a core self: an array of individual preferences, beliefs, commitments, and affinities that partly distinguish one personality from another. From this perspective, life-span stability and change in values can be understood (at least partly) as a function of psychological processes that promote or inhibit intrapsychic consistency over time. On the other hand, value orientations cannot be reduced completely to individual psychology because conceptions of the desirable are learned socially, shaped under the press of influences spanning one's interpersonal relationships, social statuses, historical period, and cultural milieu. Thus, value consistency and change over the life-span is subject to numerous structurally situated influences, including individual developmental processes, interpersonal relationships, local social conditions, and far-reaching sociocultural and historical contexts. Moreover, the processes that underlie these influences unfold along the asynchronous timelines described above.

TOWARD A METHODOLOGICAL SOLUTION: MULTI-LEVEL MODELING OF LONGITUDINAL DATA

In this section, we describe in greater detail the methodological challenges faced by investigators studying intersections between self and society in aging processes. Specifically, we outline implications for data gathering and statistical analysis resulting from the temporal and structural complexity underlying the life-span development of values. We conclude by offering a partial solution to these methodological difficulties based on a novel combination of multi-cohort, longitudinal data gathering and multi-level statistical modeling techniques.

Temporal Complexity and Cohort-Sequential Designs

The methodological difficulties posed by temporal complexity are best exemplified by the well-known confounding of age/period/cohort effects in gerontological research (Riley, 1973; Schaie, 1994). In this context, aging effects encompass individual-level processes that promote change; period effects subsume transformative influences of sociohistorical events; and cohort effects refer to the lingering imprint of sociohistorical events on individuals born during the same historical epoch (Ryder, 1965). The synchronicity of biographical and historical time thus creates multiple plausible explanations for patterns found in a set of observations obtained across age groups and/or over time (Alwin et al., 1991). For example, observed age differences in a cross-sectional study confound the potential effects of aging and cohort differences. Moreover, results from such a design cannot be generalized beyond the specific historical period during which the observations were made.

A number of design refinements have been suggested for partially untangling age, period, and cohort confounds. One approach is to pool repeated cross-sections (Alwin, 1990; Glenn, 1977) in order to compare different cohorts measured at similar ages during different periods. This design affords some leverage over the aging/cohort confound and may allow tenuous generalization beyond a single historical period. However, because individuals are not followed over time, it is impossible to draw conclusions about age change over the life course. An alternative strategy is the longitudinal (panel) design, which does allow tracking of age changes. However, longitudinal designs are plagued by aging/period confounds that invalidate generalizations beyond the period of the study.

Several researchers have argued that the optimal developmental design is a hybrid of the repeated cross-section and longitudinal protocols (Mekos & Clubb, 1997; Schaie, 1994). The so-called cohort-sequential or generation-sequential design obtains repeated measures of multiple cohorts over time such that one can compare age changes for different cohorts measured during identical developmental stages, which necessarily occur in different periods.

The primary drawback of these sequential designs is that they require a large investment in time and resources to complete successfully. Very few studies provide the requisite multi-cohort panel data necessary to untangle age, period, and cohort effects. One such study—The University of Southern California Longitudinal Study of Generations (LSOG)—forms the basis for the analyses we will further elaborate and present below.

Structural Complexity and Multi-Level Modeling

The structural complexity of human development has been only marginally easier to sort out methodologically than has temporal complexity. Although research designs that capture data across levels of social structure can be developed easily (e.g., by aggregating individual-level data and/or by including measures of higher-order levels of analysis), it has been more difficult to model accurately effects across structural levels with extant statistical methods. The primary problem has been that estimation of structural effects in traditional linear modeling approaches has been plagued by aggregation biases, imprecise estimation, and confusion over levels of analysis (Bryk & Raudenbush, 1992).

Much of the difficulty in estimating multi-level models has resulted from the need to incorporate measures gathered at different levels of analysis (e.g., individual, contextual, and sociohistorical) into single-level prediction equations. For example, researchers interested in multi-level analysis were faced with two less than satisfactory options. First, one could disaggregate higher level variables in order to include them in individual-level equations. However, this strategy violated the assumption of independent observations because individuals sharing a higher-order context (e.g., they are in the same family, school, or workplace) have the same value for the variable(s) measuring that context. Second, the alternative option was to aggregate the individual-level data and perform the analysis at the higher level (e.g., at the level of families). This option was also unsatisfactory because most of the within-individual variation was lost to the analysis.

Relatively recent innovations in the statistical analysis of hierarchically structured data—variously referred to as multi-level models, mixed-effects models, random-coefficients regression models, and hierarchical linear models (HLM)—have rendered the aforementioned problems more tractable (Bryk & Raudenbush, 1992; Goldstein, 1987; Laird & Ware, 1982; Longford, 1987). (We will use the designation "HLM" as a shorthand for these modeling strategies throughout the remainder of this chapter). The central improvement is that rather than forcing aggregation or disaggregation to a single linear model, HLM allows one to represent each level of a hierarchical data structure by its own submodel, which is linked to the other submodels. Thus, in addition to expressing relationships among variables within each level of analysis, one can model relationships between variables across levels of the hierarchical structure.

To illustrate the logic of HLM, let us return to the three-level example of social psychological development described above. Each set of influences in the example can be represented formally by a series of three hierarchical equations. The first would model the individual's attribute(s) as a function of individual-level variables, such as age, the occurrence of certain life-events and/or transitions, educational level, or occupation. A second model would specify effects of variables representing contextual factors (e.g., family size, household income, or intergenerational solidarity) on the level-one parameter estimates. A third model could then be specified effects of population variables (e.g., GDP, percent college-educated) on each of the parameters estimated at levels one and two. This multi-level approach makes maximum use of the available data while being sensitive to the nested nature of the multi-level observations. HLM promises to be an important tool for understanding the ways in which influences are transacted across levels of social realty (for a more complete discussion of HLM, see Bryk & Raudenbush, 1992).

In this chapter, we use a novel combination of generation-sequential data and multi- level statistical modeling to disentangle age/period/cohort confounds while simultaneously estimating multiple social-structural influences on stability and change in individualism and materialism in adulthood. We will explain this analytic approach in greater detail in the next section.

METHODS

Sample

The analysis was based on data from the first five waves (1971, 1985, 1988, 1991, 1994) of the University of Southern California Longitudinal Study of Generations (LSOG), an ongoing study that has examined adult development in members of more than 200 three-and four-generation families over a quarter century (for details, see Bengtson, 1975; Roberts & Bengtson, 1990, 1993, 1996).[3] The current analyses were based on a subsample of the three oldest generations—G1, "Grandparents," G2, "Parents," and G3, "Grandchildren,"—who averaged 64, 44, and 19 years of age when the study began in 1971. Inclusion in the subsample was limited to participants from families for which at least one member from each generation provided data during two or more survey waves. This resulted in a final sample of 629 (143 G1s; 235 G2s; 251 G3s) individuals representing 116 families.[4] Table 16.1 presents information about respondents' age and sex distribution within each generation.

By Waves 4 and 5 (1991/1994), there was considerable intergenerational overlap in respondents' "age at measurement," reflecting the achievement of a fully generation-sequential design. For example, G2s ranged in age from 31 to 67 years in 1971. In the 1991, the G3s ranged from 35 to 45. This age overlap is advantageous in trying to disentangle

3. Participating families were sampled from an 840,000-member HMO in southern California. The membership list was used to identify three-generation families (with grandchildren between 16 and 26 years of age), from which the study pool was sampled random. In 1971 the HMO provided service primarily to labor unions. Thus the resulting sample was mostly White, working- and middle-class, and somewhat better educated than national norms (reflecting the union memberships).
4. The longitudinal retention rate over 23 years was approximately 50%, with G2s, women, and members of middle-income families being somewhat more likely than others to participate in all waves. Despite these minor selection biases, we found no significant differences between longitudinal respondents and dropouts on baseline value orientations. Following procedures suggested by Heckman (1976, 1979), we concluded that non-random attrition processes were not major sources of bias for the analyses reported below.

Table 16.1 Age and Sex Distribution of the LSOG Sample

	Generation					
	G3		G2		G1	
	Year					
	1971	1994	1971	1994	1971	1994
AGE						
Mean	19.2	42.3	42.7	65.8	64.5	85.2
Sd	2.6	2.7	4.8	4.8	5.4	4.7
Min	16.0	38.0	31.0	54.0	50.0	73.0
Max	26.0	48.0	67.0	90.0	86.0	92.0
SEX						
Female						
N	150	118	136	119	93	45
%	60	62	59	60	65	82
Males						
N	101	74	99	81	50	10
%	40	38	42	40	35	18
Total *N*	**251**	**192**	**235**	**200**	**143**	**55**

developmental and historical influences because it allows comparisons of measurements taken at similar developmental stages during different historical periods.

Measures

Value Orientations

Individualism and materialism were assessed with a ranking scheme adapted from Rokeach (1968). In each survey wave, respondents were asked to rank-order 16 desired "ends" in order of personal importance. Each of the items had been selected originally to reflect one of four value orientations: individualism (skill, exciting life, freedom, and accomplishment); collectivism (religious affiliation, loyalty, patriotism, and friendship); materialism (financial comfort, possessions, attractiveness, recognition); and humanism (service, equality, world peace, ethical life).

A factor analysis of the 1971 data revealed that much of the item response variability could be accounted for by two bipolar factors: one juxtaposing individualism and collectivism, the other contrasting materialism and humanism (Bengtson, 1975). Further analyses demonstrated factorial invariance across generations (G1, G2, G3) and time (1971–1994), enabling tests of generational and temporal differences in these values.[5] The measures of individualism and materialism were constructed by summing the numerical ranks of the eight items with substantive loadings on the corresponding factor. Prior to summing, items corresponding to the collectivist and humanist poles of the factors were recoded so that higher scores corresponded to more individualist or materialist values, respectively. The summed scores were then centered about the midpoint of each scale so that greater individualism and materialism were reflected by positive scores.

Independent Variables

We examine value orientations in relation to several markers of time and social-structural location.

Time was measured in two metrics: biographical (age) and historical (period). Biographical time was operationalized by the respondent's *age at measurement* centered about the grand mean (53.1) for the five waves.[6] Historical time was measured by two dummy variables that allow estimation of secular trends in each value orientation across the decades of the study. The first variable (*Trend80s*) received a score of "1" for observations in Waves 2 through 5 (1985–1994); the second (*Trend90s*) was coded as "1" when observations were from Waves 4 and 5 (1991 and 1994). Both variables were coded as "0" otherwise. Including both variables in the multivariate analyses enabled estimation of any secular trend between 1971 and the 1980s (Trend80s) and any change between the 1980s and 1990s (Trend90s).

Social-structural location was operationalized in three ways. First, location in the social age structure was operationalized via generational posi-

---

5. We assessed the extent of factorial invariance across generations and time by comparing a series nested measurement models using LISREL 8 (Jöreskog & Sörbom, 1993). Because the ranked data were ipsative, weighted least-squares estimates of the factor models were obtained from a matrix of polychoric correlations (weighted by the full sample asymptotic covariance matrix). A model specifying pattern invariance in the factor structure over time and across generations provided an adequate fit to the data, suggesting the items had similar meanings over time and across generations.

6. Age was centered about the grand mean for the sample for two reasons. First, we chose this strategy to decrease collinearity between age and indicators of period. Marking the passage of age-time relative to a hypothetical life span centerpoint (as opposed to Year 1 of the survey) enabled us to make period comparisons in relation to time marked from the baseline wave. Second, we chose the grand mean as our centering point because it provided a closer approximation of a normal distribution for age than, say, centering around one of the generational means.

tion in the family.[7] Two dummy variables were constructed, with a value of "1" assigned to G1s (*Gen1*) and G3s (*Gen3*), respectively. Thus, G2 represents the omitted category in multivariate analyses that include both dummy variables. Second, gender was operationalized via a dummy variable (female = 1). Third, an identifier variable indicating common family membership was used to link observations of individuals nested within the same generational lineage in families.

Analysis Strategy

Our research questions address the effects of developmental and social change on trajectories of value orientations over the life-span. We couple these questions with a concern with the potential mediating roles played by the social-structural contexts marked by age and gender. The analysis strategy we employed was to apply hierarchical linear modeling to our repeated measures data (Bryk & Raudenbush, 1992; Laird & Ware, 1982). We used these models to estimate both temporal and structural effects accounting for individual and group variability in individualism and materialism over 23 years. We modeled temporal trajectories (i.e., the extent of stability and change over time) by estimating individual and group growth curves in values. We assessed structural effects via estimating higher-order effects of generation, gender, and family on these growth curves. Three levels of linear equations were specified, wherein temporal effects were modeled at Level 1 and structural influences on those temporal effects were modeled at Levels 2 and 3. The three levels of analysis reflected the nesting of 3135 time-varying observations (Level 1) within 659 individuals (Level 2), who are themselves nested within 116 family lineages (Level 3).

Level 1

The most fundamental level of analysis involved estimating each respondent's trajectory of value endorsements over the 23-year period. We mod-

---

7. This strategy admittedly strains the usual emphasis placed on birth cohorts in conceptualizations of age structure because of the fairly large age range within each generation. However, despite the wide age range within generations, the fairly large age gap between generations yields primarily distinct, though large, birth cohorts. Moreover, most respondents within each generation were born within a particular decade. For example, about two-thirds of the G1s were born between 1902 and 1912. A similar proportion of G2s were born between 1928 and 1938 (Depression era children). And all of the G3s were born between 1945 and 1955 (baby boomers). Finally, we conducted parallel analyses that substituted dummy variables identifying 5-year birth cohorts for the generation indicators. Because we found no substantive differences across measurement strategies, we present results from models employing the generational contrasts.

eled the observed value orientation at time t for individual i as a function of a systematic growth trajectory (change over the five measurement occasions) and random error. Developmental contributions to the change rate were modeled as a function of a respondent's age at measurement (centered around grand mean of 53.1). Sociohistorical influences were modeled as a function of the decade within which the observation was obtained. Thus the Level 1 equation was:

$$Y_{tij} = \pi_{oij} + \pi(Age)_{ij} + \pi(Trend80s)_{ij} + \pi(Trend90s)_{ij} + e_{tij}$$

where the intercept parameter, π_{oij}, represents the true value orientation of a hypothetical person I who was 53.1 years old in 1971. The developmental change rate (corresponding to the time-varying covariate *age*) is given by $\pi(Age)_{oij}$. The parameters, $\pi(Trend80s)_{ij}$ and $\pi(Trend90s)_{ij}$, represent the secular change rate from 1971 to 1985/88 and any increment/decrement to that rate in the 1990s, respectively. The errors, e_{tij}, are assumed to be independent and normally distributed with a common variance.

Because observations are treated as nested within persons, HLM allows for variability in the number and spacing of observations provided by each person. This feature maximizes the number of cases that can be included in the analysis because it is not necessary to have complete data for each respondent across all waves (Raudenbush & Chan, 1993). Thus our estimates of the developmental and historical change rates are based on all available longitudinal data, some of which is from respondents (e.g., older G1s) who did not participate in all waves of the study.

Level 2

The individual change rate parameters estimated in Level 1 become the dependent variables in equations estimated at Level 2. We assume that the baseline value orientation, $\pi(Age)_{oij}$, and developmental change rate, π_{1ij}, may be influenced by a set of individual-level variables reflecting a person's social-structural contexts. Our analyses model these Level-1 parameters as a function of generational placement (as a proxy for age-cohort) and gender. We also assume the effects of sociohistorical change, as reflected by π_{2ij} and π_{3ij}, to reflect true period effects, exerting a consistent impact on all persons in the population (only fixed effects). We therefore, do not model period effects at Level-1 as a function of individual social structural characteristics at Level 2. The Level 2 equations are as follows:

$$\pi_{oij} = \beta_{00j} + \beta_0 \text{Female}_j + \beta_0 \text{Gen1}_j + \beta_0 \text{Gen3}_j + r_{oij}, \text{ and}$$

$$\pi(\text{Age})_{ij} = \beta_{10j} + \beta_1 \text{Female}_j + \beta_1 \text{Gen1j} + \beta_1 \text{Gen3j} + r\text{1ij}, \text{ and}$$

$$\pi(\text{Trend80s})_{ij} = \beta_{20j}, \text{ and}$$

$$\pi(\text{Trend90s})_{ij} = \beta_{30j},$$

where the parameters associated with the variables Female, Gen1, and Gen 3 represent effects of each variable on either the initial value orientation (π_{oij}) or the developmental change rate (πAge_{ij}). The intercept parameters (β_{0-1j}) correspond to average levels for the initial value orientation and developmental change rate, respectively, and are estimated after taking into consideration between family variability at Level 3.

Level 3

A third level of equations is specified in order to partition value orientation variability in initial value orientation and the developmental change rate between families in the sample. Thus, these equations are specified as:

$$\beta_{00j} = \gamma_{000} + \mu_{00j}, \text{ and}$$

$$\beta_{10j} = \gamma_{100} + \mu_{10j}.$$

To summarize, our models estimate effects of developmental and social change on value orientations via individual and group growth curves. The models assume that variability in initial value orientations and developmental change rates contain both random and systematic sources of variability. Systematic variability in initial orientations and developmental change rates is modeled as a function of a person's generation, gender, and family membership.

RESULTS

Descriptive Patterns

As prelude to our presentation of the HLM results, consider the means for individualism and materialism, cross-classified by measurement wave and generation, in Table 16.2. Results from one-way unbalanced ANOVAs (evaluating mean differences across waves and generations) appear in the

Table 16.2 Mean Individualism and Materialism Scores by Generation and Year of Measurement

INDIVIDUALISM		Generation				
	G3	G2	G1			
Year	Mean	Mean	Mean	Total	F	p
1971	3.45	1.56	−3.76	1.11	39.7	<.001
1985	3.58	.29	−3.17	.71	28.9	<.001
1988	1.51	−0.05	−3.86	−0.02	13.9	<.001
1991	2.34	.38	−3.29	.67	12.6	<.001
1994	1.92	.56	−3.83	.61	11.9	<.001
Total	2.62	.60	−3.56			
F	3.1	1.3	.17			
p	.016	.268	.958			

MATERIALISM		Generation				
	G3	G2	G1			
Year	Mean	Mean	Mean	Total	F	p
1971	−2.66	−2.63	−3.62	−2.87	.6	.572
1985	.09	−1.53	−0.82	−0.74	1.7	.191
1988	−2.17	−2.54	−1.01	−2.12	.8	.432
1991	−3.01	−1.93	−1.35	−2.30	1.1	.345
1994	−2.93	−0.76	−0.47	−1.65	3.36	.036
Total	−2.12	−1.89	−1.73			
F	4.28	1.43	2.14			
p	.002	.223	.025			

marginals. These data suggest some preliminary answers to our three research questions. For example, the individualism means reveal little movement over time, but are considerably different across generations. Only the G3s experienced a statistically significant change in individualism, becoming slightly more collectivist over time ($F = 3.08$, $p = .016$). Despite the change experienced by G3s, a pattern of significant intergenerational differences—with endorsements of individualism declining from G1 to G3—was maintained across all time points. The latter pattern suggests that a strong cohort effect is present in the observed endorsements of individualism.

The materialism means provide nearly the opposite picture. First, there appears to be somewhat more temporal variability in these data. Again, the G3 means appear least stable ($F = 4.28$, $p = .002$), but they are joined in this case by the G1s, whose means demonstrate marginally significant levels of instability ($F = 2.14$, $p = .075$). However, the pattern of instability varies for each generation, with the G3s appearing to have remained consistently humanistic, except for a turn toward materialism in 1985 (perhaps reflecting "yuppie" culture), and G1s appearing to move steadily in a materialist direction. Second, the generations do not appear to differ substantially in their endorsements of materialism over time. The only significant intergenerational contrast occurs for the 1994 data, with G1s and G2s appearing more materialistic than their G3 offspring.

Thus, the preliminary data suggest somewhat greater temporal stability in average levels of individualism as compared to materialism. Moreover, the temporal stability in average levels of individualism gives the impression of strong cohort differences. Although the generations were more similar in their endorsements of materialism, intragenerational instability in the means suggests the possibility of developmental and/or sociohistorical influences. Obviously, these data are limited for our present purposes, insofar as one cannot make inferences about individual-level stability and change from patterns of group means. In order to draw firmer conclusions, we turn now to the HLM results, which provide greater leverage in exploring the effects of developmental and social processes as they pertain to our primary research questions.

Stable Value Orientations Over the Life Span?

We address the question of individual stability in value orientations by using the observed change rates for each of the respondents to estimate an average rate of change for each value orientation. This procedure involves estimating a simplified Level-1 model that describes the average temporal trajectories of individualism and materialism. We perform this estimation in two stages. First, we model the average trajectory as a function of an average initial level (π_{ojk}) and an average change rate ($\pi(\text{Age})_{ij}$). Second, we re-estimate this model after including control terms for period effects ($\pi(\text{Trend80s})_{ij}$ and $\pi(\text{Trend90s})_{ij}$). Note that these models—referred to below as M1 and M2, respectively—are unconditional because neither specifies any Level-2 or Level-3 effects on the value trajectory parameters.

Table 16.3 presents estimates of the fixed (average) and random (varying across individuals) effects produced by the unconditional models. The estimates from the more parsimonious specification (M1) produce the first glimpse of the life-span value trajectories we elaborate more fully as we proceed through the analysis. This model describes a life-course trajectory for both individualism and materialism in terms of an average value for a hypothetical 53-year-old and a change coefficient that indicates the magnitude of change in values one can expect given a 1 year change in age. The coefficient estimates for M1 (column 1) describe a life-span trajectory characterized by a .066 decrease in one's true score on the individualism scale and a .461 increase in materialism for every 1 year of age. Both trajectories run through a life-span "midpoint" (at age 53) of .678 and -1.826, respectively.

The fact that the magnitude of each change rate reaches statistical significance suggests that individualism and materialism are not static over the adult life-span. Comparing the magnitude of Level-1 error variance for M1 versus a random effects ANOVA specification (omitting the age-change coefficient) reveals that "age at measurement" explains 7.4 and 9.3 percent of the variance in individualism and materialism, respectively.[8] These findings suggest that there is a modest degree of predictability (i.e., non-randomness) in change over time.[9] However, at this stage of the analysis, we can not determine how much of this explained variance is due to developmental versus sociohistorical change and/or the masked effects of cohort differences.

Effects of Sociohistorical Change

We begin our decomposition of developmental and sociohistorical influences by adding the control terms for historical period, Trend80s and Trend90s, to the first model (M2). The results, presented in Table 16.3, indicate significant secular trends in both individualism and materialism. First, the individualism estimates reveal a strong shift toward individualism from the early 1970s to the mid-to-late 1980s (π(Trend80s) = 1.43, $p < .001$). The estimates also show a further shift toward individualism from the 1980s to the 1990s (π(Trend90s) = .97, $p < .001$). Interestingly, including the controls for period effects doubled the age change estimate (π(age) = $-.133, p < .001$) for individualism. These findings suggests that individuals

---

8. The random effects ANOVA error variances for individualism and materialism were 24.52 and 33.38, respectively. The proportion of variance explained is equal to the difference between the error variances for the random effects model and the mixed model divided by the error variance for the random effects model (e.g., the equation for individualism would be ((24.52–22.71) / 24.52) = 7.4%).
9. Note that the significant random variance components associated with the intercept and age change coefficient indicate substantial variability of individual trajectories around the average trajectory. The fairly high reliabilities for each of the regression coefficients suggests that individual variability around each estimate is largely systematic, as opposed to random. The presence of such systematic variation encourages further exploration of the data for explanatory factors.

Table 16.3 Linear Models of Temporal Change in Individualism and Materialism (Unconditional Specification at Levels 2 and 3)

Fixed Effect	Coefficient		s.e.		p-value	
	M1	M2	M1	M2	M1	M2
Individualism						
Mean Orientation at 53	0.678	−0.936	.366	.457	.064	.040
Trend for 1985–88		1.427		.310		<.001
Trend for 1991–94		0.973		.205		<.001
Mean Age Change Rate	−0.066	−0.133	.010	.015	<.001	<.001
Materialism						
Mean Orientation at 53	−1.826	−3.487	.396	.504	<.001	<.001
Trend for 1985–88		2.276		.360		<.001
Trend for 1991–94		0.511		.236		.031
Mean Age Change Rate	0.461	−0.007	.013	.018	<.001	.683

Random Effect	Variance Component		df	Chi-Square		p-value	
	M1	M2		M1	M2	M1	M2
Individualism							
Orientation at 53	30.576	28.990	513	1900.8	1831.8	<.001	<.001
Age Change Rate	0.015	0.015	513	1116.8	1115.6	<.001	<.001
Level–1 Error	22.713	22.448					
Materialism							
Orientation at 53	40.961	40.746	513	1957.8	1975.1	<.001	<.001
Age Change Rate	0.022	0.024	513	1104.2	1124.3	<.001	<.001
Level–1 Error	30.248	29.587					

Reliability of OLS Regression Coefficient

	M1	M2
Individualism		
Orientation at 53	.957	.961
Age Change Rate	.681	.702
Materialism		
Orientation at 53	.956	.955
Age Change Rate	.863	.859

tended to become more collectivistic as they aged, although the sample as a whole was becoming more individualistic over time due to cohort replacement (i.e., there was greater attrition among the oldest generations, who were more collectivistic to begin with than the younger generations, especially the G3s). Looking at this another way, the tendency for individuals to become more collectivistic with age actually reduced the magnitude of the secular trend toward individualism from what one would have expected given the large cohort differences at baseline.

Second, the secular trends in materialism were similar to those of individualism. First, there was a large shift toward materialism from 1971 to the 1980s (π(Trend80s) = 2.28, $p < .001$) followed by a smaller increment moving to the 1990s (πTrend90s) = .51, $p = .031$). However, including the time period controls has the opposite effect on the age change rate estimate we saw with individualism, effectively decreasing its magnitude to zero (π(age) = −.007, $p = .683$). This indicates that most of the change in materialism reflects a sociohistorical trend not reducible to developmental change. However, unlike the trend toward greater individualism, the secular increase in materialism does not appear to be due to cohort-replacement. Recall from Table 16.2 that the G1s were not significantly more humanist in their orientations than the younger generations. In fact, over time the G1s became more materialistic than the younger family members. Further perusal of Table 16.2 indicates that the significant period effects found in the HLM modeling were most likely due to: (1) a large, but temporary, move toward greater materialism among the G3s in 1985 (perhaps again reflecting the popularization of yuppie culture); and (2) a significant move toward greater materialism among G1s in the later years of the study. This latter finding may reflect increasing concerns with financial security as the G1s live longer into retirement.

Conditional Models

Prior to drawing conclusions based on the estimates from M2, we consider the possibility that these temporal patterns can be explained by structural factors related to generational membership and gender. As discussed above, we treat generational membership as an indicator of the respondent's placement in the social age structure, reflecting the shared biographical and contemporaneous experiences of people of similar ages. In this stage of the analysis, we augment M2 with a Level-2 equation that models variability in each of the Level-1 parameters as a function of generation and gender. Thus, we are able to ascertain whether individual variation around the "average" trajectory varies systematically with one's location in age and gender structures. One advantage of this two-stage approach is that it allows estimation of potential cohort effects that might be embedded within the average trajectory estimates provided by M2.

Table 16.4 presents the conditional model estimates for individualism. It is important to keep in mind that the outcome variables in these equations are estimates of the Level-1 parameters. Thus, a set of Level-2 coefficients are provided for each parameter estimated in M2. Further, the intercept in each equation reflects the mean of the individual growth parameters for members of the omitted category as specified by the dummy variables at Level- 2. For example, the intercept for "orientation at 53" is the expected individualism score for 53 year old G2 males. Note that the value of this intercept (3.36) indicates that G2 men were relatively high in their endorsements of individualism around age 53. Further examination of Level-2 estimates for "orientation at 53" reveals a significant gender gap in expected values, with women, on average, much more collectivistic than men ($\beta= -2.25$, $p < .001$). In addition, the estimates for generational placement reveal less expected endorsement of individualism among G1s and G3s at midlife, though the differences fail to reach statistical significance.[10] Thus, while cohort differences account for some of the variability in estimates of midlife individualism, it appears that gender is a more powerful explanatory variable.

Perusal of the estimates for Level–2 predictors of developmental change reveals that, similar to the overall findings from M2, G2 males experienced declines in their endorsements of individualism with age ($\beta = -.210$, $p < .001$). Moreover, women and G1s experienced slightly lower change rates (incremental b's = .028 and .055, respectively), although the coefficients only approached statistical significance. Again, these findings suggest little effect of cohort membership on the rate of age-based change in individualism.

Table 16.5 presents the Level–2 estimates for materialism. We consider first the models for "orientation at 53." Note that the expected average for G2 males at age 53 is substantially higher than the estimate for the overall sample (i.e., -.466 versus -3.487). It appears that the G2 men were more materialistic as well as individualistic than other respondents. Again, we

---

10. If cohort effects accounted for variability in these data, one would expect to find substantive generational differences in the intercept terms for the equations. The weak generational differences discovered here increase our confidence in inferences about developmental versus social change effects on individualism.

Table 16.4 Effects of Generation and Gender on Age-Based Change in Individualism (a three-level HLM analysis of the LSOG sample)

Fixed Effect	Coefficient	se	*p*-value
Model for midlife orientation			
Model for G2 males			
Intercept	3.357	1.02	.001
Model for gender gap			
Intercept (females)	−2.246	.50	<.001
Model for G1 increment			
Intercept	−2.221	1.31	.090
Model for G3 increment			
Intercept	−1.880	1.26	.136
Model for 1980s trend			
Intercept	1.711	.771	.026
Model for 1990s trend			
Intercept	1.083	.342	.002
Model for age change rate			
Model for G2 males			
Intercept	−.210	.058	<.001
Model for gender gap			
Intercept (females)	.028	.020	.165
Model for G1 increment			
Intercept	.055	.030	.072
Model for G3 increment			
Intercept	.003	.026	.907

find a significant gender gap, with women tending toward more humanist orientations ($\beta = -2.29$, $p < .001$). We also find evidence of a modest cohort effect, with G3s endorsing more humanist orientations ($\beta = -2.90$, $p < .046$).

Next, we turn to the Level–2 models for the age change rate. As with individualism, we find the G2 male change rate to be substantively similar to the overall rate estimated in M1 (neither estimate is statistically different from zero). We also find no evidence of a gender difference in the age change rate ($\beta = -.015$, $p = .522$), but do find a suggestion of a cohort difference. Though only approaching statistical significance, the estimates for the G1 and G3 increments indicate that G1s gravitated toward more

Table 16.5 Effects of Generation and Gender on Age-Based Change in Materialism (a three-level HLM analysis of the LSOG sample)

Fixed Effect	Coefficient	se	*p*-value
Model for midlife orientation			
Model for G2 males			
Intercept	–.466	1.19	.696
Model for gender gap			
Intercept (females)	–2.289	.60	<.001
Model for G1 increment			
Intercept	.220	1.52	.886
Model for G3 increment			
Intercept	–2.901	1.46	.046
Model for 1980s trend			
Intercept	3.501	.89	<.001
Model for 1990s trend			
Intercept	–0.037	.39	.926
Model for age change rate			
Model for G2 males			
Intercept	–.060	.068	.375
Model for gender gap			
Intercept (females)	–.015	.024	.522
Model for G1 increment			
Intercept	.065	.036	.068
Model for G3 increment			
Intercept	–0.043	.031	.165

materialist orientations with age, while G3s tended to become more humanistic with age. A test of the contrast between G1s and G3s revealed the difference in age-change rates between these groups to be statistically significant.

Shared Family Trajectories?

We address our third research question by evaluating how much of the overall variability in value trajectories can be explained by family membership. In this analysis, family serves as an imperfect, but useful, marker of intergenerational transmission via shared social structural placement, socialization experiences, and genetic makeup across individuals. Although our design does not allow us to isolate effects within each of these categories, we are able to assess the overall degree of intergenerational similarity in the adult value trajectories within families.

Table 16.6 presents a decomposition of the random variance in individualism and materialism within each level of analysis. The significance tests associated with the Level–2 and Level–3 variances correspond to the null hypothesis of no between-individual or between-family variability in value trajectories. Thus the low probabilities associated with the Level–2 variances indicate that there was significant individual variability in midlife orientations and developmental change rates. Examining the Level–3 results indicates that there was also substantial between–family variability in the value orientations expected of family members at midlife. This finding provides evidence of substantive intergenerational transmission in value orientations, at least in terms of promoting similarity among family members in overall outlook. However, further examination of the Level–3 results indicates no effect of family membership on individual value trajectories over the life-span. This result suggests that the developmental and social change influences documented in the earlier analyses did not differ across families. Thus, while families may cultivate more or less individualistic or materialistic orientations in their members, the individual tendencies toward greater collectivism and materialism over time were not greatly affected by one's family ties.

Examining the decomposition of within- versus between-family variation further clarifies the picture. For instance, the relative contribution of family membership to the overall variance in expected midlife endorsements of individualism and materialism are moderately high: within-family similarity (between-family difference) accounts for 25.4% and 17.5% of the overall variation in the average orientation of individualism∂ and materialism, respectively. As one would expect from the general tests of the Level–2 and Level–3 hypotheses, the contribution of family membership to variation in the change rates is smaller, accounting for only 5.1% and 11.1% of the variation in individualism and materialism, respectively.

DISCUSSION AND CONCLUSION

This study sheds light on the effects of developmental and social change on endorsements of individualism and materialism over the adult life-span. Moreover, our analyses document the extent of family resemblance in value orientations over time. Prior to summarizing the results and dis-

Table 16.6 Variance Decomposition From the Three-Level Analysis of Individualism and Materialism Over the Life Span

Random Effect	Individualism		Materialism	
	Variance Component	p-value	Variance Component	p-value
Level–1 variance				
Temporal variation	29.42		22.42	
Level–2 (ind. within family)				
Midlife orientation	39.53	<.001	26.91	<.001
Individual change rate	.024	<.001	.015	<.001
Level–3 (between families)				
Avg. midlife orientation	8.40	<.001	9.15	<.001
Family change rate	.003	.172	.001	.161
Proportion of Variance (percentages)				
Midlife orientation				
Within families	82.5		74.6	
Between families	17.5		25.4	
Change rate				
Within families	94.9		89.9	
Between families	5.1		11.1	

cussing their implications, we suggest that inferences to the larger population and other value orientations be drawn with caution. Although our sample provides many advantages for developmental research, it is limited in that it is not representative of the U.S. population. While the LSOG sample has been shown to be quite similar to U.S. norms in terms of psychological well-being, family relationship quality, and sociopolitical attitudes, the sample does not represent well the low and high extremes on socioeconomic status or people of color. This artifact of sampling from a southern California HMO in the early 1970s limited the extent to which we could explore the effect of socioeconomic status and race/ethnicity on value trajectories. Despite these limitations, our analyses contribute to emerging understandings of life-span developmental processes in several ways.

First, we have demonstrated the effectiveness of combining a generation-sequential design with dynamic hierarchical modeling techniques to overcome somewhat the classic problems of temporal and structural confounds in developmental research. Our analyses provided unique estimates of aging, period, and cohort effects on individualism and materialism over the life-span. These analyses allowed us to evaluate whether value orientations were static or fluid in adulthood and to estimate the unique influence of age-based versus sociohistorical factors in promoting change. Moreover, by utilizing a hierarchical design that recognized individuals as nested within family structures, we were able to assess the total effect of one microsocial context—the intergenerational family—on an individual's value trajectory in adulthood.

Second, our findings document considerable fluidity in both individualism and materialism over the life-span. The malleability of these value orientations was reflected in three ways: (1) in terms of a predictable life-span developmental trajectory across individuals, (2) as a function of sociohistorical change, and (3) as unexplained systematic and random variation over time. We found significant unique age (negative) and cohort effects on individualism in this sample, as well as an interesting joint effect of development and cohort replacement reflected in period shifts in the larger cultural context. Thus, the tendency for individuals to become more collectivistic with age diminished the secular trend toward individualism that would have been expected, given cohort differences in endorsements of individualism in 1971. Our analyses of materialism also documented individual change over time. However, we found only limited evidence of a developmental trajectory, with most of the change in materialism due to a secular increase in materialism among G3s in 1985, and a general trend toward greater materialism among G1s over time.

Third, we were able to explore whether location in the social age and gender structures altered the expected trajectory of value orientations over time. We found only weak evidence that generational placement (a proxy for age cohort) influenced the trajectory of each value orientation over time. Gender was a more important factor, influencing the average level, but not the rate of developmental change, in both individualism and materialism. Though women experienced a parallel age-change trajectory to men, they were, on average, more collectivistic and humanistic than their male counterparts.

Fourth, our findings speak to lingering questions about the importance of the intergenerational family as a context for adult value development. We found evidence of intergenerational transmission reflected in greater value similarity among family members than among unrelated persons. This suggests that families remain an important context for value socialization, explaining a modest amount of individual differences in the population. Yet there was no evidence, beyond establishing initial orientations, that intergenerational ties altered the general life-span developmental trajectories we discovered. This latter finding increased our confidence in concluding that increasing age promotes a decrease in individualism over the adult life-span—consistent with the developmental stake phenomenon hypothesized by Bengtson and Kuypers (1971).

To summarize, our findings provide a clearer view of the connections between self and society in shaping value orientations over the life-span. By isolating influences across three levels of analysis—individual, familial, and sociohistorical—we were able to document how stability or change in individual orientations was related to stability and change in the others. Most importantly, our findings illuminate bidirectional flows of influence linking individuals and their sociohistorical contexts. For example, we were able to trace sociohistorical period effects on individuals that led to age-cohort differences in individualism. We were then able to show that the long-term effects of these cohort differences on the sociocultural milieu was mitigated by the developmental tendency for individuals to become more collectivistic with age.

In conclusion, we note that although we provide novel empirical evidence of the interconnectedness of self and sociohistorical processes, our study raises at least as many questions as it answers. Chief among them are questions concerning lines of influence among the macro-, meso-, and micro-social contexts wherein value socialization takes place. While our analyses show that stability and change at the individual level is related to both biographical and sociohistorical change, we were able to glean only limited information about family-level change in response to social change. Moreover, we did not explore the roles played by other meso-level contexts (e.g., the workplace) in connecting individual life-span and socialhistorical trajectories of value orientations. Clearly, a more holistic understanding of micro-macro linkages in development rests on further investigation of the role that meso-level contexts serve as "conduits" for bidirectional influences. Resolution of this issue requires data-gathering strategies that allow assessments of stability and change across multiple dimensions of the meso- and macro-level contexts.

REFERENCES

Abrahamson, P. R., & Inglehart, R. (1987). Generational replacement and the future of post-materialist values. *Journal of Politics, 49*, 231–241.

Abrahamson, P. R., & Inglehart, R. (1995). *Value change in global perspective.* Ann Arbor, MI: University of Michigan Press.

Acock, A. C., & Bengtson, V. L. (1978). On the relative influence of mothers and fathers: A covariance analysis of political and religious socialization. *Journal of Marriage and the Family, 40*, 519–530.

Alwin, D. F. (1984). Trends in parental socialization values: Detroit 1958 to 1983. *American Journal of Sociology, 90*, 359–382.

Alwin, D. F. (1990). Cohort replacement and changes in parental socialization values. *Journal of Marriage and the Family, 52*, 347–360.

Alwin, D. F., Cohen, R., & Newcomb, T. (1991). *Political attitudes over the life span: the Bennington women after 50 years.* Madison, WI: University of Wisconsin Press.

Bellah, R. H., Madsen, R., Sullivan, W. M., Swidler, A., & Tipton, S. M. (1985). *Habits of the heart.* Berkeley, CA: University of California Press.

Bengtson, V. L. (1975). Generation and family effects in value socialization. *American Sociological Review, 40*, 358–371.

Bengtson, V. L., & Kuypers, J. A. (1971). Generational difference and the "developmental stake." *Aging and Human Development, 2*, 249–260.

Bronfenbrenner, U. (1979). *The ecology of human development: Experiments by nature and design.* Cambridge, MA: Harvard University Press.

Bryk, A. S., & Raudenbush, S. W. (1992). *Hierarchical linear models: Applications and data analysis methods.* Newbury Park, CA: Sage.

Connell, R. W. (1972). Political socialization in the American family: The evidence re-examined. *Public Opinion Quarterly, 68*, 232–333.

Converse, P. E. (1964). The nature of belief systems in mass publics. In D. E. Apter (Ed.), *Ideology and discontent* (pp. 206–261). New York: Free Press.

Converse, P. E. (1987). The enduring impact of the Vietnam War on American public opinion. In *After the storm: American society a decade after the Vietnam War*. Taipei, Republic of China: Institute of American Culture.

Elder, G. H. (1974). *Children of the Great Depression*. Chicago: University of Chicago Press.

George, L. K., & Gold, D. T. (1991). Life course perspectives on intergenerational and generational connections. In S. P. Pfeifer & M. B. Sussman (Eds.), *Families: Intergenerational and generational connections* (pp. 67–88). New York: Haworth.

Glass, J., Bengtson, V. L., & Dunham, C. C. (1986). Attitude similarity in three-generation families: Socialization, status inheritance or reciprocal influence? *American Sociological Review, 51*, 685–698.

Glenn, N. D. (1977). *Cohort analysis*. Beverly Hills, CA: Sage.

Goldstein, H. I. (1987). *Multilevel models in educational and social research*. London: Oxford University Press.

Hagestad, G. O., & Neugarten, B. L. (1985). Aging and the life course. In R. H. Binstock & E. Shanas (Eds.), *Handbook of aging and the social sciences* (2nd ed., pp. 36–61). New York: Van Nostrand Reinhold.

Heckman, J. S. (1976). The common structure of statistical models of truncation, sample selection and limited dependent variables and a simple estimator for such models. *Annals of Economic and Social Measurement, 5*, 475–492.

Heckman, J. S. (1979). Sample selection as a specification error. *Econometrica, 45*, 153–161.

House, J. S., & Mortimer, J. (1990). Social structure and the individual: Emerging themes and new directions. *Social Psychology Quarterly, 53*, 71–80.

Jennings, M. K. (1987). Residues of a movement: The aging of the American protest movement. *American Political Science Review, 81*, 367–382.

Jennings, M. K., & Niemi, R. G. (1968). The transmission of political values from parent to child. *American Political Science Review, 62*, 169–184.

Jöreskog, K. G., & Sörbom, D. (1993). *LISREL 8 User's Guide*. Chicago: Scientific Software, Inc.

Kohn, M. (1969). *Class and conformity: a study in values*. Homewood, IL: Dorsey.

Kohn, M., & Schooler, C. (1983). *Work and personality: An inquiry into the impact of social stratification*. Norwood, NJ: Ablex.

Laird, N. M., & Ware, H. (1982). Random-effects models for longitudinal data. *Biometrics, 38*, 963–74.

Longford, N. T. (1987). A fast scoring algorithm for maximum likelihood estimation in unbalanced mixed models with nested random effects. *Biometrika, 74*, 817–27.

Mannheim, K. (1952). The problem of generations. In K. Mannheim (Ed.), *Essays in the sociology of knowledge* (pp. 276–322). London: Routledge and Kegan Paul. (Originally published 1922).

Marwell, G., Aiken, M. T., & Demerath, N. J., III. (1987). The persistence of political attitudes among 1960s civil rights activists. *Public Opinion Quarterly, 51*, 359–375.

McBroom, W., Reed, F., Burns, C., Hargraves, J., & Trankel, M. (1987). Intergenerational transmission of values: A data-based reassessment. *Social Psychology Quarterly, 50*, 150–161.

Mekos, D., & Clubb, P. A. (1997). The value of comparisons in developmental psychology. In J. Tudge, M. J. Shanahan, & J. Vaalsiner (Eds.), *Comparisons in human development: Understanding time and context* (pp. 137–161). Cambridge: Cambridge University Press.

Putnam, R. D. (1996). The strange disappearance of civic America. *American Prospect, 24*, 34–48.

Raudenbush, S. W., & Chan, W. S. (1993). Application of hierarchical linear modeling to the study of adolescent deviance in an overlapping cohort design. *Journal of Consulting and Clinical Psychology, 61*, 941–951.

Riley, M. W. (1973). Aging and cohort succession: Interpretations and misinterpretations. *Public Opinion Quarterly, 37*, 774–787.

Roberts, R. E. L., & Bengtson, V. L. (1990). Is intergenerational solidarity a unidimensional construct? A second test of a formal model. *Journal of Gerontology: Social Sciences, 45*, S12–20.

Roberts, R. E. L., & Bengtson, V. L. (1993). Relationships with parents, self-esteem, and psychological well-being in adulthood. *Social Psychology Quarterly, 56*, 263–277.

Roberts, R. E. L., & Bengtson, V. L. (1996). Affective ties to parents in early adulthood and self-esteem across 20 years. *Social Psychology Quarterly, 59*, 96–106.

Rokeach, M. (1968). *Beliefs, attitudes and values: A theory of organization and change*. San Francisco: Jossey-Bass.

Ryder, N. B. (1965). The cohort as a concept in the study of social change. *American Sociological Review, 30*, 843–861.

Schaie, K. W. (1994). Developmental designs revisited. In S. H. Cohen & H. W. Reese (Eds.), *Life-span developmental psychology: Theoretical issues revisited* (pp. 45–64). Hillsdale, NJ: Erlbaum.

Schuman, H., & Rieger, C. (1992). Historical analogies, generational effects, and attitudes toward war. *American Sociological Review, 57*, 315–326.

Schuman, H., & Scott, J. (1989). Generations and collective memories. *American Sociological Review, 54*, 359–381.

Sears, D. O. (1983). On the persistence of early political predispositions: The roles of attitude object and life stage. In L. Wheeler (Ed.), *Review of Personality and Social Psychology* (pp. 79–116). Beverly Hills, CA: Sage.

Tudge, J., Gray, J. T., & Hogan, D. M. (1997). Ecological perspectives in human development: A comparison of Gibson and Bronfenbrenner. In J. Tudge, M. J. Shanahan, & J. Vaalsiner (Eds.), *Comparisons in human development: Understanding time and context* (pp. 72–105). Cambridge: Cambridge University Press.

Index

Accentuation principle, 18
Accommodation, 129, 134, 139–141
Acculturation, impact on well-being,
 426–429, 440
Adaptation:
 aging process and, 130–131
 continuity theory, 98–99, 103–104
 to normal aging, 123–124
 significance of, 68
Adaptive capacity, 98
Adaptive change, 97
Adjustment, 68
Adolescence:
 naturalization and, 82–83
 self-image, 104
Adult children, as caregivers,
 379–380, 382–383, 386–388
Adulthood, generally:
 naturalization and, 82
 transition to, 54
Age-appropriate behavior, 212
Age-integrated society, 79
Age-irrelevant society, 79
Ageism, 142
Ageless Self: Sources of Meaning in
 Late Life, The (Kaufman),
 311–312
Age-status synchronization, 199
Age stratification, 13–14, 310
"Aging and society" paradigm, 307
Aging patterns, 68

Aging research, generally:
 human agency in, 310–318
 social structure, 306–309, 313–318
Alzheimer's Disease (AD), caregivers
 of, 399–400, 403, 405–406, 414
Anxiety, 126, 138, 259
Apprehension, 189–190
Aspired self, 57
Assimilation, 128–129, 139–140
Authenticity, 168
Authoritarian personality, 8
Autonomy, 52, 173, 209, 251, 267, 272
Avoidance, 138

Belief systems, gender and, 340, 345
Biographical meaningfulness, in aging
 self, 165

Career mobility, 79
Caregiver(s), *see* Caregiving
 burden, 196–197
 family as, generally, 363, 365, 399
 stress, 72
Caregiving
 as function of kinship relationship:
  future research directions,
   388–391
  research methodology, 384–385
  social support, 380–383, 386–388
  wife and daughter caregivers,
   378–380, 386–388

Caregiving *(continued)*
  as function of type of disability:
    coping issues, 369–378
    mental retardation, 367–368
    mother's role in, 369
  gender differences, 364
  as mediator:
    between income and mastery,
      401, 410–412
    between socioeconomic status
      and mastery, 405–406
Center for Epidemiological
    Depression Scale (CES-D),
    348, 371, 384
Childhood, socioeconomic status
    and, 264
Chronological age, 207
Cognitive development, 129, 155
Cognitive dysfunction, 123
Cognitive Reframing, 410–411, 415
Competency, later-life, 15
Constructionist perspective, 98, 191
Content domains, identity,
    125–127
Context characteristics, critical
    life events model, 162–163
Continuity, in aging self, 165
Continuity theory:
assumptions, 101
elements of:
    adaptive capacity, maintenance
      of, 103–104
    external structure, 102–103
    goal setting, 103
    internal structure, 100, 102
historical perspective, 95–97
personal agency, social structural
    attributes, 107, 109–110, 112, 117
propositions, 101
research examples, 106–107
self:
    functional disability and, 109–119
    social structure and, 104–106

as theory, 97–100
Control:
    critical life events and, 167–169
    cycle, 18
    interactionist/proactive perspective,
      45
    locus of, *see* Locus of control
    mastery and, 415
    processes, identity and, 135–137
Coping:
    adaptation distinguished from,
      137–139
    caregiver strategies, 369–378
    critical life events model, 163–164,
      168
    identity and:
      generally, 135–137
      interaction with, 139–142
    stress research, 406–412
Creativity, 209
Critical life events:
    comprehensive model of, 159
    impact of, generally, 17
    life-span development, 152–158
    self-development:
      adult, 164–174
      overview, 159–164
Cultural influences, on personality, 9
Current Population Survey, 288

Daughter, as caregiver:
    burden of, 378–380
    social support for, 386–388
Death, social structure and, 314
Depression, 123, 142, 253, 259, 262,
    348–349, 369, 374, 376, 414,
    436
Developmental asynchrony, 155–156
Developmental psychology, 6–7
Discrimination, impact on well-being,
    447
Discriminative relevance, in aging
    self, 165

Disengagement theory, 4–6, 12
Disequilibrium, 155
Divorce, impact of, 105

Ecological perspective, 200–208
Educational attainment, generally:
   impact on self, 225, 228–230,
      241–242
   midlife, comparison with, 265–271
   self-making in older age, 231–240
   socioeconomic standing, as marker
      of, 263–264
   well-being, influence on, 254–256,
      258
Ego integrity, 127
Emotion-focused coping, 136–137,
   139–140, 372
Emotional resilience, 108, 112, 117
Employment:
   lifelong, *see* Lifelong employment
   marital status and, 341–342
   mental health, implications for,
      347–354
Equilibration process, 129
Equilibrium, self-regulation, 12
Erikson's theory, 127
Ethnography, 195
Event characteristics, critical life
      events model, 163
Event outcomes, critical life events
      model, 163–164
Experimental psychology, 8
Exterogestation, 70–71

Familism, cultural, 429, 436
Family attitude, impact on well-being,
   445–446
Family structure, impact on well-
      being, 429–430, 440, 443
Fecundity, 86
Feedback systems theories, 97
Field theory, 192
Fruhjahr, 70–71

Functional disability, 109–119
Functional impairment, 229

Gatekeeping, 59
Gender:
   age relations, 343–344
   belief systems, 340
   differences in, *see* Gender differences
   historical factors and life course,
      344–347
   marriage and, 341–342
Gender differences:
   educational attainment, 267, 270
   Hispanic population, well-being in,
      436
   midlife, 73
   value orientation, generally, 479
   in well-being, 252–254, 256
Gender identity, 55
General Social Survey, 286
Generativity, 127
Genotypes, 68–69
Gestation, 70
Goal setting, 103
Goodness-of-fit, 69
Grounded theory, 46

Happiness:
   Hispanic population study, 436,
      440, 443
   life cycle patterns, 286–289, 293,
      299–300
Health, socioeconomic status and,
   258–260
Heterogeneity, 207–208
Hispanic Health and Nutrition
      Examination Survey (H-
      HANES), 198, 447
Hispanic population, well-being
      studies:
   acculturation, culture and self,
      426–429
   conceptual framework, 430–433

Hispanic population, well-being
    studies *(continued)*
  cultural familism, self and, 429
  family structure, support, and inter-
      action, 429–430
  gender differences, 436
  happiness, 436, 440, 443
  research methodology, 433–436
  societal barriers to, 425–426
Human agency, 310–313, 316–318
Human development:
  distinctives of:
    exterogestation, 70–71
    neoteny, 71–73, 87
    world construction, 73–74, 87
  naturalization, 81–87
  social legitimation and, 81–87
  social relations, co-constitution of:
    micro-macro linkage, 80–81
    social allocation, 78–80
    social reality production (SRP),
        74–81

Ideal self, 102
Identity, generally:
  aging process model, *see* Identity
      model of aging process
  crisis, 140
  gender, 55
  job-related, 55–56
  processes:
    measurement of, 131–132
    overview, 127–130
  social roles, impact on, 399
  structural/deterministic perspective,
      44
Identity and Experiences Scale:
  General (IES-G), 131–132
  Specific Aging Form (IEG-SA),
      132
  Ways of Coping scale, 141–142
Identity model of aging process,
    applications of:

identity content domains, 125–127
identity processes:
  measurement of, 131–132
  overview, 127–130
  identity in relation to aging process,
      130–131
Income, link with mastery:
  through caregiver role, 410–412
  overview, 402–403
Individual, generally:
  aging research, interpretation in,
      196–199
  linkage to social structure, 4–7
  mediated experience, 190–196
Individualism, 473–474, 476, 478
Inequalities, perceived, 271–274
Intentionality, 189–190, 204
Interactionist paradigm:
  proactive paradigm, 45–47
  social structure, perspective of,
      57–59
Internal control, 136
Interpretative meaning, 197–199
Intimacy, 127

Kinship relationships, 364, 380–391

Labelling theory, 77–78
Learning disabilities, 83
Life course development, 6–7
Life course themes, aging of self,
    123–124
Life events, 17–19
Life-span development:
  adult development, 154–157
  critical life events:
    dialectical view of adult develop-
        ment, 154–156
    individuals as proactive producers
        and reactive responders in
        developmental processes,
        156–157
    triarchic model of developmental

influences, 152–154, 157–158
Life-span developmental psychology, traditional, 150–151
Lifelong employment:
  coefficients of distress, 352, 356–357
  gender differences, 345, 349–350, 354–355
  mental health and, 347–355
  micro/macro linkage, 357–358
Lifestyle, well-being and, 274
Likert scale, 118
Linkage mechanisms:
  life events, 17–19
  meso-structures, 12–13
  role allocation and socialization, 13–15
  self-processes, 16–17
LISREL VIII, 236–237
Locus of control, 52–53, 137

MacArthur Foundation Research Network on Midlife Development, 271
Macro-micro linkages, 259
Marital status, *see* Marriage, impact of
  continuity theory and, 105
  self-selection and, 50–51
Marriage, impact of:
  age relations, 343–344
  caregiving burden, 365
  employment issues, 341–342
  gender inequality in, 342
Marxism, 309
Mastery:
  defined, 401–402
  future research directions, 413–416
  implications of, generally, 52, 251–252, 254, 256, 267–268, 368, 378
  predictors of, 417
  social roles and, 400, 403–404

social structure linked with, 402–403
  socioeconomic status and, 400–401
  stress, impact of, 405
Materialism, 472–473, 475–476
Mediated experience:
  constructing self, 190–193
  origins of meaning, 193–196
  personal agency, 193–196
  practical consciousness, 194–195, 213
Menopause, 72
Menses, 207
Mental health, 259, 262, 369
Mental illness, mental retardation distinguished from, 367–368
Mental retardation, 367–368
Meritocratic society, 225
Meso-level social structures, 12–13
Meso-sphere, well-being and, 449
Midlife:
  parental experiences, 254
  social comparisons, 265–271
  women and, 72–73
Modernization theory, 4–5
Mortality, 348
Mothers, as caregivers, 369
Multiple threshold model of aging, 132–135

National character studies, 8
National Survey of Families and Households (NSFH), 260, 262, 348
Naturalization:
  defined, 81
  inter-age differences, 82–83
  intra-age/intracohort differences, 83–87
  significance of, 84–85
Natural selection process, 67
Neoteny, 71–73, 87
Normal aging, 123–124

Old-age heterogeneity, 208

Pain management, 138
Parallel process model, 69, 83
Pearlin mastery scale, 407
Permanence, in aging self, 165
Person characteristics, critical life
    events model, 161–162
Personal agency, 107, 109–110, 112,
    117, 188
Personal goals, indicators of, 108,
    112, 117
Personality and Social Systems
    (Smelser/Smelser), 11
Personality development theories, 161
Personality theory, historical perspec-
    tives, 7–8
Phenotypes, 68–69
Physical identity, 126, 137–138, 141
Piaget's theory, 129, 155
Political economy, aging and,
    308–309
Possible selves, 15–16, 57, 126
Poverty, impact of, 143–144. *See also*
    Socioeconomic status (SES)
Practical consciousness, 187, 192,
    194–195, 213
Primary control, 136
Problem-focused coping, 136–140,
    372, 414
Protean Self, 52
Psychological well-being:
    age differences, 249, 251–252
    defined, 248–249
    formulations, 248–249
    gender differences, 252–253
    perceived inequalities, 271–274
    social class and, 258–263
    social structure and, 253–258
    socioeconomic status:
        educational attainment, 263–266
        social comparison process, 264–265
    theory-guided dimensions, 250

Psychoneuroimmunology, 72
Psychosocial well-being, 424
Purpose in life, 267, 272

Quantity-quality distinction, 86
Quebec, retirement policy in, 324–326

Racism, 142
Reality maintenance, 18
Reflexive processes, 189
Reflexivity, 189
Religious switchers, 51
Relocation, impact of, 256
Reproductive fitness, 84–85
Retirement process, Montreal garment
    workers case study:
    market conditions and, 333–334
    methodology, 319–320
    retirement timing, 326–332
    social factors, 334
    structure and agency, 320–324
Role allocation, socialization and,
    13–15, 310
Role-based identities, 55–57
Role changes, structural/deterministic
    perspective, 44

School:
    age-grading and ability grouping,
        81
    social reality production (SRP)
        process, 74–78
Secondary control, 406
Selection, 69. *See also* Natural
    selection
Self, generally:
    aging of, 123–124
    interactionist/proactive perspective,
        45
    social class, ecological perspective,
        200–208
    sociological perspectives, 43–59
    structuralist view of, 55–57

successful aging, 225–227
view of, generally, 55–57
Self Portraits study, 231–232, 237, 239
Self-acceptance, 254, 267
Self-appraisals, 206
Self-attributions, 127
Self-authenticating, 191
Self-concept:
  age and health factors, generally,
    198–199
  in aging self, 165
  critical life events and, 167
  positive changes, 174
  significance of, generally, 15, 102
  social roles and, 400
  structural/deterministic perspective, 43
Self-consciousness, 55
Self-determination, 169, 173–174
Self-development, in adults:
  aging process, 164–167
  critical life events and, 167–170
  developmental effects on, 159
  individual and social structure links,
    159, 161–164
  self-determined life events and,
    173–174
  uncontrollable life events and,
    171–173
Self-direction, 52–55, 210
Self-efficacy, 52, 126–127, 142, 169
Self-enhancement, 16, 169–170, 205
Self-esteem:
  continuity theory, 102, 104
  cultural influences, 448
  Hispanic population study, 43
  interactionist/proactive perspective, 45
  significance of, 161–162
  social class and, 9, 264
Self-evaluation, 16, 18, 102, 205
Self-fulfilling prophecies, 77
Self-identity, 194
Self-improvement, 205
Self-making:

influential factors, 228–229
in older age, 231–240
Self-perception, 46, 48, 51, 59, 116,
  253, 414
Self-Perception Scale (SPS), 134–135
Self-processes, 16–17
Self-protection strategies, 58
Self-realization, 169
Self-referent dimensions, indicators
  of, 108, 113–114
Self-regulation, 169
Self-representation, 241
Self-selection, into social environments,
  48–51
Self-society linkage, 18
Self-striving, 102–103
Self-system, characteristics of, 224,
  227–228
Self-validation, 195
Self-values, 102
Seratonin levels, implications of, 72
Sexism, 142
Social allocation processes, 78–79
Social breakdown syndrome, 4, 14
Social class, *see* Socioeconomic status
  (SES)
  differentiation, 202–203
  sense of self and, overview,
    200–208
  social relativity and, 203
  social stratification, 204–206
Social comparison processes,
  264–268, 414
Social Construction of Reality, The
  (Berger/Luckmann), 18
Social constructionist perspective, 342
Social contingencies, transitions and
  social class, 218–222
Social differentiation, 52
Socialization:
  role allocation and, 13–15
  structural/deterministic perspective,
    43–44

Social legitimation, 81–87
Social norms, personality and, 9
Social physique anxiety, 126
Social-psychological paradigm,
    196–197
Social-psychological theory, 298
Social reality production (SRP)
    process, 74–78
Social relations, human development
    and, 74–81
Social relativity:
    heterogeneity and, 207–208
    social class and, 203
Social roles:
    interpretation of, 200
    link between socioeconomic status
        and mastery, 403–404
Social Sciences Research Council
    Committee, 5
Social status, 400
Social stratification, 204–206
Social stress model, 447–448
Social structure:
    in aging research, 306–309
    future research directions, 413–416
    individuals, linkage of, 4–7, 10–19
    influence on self, 312
    mastery and, 402–403
    personality and, 7–10
    value orientation, influence on,
        456–458
Social support:
    caregiving and, 380–382, 385–388,
        413
    implications of, generally, 242
Sociodemographics, 253, 258
Socioeconomic status (SES):
    caregiving role, effect on, 400–401
    employment issues, 346
    health and, 258–260
    personality and, 9, 167
    social roles, link with mastery,
        403–404

stress and, 404
    well-being and, 255–256, 445–446
Sociological aging, 311
Sociological perspectives of self:
    integration of structural and
        interactionist paradigm:
        interactionist perspective of social
            structure, 57–59
        overview, 47–48
        self-direction, environmental
            assessment, 52–55
        self-selection into social
            environments, 48–51
        structuralist view of self, 55–57
    interactionist/proactive paradigm,
        45–47
    overview, 42–43
    structural/deterministic paradigm,
        43–45
Stereotypes, cultural, 142–144
Stigmatization, 390
Stress:
    caregiving, 384, 389
    coping research, 136–137, 406–412
    mastery and, 405
    socioeconomic status, impact of, 404
Structural/deterministic paradigm,
    43–45
Structural-functionalism, 11, 13–14,
    307, 309, 311
Subjective well-being:
    implications of, generally, 49–50, 119
    income and:
        income measurement, 286–287
        research studies, 285–286
        theory, 280–285, 293–299
Successful aging, 142, 207, 225–227

Temporal complexity, in social
    psychology, 456–459
Three boxes of life, 82
Traditional classroom, effects of, 77–78
Transitions, social class and, 218–222

Uncontrollable life events, impact of, 171–173
Use it or lose it principle (UIOLIs), 124, 130–131, 133, 136, 140

Value orientation:
gender differences, 479
impact of, 454–455
stability over life span, 468–469

Values, social psychology of:
gender differences, 479
individualism, 473–474, 476, 478
intergenerational transmission, 475–476, 478
materialism, 472–473, 475–476
multi-level modeling, longitudinal data:
structural complexity, 459–460
temporal complexity and cohort-sequential designs, 458–459
research methodology, 461–466
social structure, problems of:
structural complexity, 457–458
temporal complexity, 456–458

sociohistorical change, effects of, 469, 472
stability over life span, 468–469, 476

Voluntarism, 311
Vulnerability, mastery and, 415

WAIS-R, 238
Well-being, *see* Psychological well-being; Subjective well-being
macro-sphere influence on, 446–447
self and, 424–425
Whitehall II Study of British, 260, 262
"Who Are You?," 55
Widowhood, 44, 105, 343–344
Wife, as caregiver:
burden of, 378–380
social support for, 386–388
Wisconsin Longitudinal Study (WLS), 260, 262, 265–267, 270
Work-based identity, 55-56
Working self-concepts, 213
World construction, 73-74, 87
World-view, well-being and, 274